FUNDAMENTALS OF FOODS, NUTRITION AND DIET THERAPY

FUNDAMENTALS OF
FOODS, NUTRITION
AND
DIET THERAPY

EIGHTH EDITION

SUMATI R MUDAMBI
MSc., MS (Wisc.), PhD (Wisc.)

M V RAJAGOPAL
MSc., PhD (Wisc.), FIFST (UK)

NEW AGE
TECHNO
PRESS

An Imprint of

NEW AGE INTERNATIONAL (P) LIMITED, PUBLISHERS
LONDON • NEW DELHI
Bangalore • Chennai • Cochin • Guwahati • Hyderabad • Kolkata • Mumbai
Visit us at **www.newagepublishers.com**

Published by New Age International (P) Ltd., Publishers
First Edition: 1982
Eighth Edition: 2025

GLOBAL OFFICES

- **New Delhi** **NEW AGE INTERNATIONAL (P) LIMITED, PUBLISHERS**
  7/30 A, Daryaganj, New Delhi-110002, (INDIA), **Tel.:** (011) 23253472, 23253771
  Visit us at www.newagepublishers.com • e-mail: contactus@newagepublishers.com
- **London** **NEW AGE INTERNATIONAL (UK) LTD.**
  27 Old Gloucester Street, London, WC1N 3AX, UK
  Visit us at www.newacademicscience.co.uk • e-mail: info@newacademicscience.co.uk

BRANCHES

- **Bangalore** 37/10, 8th Cross (Near Hanuman Temple), Azad Nagar, Chamarajpet, Bangalore- 560 018
  Tel.: (080) 26756823, **E-mail: bangalore@newagepublishers.com**
- **Chennai** 26, Damodaran Street, T. Nagar, Chennai-600 017, **Tel.:** (044) 24353401
  E-mail: chennai@newagepublishers.com
- **Cochin** CC-39/1016, Carrier Station Road, Ernakulam South, Cochin-682 016, **Tel.:** (0484) 4051304
  E-mail: cochin@newagepublishers.com
- **Guwahati** Hemsen Complex, Mohd. Shah Road, Paltan Bazar, Near Starline Hotel, Guwahati-781 008,
  Tel.: (0361) 2513881, **E-mail: guwahati@newagepublishers.com**
- **Hyderabad** 105, 1st Floor, Madhiray Kaveri Tower, 3-2-19, Azam Jahi Road, Near Kumar Theater, Nimboliadda Kachiguda, Hyderabad-500 027, **Tel.:** (040) 24652456, **E-mail: hyderabad@newagepublishers.com**
- **Kolkata** RDB Chambers (Formerly Lotus Cinema) 106A, 1st Floor, S N Banerjee Road, Kolkata-700 014
  Tel.: (033) 22273773, **E-mail: kolkata@newagepublishers.com**
- **Mumbai** 142C, Victor House, Ground Floor, N.M. Joshi Marg, Lower Parel, Mumbai-400 013
  Tel.: (022) 24927869, 24915415, **E-mail: mumbai@newagepublishers.com**
- **New Delhi** 22, Golden House, Daryaganj, New Delhi-110 002, **Tel.:** (011) 23262368, 23262370
  E-mail: sales@newagepublishers.com

C-24-11-14387

Printed in India at Ess Enterprises, Rai, Haryana.
Typeset at Aakriti Graphics, Delhi.

NEW AGE INTERNATIONAL (P) LIMITED, PUBLISHERS
7/30 A, Daryaganj, New Delhi - 110002
Visit us at **www.newagepublishers.com**
(CIN: U74899DL1966PTC004618)

Foreword

FOODS AND NUTRITION are essential for maintaining good health and to prevent disease. Although food occupies the first position in the hierarchical needs of man, ignorance of many basic facts relating to foods and nutrition is still widespread. Consequently, various nutritional disorders for which there are simple remedies such as blindness caused by vitamin A deficiency persist. Good nutrition is a function of both economics and education. In our country, the most serious form of nutritional disorder is undernutrition arising from inadequate purchasing power. However, even when purchasing power is adequate to access balanced nutrition, various forms of imbalance in dietary intake occur due to lack of knowledge.

The culinary art of which we are justifiably proud, has placed organoleptic considerations as the sole criteria of excellence. The various opportunities for accomplishing balanced nutrition through synergistic interaction within the components of diet have not received the consideration they deserve. The book covers all the important areas which ought to be taken into consideration while promoting good nutrition in health and disease.

The knowledge of foods and nutrition is essential for teachers, health professionals, students of home sciences and health sciences and civil society organizations engaged in fighting endemic and hidden hunger.

The revised edition with the addition of diet therapy will be a valuable book for the use of dietetics and nursing students. It will also be a valuable guide and reference book for physicians and other health professionals. The book of Dr. Mudambi and Dr. Rajagopal will make an important contribution to accelerating the pace of achieving good nutrition in health and disease.

Dr. M.S. Swaminathan
UNESCO Cousteau Chair in Ecotechnology & Chairman,
M.S. Swaminathan Research Foundation,
Chennai 600113.

Preface to the Eighth Edition

WE ARE HAPPY to present the 8th edition of *Fundamentals of Foods, Nutrition and Diet Therapy*. This book is an introduction to Foods, Nutrition and Diet Therapy. The science courses studied at high school level are sufficient background for this course.

This book has consistently been used by students studying the first course in Food Science and Nutrition. In several universities the topics food and environment and diet therapy topics have been added in the curricula of this course. Therefore these have been added in this revision. We hope it meets the altered needs of our readers.

The revised book is intended to meet the needs of students in a number of faculties in which Foods, Nutrition and Diet Therapy is a **major, elective or ancillary** subject. These include Home Science, Nursing, Medical and Paramedical, Agriculture, Food Technology, Education, Arts, Social Sciences, Community Health, Pediatrics, Environmental Health and Allied areas.

The contents of this edition have been revised in view of the recent developments in the area, logical sequence of subject matter, changes in the syllabi of universities and the feedback from teachers and students.

The book covers the following aspects:

I. Introduction to the Study of Nutrition (Chapters 1 to 3)
II. The Nutrients and Energy (Chapters 4 to 13)
III. Meal Planning and Management (Chapters 14 to 17)
IV. Foods (Chapters 18 to 23)
V. Diet Therapy (Chapters 24 to 37)

As in earlier editions, this book covers the principles of nutrition and food science and discusses the application of this knowledge in practice. In addition, eighth edition covers the topic food environment and the principles of diet therapy, the changes in body that occur due to disease, the altered needs of the body due to disease and how to meet these through modification of the normal diet. Figures and tables have been used to help visualise practical information. The contents of the book have been developed out of continuous study and teaching of these subjects and use of the knowledge in consultation with patients and use in practical situations.

Each chapter opens with an outline of its contents. Any abbreviations used are explained, and all terms, which need explanation are included in the Glossary at the end of the book.

In the Appendices, Food Exchange Lists, Recommended Dietary Allowances for Indians and Food Composition Tables have been included. In addition, Table of Indian names of foods, height and weight of girls and boys from birth to eighteen years, low and high calorie vegetables and fruits, calorific value of some cooked preparation, energy expenditure and cost on various Physical activities and other useful information is given.

We hope this edition helps towards making the goal of good nutrition for all, in health and disease, a reality.

Any suggestions for improvement of the book in later edition are very welcome, for it indicates a shared interest in the study, development and use of this fascinating subject.

Great care has been taken to ensure that mistakes do not crept into the book. However, if there are any which have escaped our scrutiny, we would welcome corrections from our readers.

Several figures have been altered to improve their clarity. We appreciate the help given by the Dr. P.S. Sindhu in this respect.

We are grateful to the staff of New Age International (Private) Limited for their contribution to the development and completion of the eighth edition.

Sumati R. Mudambi

M.V. Rajagopal

Preface to the First Edition

THERE HAS been a long felt need for a book on the fundamentals of foods and nutrition for the students preparing for the Higher Secondary School of Certificate Examinations of both the Central and State Boards of Education. Neither do the students of nutrition in the first year of Home Science colleges have any compact Indian book on this subject. Most of the colleges usually recommend American textbooks because of the absence of any suitable Indian book in this area. The American books, however, discuss the subject with reference to the needs of an economy different from ours with the result that students do not learn anything about the applications of nutrition to Indian conditions.

This book covers the subjects of applications of the findings of the food science and nutrition to Indian conditions and at the same time discusses in simple language all the basic principles of foods and nutrition. Figures and tables have been used profusely to bring home to the beginner all aspects of foods and nutrition. For the more inquisitive and interested student references to advanced books are given in the bibliography. Through painstaking research, knowledge has been acquired about the nutrition needs of people. It is the aim of this book to motivate teachers and students to make use of this knowledge and bring about a change in the health and welfare of our people.

(i) Basic Nutrition (Chapters 1 and 2).
(ii) Food Selection and Preparation (Chapters 3, 4 and 5)
(iii) Meal Planning (Chapters 6, 7 and 8)
(iv) Disorders of Malnutrition (Chapter 9)
(v) Food Preservation (Chapters 10 and 11)
(vi) Safeguarding the Food Supply (Chapters 12, 13 and 14)

It is hoped that this book will help our readers to understand:

1. Functions of foods, which supply our nutritional needs.
2. How to meet human need of nutrients in terms of available foods.
3. Prices are guides of supply and demand and not of their nutritive value.
4. Techniques of preparation which help us meet our needs in an enjoyable manner.
5. Meal planning as a tool in meeting nutritional needs of the family through acceptable enjoyable meals.
6. Preservation as an aid to improved food availability.
7. Safeguarding the supply through proper selection, careful storage and preparation.
8. One's responsibilities as a consumer.

The difficulties encountered by foods and nutrition teachers, due to lack of an appropriate Indian text, were brought to our notice by the teachers, who attended the NCERT Summer Workshops conducted by one of us (SRM) at the Lady Irwin College in 1978. It prompted us to complete this book, which we had started writing, on a priority basis.

Great care has been taken to ensure that no mistakes have crept into the book. However, if there are any which have escaped our scrutiny, we would welcome corrections from our readers.

We are grateful to the Director, National Institute of Nutrition for supplying the figures 9.2, 9.3, 9.4, 9.5, 9.6, and 9.7, to Messrs Voltas Limited for figures 3.1, 10.2, 10.3, 10.4, 12.4 and 14.1 and to Messrs Balsara & Company for figure 12.2.

We are grateful to late Dr. Leela Phadnis, Professor of Foods & Nutrition, Vanasthali Vidyapeeth, Vanasthali, Rajasthan, Dr. S.S. Ajagaonkar, former President, All-India Institute of Diabetes, Bombay and to late Dr. V. Nagarajan, Assistant Director-General, Indian Council of Agricultural Research, New Delhi, for their careful appraisal of the manuscript and valuable suggestions.

We sincerely appreciate the assistance of our sons Anand and Shyam, who corrected typescripts and prepared the glossary for us.

Bombay
September, 1982

SRM
MVR

Contents

Part V: Diet Therapy

Appendices

PART - I

Introduction to the Study of Nutrition

CHAPTER

1

Foods, Nutrition and Health

Definitions
- Food
- Nutrition
- Adequate Nutrition
- Nutritional Status
- Malnutrition
- Nutritional Care
- Health

Functions of Food
- Physiological, Social and Psychological Functions

Functions of Nutrients
- Carbohydrates, Fats, Proteins, Vitamins, Minerals and Water

Food Composition
- Food Exchange Lists
- Nutrient Density
- How Will you be a Responsible Nutrition Student?

Study Questions

FOOD HAS been a basic part of our existence. Through the centuries we have acquired a wealth of information about the use of food to ensure growth of children and youth, to maintain good health through life, and to meet special needs of pregnancy and lactation and to use it to recover from illness.

When you study food composition you will know the nutritional contribution of foods. You may have been told that certain foods are very important for maintaining good health, while others are harmful. As you study the science of Foods and Nutrition, you will need to examine the ideas you have about foods very carefully and accept or reject these in the light of the knowledge you will acquire. Whatever you learn in this area should be used and applied in your personal life.

A large part of our food heritage is scientifically beneficial and needs to be retained; some aspects may need to be modified in the view of the changes in our lifestyle.

Food is an important topic of conversations, articles in newspapers and magazines, as also of advertisements. Some of this information may be correct, but a large part of it may not be. As you learn this subject, you will be able to spread the knowledge gained to those around you, so that they discard false ideas about food, which interfere with their food selection and affect their health.

Food, nutrition and health are intimately connected aspects of our life. Let us start our study by defining these and related terms.

Definitions

Food is that which nourishes the body. Food may also be defined as anything eaten or drunk, which meets the needs for energy, building, regulation and protection of the body. In short, food is the raw material from which our bodies are made. Intake of the right kinds and amounts of food can ensure good nutrition and health, which may be evident in our appearance, efficiency and emotional well-being (Figure 1.1).

Nutrition has been defined as food at work in the body. Nutrition includes everything that happens to food from the time it is eaten until it is used for various functions in the body. Nutrients are components of food that are needed by the body in adequate amounts in order to grow, reproduce and lead a normal, healthy life. Nutrients include water, proteins, fats, carbohydrates, minerals and vitamins. There are several nutrients in each of the groups: proteins, fats, carbohydrates, minerals and vitamins; hence the plural form of these words has been used. Thus there are over 40 essential nutrients supplied by food, which are used to produce literally thousands of substances necessary for life and physical fitness.

The study of the science of nutrition deals with what nutrients we need, how much we need, why we need these and where we can get them. Nutrition is the result of the kinds of foods supplied to the body and how the body uses the food supplied.

Adequate, optimum and good nutrition are expressions used to indicate that the supply of the essential nutrients is correct in amount and proportion. It also implies that the utilisation of such nutrients in the body is such that the highest level of physical and mental health is maintained throughout the life-cycle.

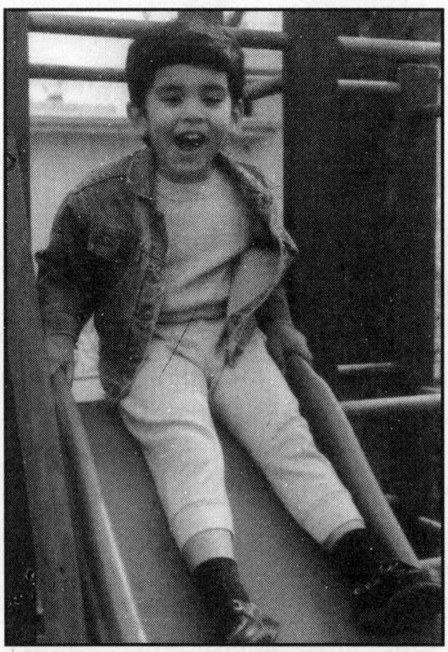

Figure 1.1: A well-nourished child engrossed in play.

Nutritional status is the state of our body as a result of the foods consumed and their use by the body. Nutritional status can be good, fair or poor.

The characteristics of **good nutritional status** are an alert, good natured personality, a well developed body, with normal weight for height, well developed and firm muscles, healthy skin, reddish pink colour of eyelids and membranes of mouth, good layer of subcutaneous fat, clear eyes, smooth and glossy hair, good appetite and excellent general health. General good health is evident by stamina for work, regular meal times, sound regular sleep, normal elimination and resistance to disease.

Poor nutritional status is evidenced by a listless, apathetic or irritable personality, undersized poorly developed body, abnormal body weight (too thin or fat and flabby body), muscles small and flabby, pale or sallow skin, too little or too much subcutaneous fat, dull or reddened eyes, lustreless and rough hair, poor appetite, lack of vigour and endurance for work and susceptibility to infections. Poor nutritional status may be the result of poor food selection, irregularity in schedule of meals, work, sleep and elimination.

The WHO (World Health Organization) has defined **health** as the 'state of complete physical, mental and social well-being and not merely the absence of disease or infirmity'.

Malnutrition means an undesirable kind of nutrition leading to ill-health. It results from a lack, excess or imbalance of nutrients in the diet. It includes **undernutrition** and **overnutrition.** Undernutrition is a state of an insufficient supply of essential nutrients.

Malnutrition can be primarily be due to insufficient supply of one or more essential nutrients; or it can be secondary, which means it results from an error in metabolism, interaction between nutrients or nutrients and drugs used in treatment.

Overnutrition refers to an excessive intake of one or more nutrients, which creates a stress in the bodily function.

Diet refers to whatever you eat and drink each day. Thus it includes the normal diet you consume and the diet people consume in groups (hostel diet). Diet may also be modified and used for ill persons as part of their therapy (therapeutic diets).

Nutritional care is the use of nutritional knowledge in planning meals and the preparation of these meals in an acceptable and attractive manner to feed people. It involves assessment of the exiting meal patterns and improving these in an acceptable manner. While the nutritional plan may be general for a group of people, the actual execution is individualized to suit the person's needs and background. Thus one has to use a lot of ingenuity to succeed in making nutritional care effective in practical terms.

Health the word health refers to the condition of the body, good health not only implies freedom from disease, but physical, mental and emotional fitness as well.

Functions of Food

Physiological functions of food. The first function of the body is to **provide energy.** The body needs energy to sustain the involuntary processes essential for continuance of life, to carry out professional, household and recreational activities, to convert food ingested into usable nutrients in the body, to grow and to keep warm. The energy needed is supplied by the oxidation of the foods consumed.

The foods we eat become a part of us. Thus one of the most important functions of food is **building the body.** A newborn baby weighing 2.7-3.2 kg can grow to its potential adult size of 50–60 kg if the right kinds and amounts of food are eaten from birth to adulthood. The food eaten each day helps to maintain the structure of the adult body, and to **replace** worn out cells of the body.

The third function of food is to **regulate activities of the body**. It includes regulation of such varied activities as:

- Beating of the heart
- Maintenance of the body temperature
- Muscle contraction
- Control of water balance
- Clotting of blood
- Removal of waste products from the body

The fourth function of food is to improve our body's **resistance to disease.**

The Social Functions of Food. Food has always been a central part of our social existence. It has been a part of our community, social, cultural and religious life. Special foods are distributed as a benediction or *prasad* in the religious functions in homes, temples and churches. Feasts are given at specific stages of life such as birth, naming ceremony, birthdays, marriages, etc. Most of the religious festivals also call for feasts and feeding of specific segments of the population. Certain menus are associated with most of these feasts in each region.

Food has been used as an expression of love, friendship and social acceptance. It is also used as a symbol of happiness at certain events in life, for example, *pedhas* are distributed to announce success in examinations, or the birth of a baby; *laddus* are associated with the celebration of Deepavali and marriages, cakes are associated with Christmas and birthdays and *tilgul* with *sankranti* the festival of friendship.

As food is an integral part of our social existence, this function is important in daily life. Refreshments served at get-togethers or meetings create a relaxed atmosphere. The menu for such get-together should bring the people together, rather than divide them. This basic aspect should be considered in planning menus for such occasions (Figure 1.2).

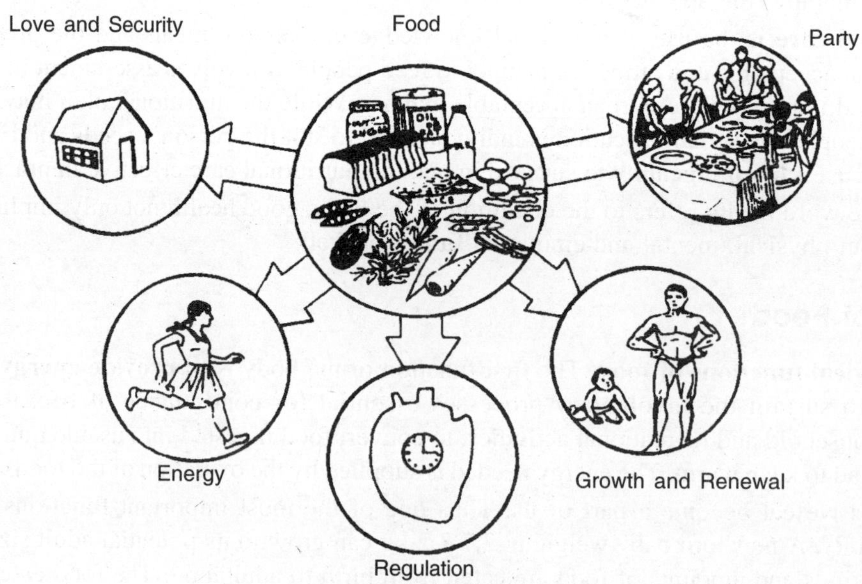

Figure 1.2: Functions of food.

The Psychological Functions of Food. In addition to satisfying physical and social needs, food must satisfy certain emotional needs. These includes a sense of security, love and attention. Thus familiar foods make us feel secure. Anticipating needs and fulfilling these are expressions of love and attention. These sentiments are the basis of the normal attachment to the mother's cooking.

Sharing of food is a token of friendship and acceptance. In a friendly gathering we try unfamiliar foods and thus enlarge our food experiences. It must be noted that even a nutritionally balanced meal may not be satisfying to the individual, if the foods included are unfamiliar or distasteful to him/her. With time and repeated experience, strange foods become familiar and new tastes are formed.

These aspects are important in food acceptance and must be considered in planning meals, which are not only nutritionally adequate, but also enjoyable for the group for whom they are intended.

Functions of Nutrients

The foods which we use daily include rice, wheat, dal, vegetables, fruits, milk, eggs, fish, meat, sugar, butter, oils, etc. These different foods are made up of a number of chemical components called **nutrients.** These are classified according to their chemical composition.

Each nutrient class has its own function, but the various nutrients must act in unison for effective action. The nutrients found in foods are — carbohydrates, proteins, fats, minerals, vitamins and water. Fibre is also an essential component of our diet. The functions of nutrients are given below.

Carbohydrates: Starch found in cereals and sugar in sugarcane and fruits are examples of carbohydrates in foods. The chief function of carbohydrates is to provide energy needed by our body. Those not used immediately for this purpose are stored as glycogen or converted to fat and stored, to be mobilised for energy supply when needed.

Fats: Oils found in seeds, butter from milk, and lard from meat, are examples of fats found in foods. Fats are concentrated sources of energy, carriers of fat soluble vitamins and a source of essential fatty acids. If excess fats are taken in the diet, these are stored as fat reserves in the body. Energy taken in excess of body needs, is stored as fat in the body.

Proteins: Casein from milk, albumin in egg, globulins in legumes and gluten in wheat, are examples of proteins occurring in foods. The main function of protein is the building of new tissues and maintaining and repair of those already built. Synthesis of regulatory and protective substances such as enzymes, hormones and antibodies is also a function of food proteins. About 10 per cent of the total energy is supplied by proteins in the diet. Protein, when taken in excess of the body's need, is converted to carbohydrates and fats and is stored in the body.

Minerals: The minerals calcium, phosphorus, iron, iodine, sodium, potassium and others are found in various foods in combination with organic and inorganic compounds. Minerals are necessary for body-building, for building of bones, teeth and structural parts of soft tissues. They also play a role in regulation of processes in the body, e.g., muscle contraction, clotting of blood, nerve stimuli, etc.

Vitamins: Fat-soluble vitamins A, D, E and K and also water-soluble vitamins C and B group are found in foods. These are needed for growth, normal function of the body and normal body processes.

Water: We get water in foods we eat and a major part from the water we drink as such and as beverages. Water is an essential part of our body structure and it accounts for about 60 per cent of our body weight. Water is essential for the utilisation of food material in the body and also for elimination of food waste. It is a regulator of body processes such as maintenance of body temperature.

All individuals need the same nutrients for the same body function. The only variation is in the amounts of each nutrient required according to age, size, activity, etc. For example, all persons need energy for work, but a man, who carries loads may need more energy than a man, who works in an office at a desk job.

As you know, we get the nutrients from the foods and the beverages we consume. Most foods contain the nutrients in varying amounts. Let us understand the nutrient composition of the foods we use everyday.

Food Composition

Most food contain more than one nutrient. The nutrient contents of foods have been determined by analysing these in the laboratory. The composition of over 650 Indian foods has been determined. Of these, the nutritive value of about 160 foods is presented in the Appendix F.

The food composition tables give the concentration of nutrients in 100 g of the edible portion (E.P.) of the food. Therefore it is important to know **how much of the food purchased is edible.** In some foods, such as milk, butter, sugar, the edible portion is 100 per cent. In fruits and vegetables, it varies from 65 per cent in bananas to 98 per cent in tomatoes.

The values for nutrients given in food composition tables are averages of the results obtained by analysing a large number of samples of each food. Therefore the figures in such tables give a fairly good idea of the composition of each food.

Foods are grouped in the food value tables, on the basis of the plant part from which the food is derived, for example, seeds, roots, leaves, fruits, etc. Animal foods are grouped on the basis of species and the product used.

It is interesting to note that there are inherent similarities in the composition of foods in each group. In Table 1.1, the composition of various foods has been presented to illustrate this point. For example, the protein content of cereals varies from 7 to 12, and that of *dals* and legumes from 17 to 25 per cent. This information has important applications in practical usage of tables. It is possible to predict the overall nutrient content of combinations used, if we know the amounts of individual foods used. If the composition of a particular food is not found in the tables, you can roughly predict its nutrient contribution, by knowing the group to which it belongs.

You may observe from Table 1.1, that cereals and *dals* do not contain vitamins A and C. Therefore you will realise how important it is to include vegetables and fruits, which are rich source of these two vitamins, in our daily menu of cereals and *dal.* Most of the vegetables and fruits, as you will observe from Table 1.1, are low in calories. Oils, fats and sugars are mainly sources of calories. Thus you get an idea of the contribution of various foods by studying Table 1.1.

Most of the analytical work on Indian foods was carried out in various laboratories under the auspices of Indian Council of Medical Research. A compilation of results is published as the *Nutritive Value of Indian Foods,* by the Indian Council of Medical Research (ICMR). A number of new varieties of food with high contents of certain nutrients, have been developed at research centres under the auspices of the Indian Council of Agricultural Research. You get a number of these foods in the market and use these in your dietary. The nutritive value of these new varieties of foods need to be included in the book on Nutritive Value of Indian Foods. There are two International Food Value tables published by the Food & Agriculture Organisation (FAO) (please refer to these books, which are listed in Further Reading at the end of this book).

It is good to remember that the nutritive value of natural foods does not vary a great deal for a particular variety of the same food from one country to another. But there is a great variation in the composition of prepared foods such as bread, biscuits, cakes, etc., due to variation in recipes and the basic ingredients used from one region to another.

Table 1.1: Food Composition at a Glance[1]

(Approx. Group Values per 100 g. E.P.)

Foods	*Moisture*	*Calories*	*Protein (g)*	*Vit. A (mcg.)*	*Vit. C (mg)*	*Minerals & Vit. B-Comp*
Cereals– rice, Wheat, bajra, Jowar	10	340	7 to 12	—	—	Some
Dals, legumes	10	340	17 to 25	—	—	Some[2]
Milk	85	70	3	48	—	Some[3]
Eggs	75	170	13	960	—	Some
Meat– fish, poultry	75	100–190	18	Some	—	Some
Leafy & Orange-yellow Vegetables & Fruits	90	20	2	1,800	30	Some
Fruits– Vit. C-rich	85	50	1	Some	50	Some
Other vegetables	90	30	2	Some	Some	Some
Other Fruits	85	50	1	Some	Some	Some
Roots & tubers	60–85	50–100	1	Some	Some	Some
Oils & Fats	0	900	—	750[4]	—	—
Sugar, jaggery	0	400	—	—	—	—

1. Please refer to Appendix F for individual composition of foods.
2. Rich source of iron and B-complex.
3. Rich source of calcium and riboflavin.
4. Ghee contains this amount and vanaspati is fortified to provide this amount of Vit. A.

Food Exchange Lists

In 1950, the American Diabetes Association and the American Dietetic Association collaboratively developed a system of food lists to help diabetic patients to select foods in their diets. Similar food lists were prepared in other countries to help diabetics to choose their foods. In India also food lists were prepared based on the foods available and our meal pattern. Since India is a large country there are three major agencies that have evolved their food exchange lists. These agencies are dietetic departments of major regional hospitals, the Home Science colleges, which train dietetic students, and the dietetics department of the National Institute of Nutrition. These are presented in Appendix B.

Each of the list includes a group of foods, which supply about the same calories in the portion indicated. Each food choice within a list is called an exchange. It represents an amount of food that has about the same macronutrient value as other foods in the same group.

The exchange lists are very useful tools in diet planning in hospitals and in personal diet management in the home.

Nutrient Density

It refers to the quantity of one or more nutrients supplied by a food in reference to its calorie content. For example, if one compares the protein content of isocaloric portions of *dal,* bread and milk, one can see that *dal* has the highest nutrient density for protein, milk next and bread the least.

	Calories	*Protein*
Dal	85	5.5
Milk	85	4.0
Bread	85	2.4

Thus, nutrient density is an important aspect to be considered in selection of foods, especially in diets of children, pregnant women, nursing mothers and in therapeutic diets for patients.

Nutrient dense foods like low-fat milk, beans, *dals*, amla, oranges, carrots, spinach, chapatti, etc., do help balance less nutrient dense choices we often make, like *mithai* and chips. The latter tend to supply energy as sugar and fat, but little else.

How will you be a responsible nutrition student?

First, use what you learn in nutrition and benefit yourself. It will help you to look better, feel better and work effectively. By practising what you learn, you will set a good example for others.

Secondly, take care of nutrition of your family. Help the children in the family to develop good food habits, the adults to make good food choices in eating and seniors to meet their changed needs.

Thirdly, as a professional you will be able to help people, who seek your advice, to make appropriate changes to improve their food choices to improve their well-being.

Lastly, as a member of the community, you can influence the choice of foods served in social events.

Study Questions

1. Explain the terms nutrition, nutrients, nutritional care, optimum nutrition and undernutrition.
2. How is food related to health?
3. Discuss the physiological functions of food.
4. "Food is also used to satisfy social and psychological needs". Explain this statement by giving examples..
5. What do you understand by adequate nutrition?
6. Explain the concept of exchange lists.
7. What is nutrient density?
8. How will you use your knowledge of nutrition?

CHAPTER 2

Digestion, Absorption and Utilisation of Nutrients

Introduction

OUR BODY is synthesised from the food we eat. It is made of a complex structure of cells, tissues and organs. How does this change from food to our body structure occur? All the changes that occur in the food from the time we eat it, to its use in the body and discarding of the waste matter are known as metabolism. One can describe metabolism of each nutrient separately to ensure ease of understanding. But actually it occurs in a correlated systematic manner.

Basic concepts of biology and chemistry need to be understood in the study of nutrition. Let us review these.

Concepts in Biology: The study of nutrition begins with the cell, the basic unit of our body. All the nutrition processes, which we refer to as metabolism, take place in the cell. Metabolism includes both **anabolism** and **catabolism.** Anabolism involves synthesis of compounds needed for use in the body. Breakdown of complex substances to simpler ones is known as catabolism. Thus cells are able to take up nutrients, synthesise substances they need and eliminate wastes. The energy release and its utilisation occurs in the cell.

There are many kinds of cells in the body, each type specialises in carrying out certain functions required by the body.

Cells are grouped together to form a tissue. Muscle, nerve, epithelial and connective tissue are examples of various tissues.

Two or more tissues are combined to form an organ, which carries out a specific function. Heart, lungs and kidneys are examples of organs.

Cells are made up of several parts. Each part has an appropriate structure and a specific function. Two main parts of the cell are the nucleus and the protoplasm, which surrounds the nucleus and is called cytoplasm (Figure 2.1).

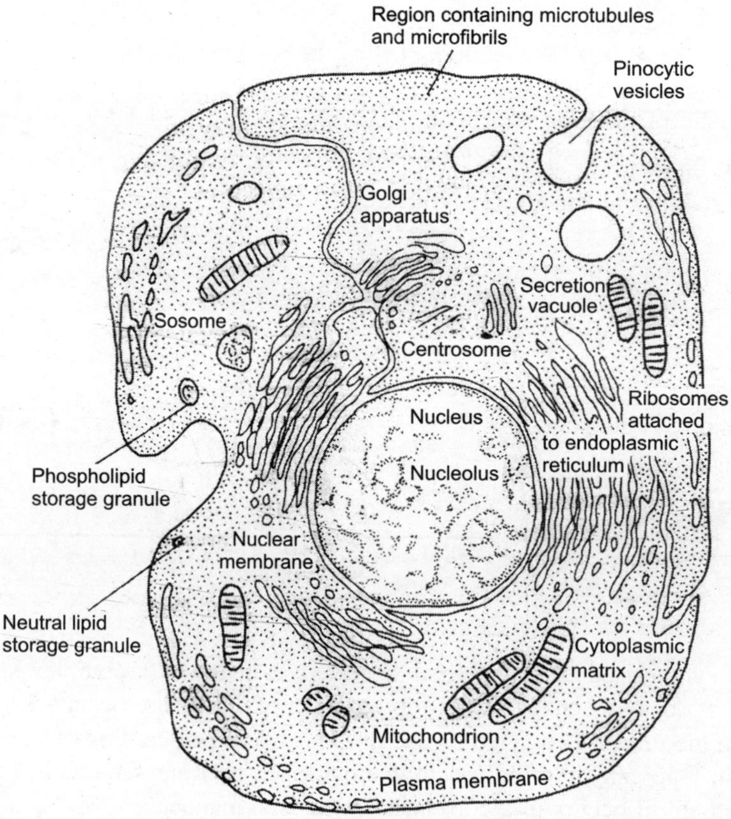

Figure 2.1: Diagram of a typical cell based on electron micrographs. (Adapted from "The Living Cell" by J. Bracket. Copyright © 1961 by Scientific American, Inc. All rights reserved.)

The nucleus controls the functions of the cell; the metabolic activities of the cell are carried out by the cytoplasm.

The deoxyribonucleic acid **(DNA)** in the cell nucleus contains the pattern for each of the different proteins in the body. The ribonucleic acid **(RNA)** directs the actual protein synthesis in the ribosomes, using the information stored in the DNA. This process, which is directed and controlled by DNA, is the key to nutrition.

All the components, which form nutrients, come from food. Our genes determine the nutrients that can be synthesised in the body and those which need to be provided preformed in the food.

The small channels in the cytoplasm, called endoplasmic reticulum, transport nutrients and their metabolites throughout the cytoplasm. The enzymes, which function in metabolism, are found in the membranes surrounding the channels.

The **mitochondria** and **lysosomes** are also present in the cytoplasm. Mitochondria release the energy provided by the carbohydrates, fats and proteins and transfer it to an energy acceptor (ATP). The ATP transfers the energy as needed wherever work is being done. Therefore the mitochondria are known as the 'power plants' of the cell.

Lysosomes contain enzymes, which function in the breakdown of proteins and other compounds. Lysosomes help to digest foreign matter that may have entered the cell and thus protect the body from their harmful effects.

Chemistry: Our body and the food that nourishes it are made of chemical elements. Therefore knowledge of the chemical elements and their behaviour is basic to the study of nutrition.

Elements: Elements are fundamental units of matter, which have characteristic properties. The Periodic Table contains all the elements. Of the 106 known elements, 92 occur in nature, the rest are of synthetic origin. Examples of elements are oxygen, carbon and iron.

Atoms: The smallest constituent part of an element is an atom. There are smaller particles, which are parts of an atom. The **proton** (+vely charged) and **neutron** (uncharged) particle are located in the nucleus of the atom. In the shells (orbits) around the nucleus, the **electron,** a negatively charged particle is found.

Atoms of one element can combine with atoms of another element to form a compound. For example, water contains two atoms of hydrogen and one of oxygen (H_2O).

Molecule: Chemical elements exist as molecules, a basic unit, which can be made up of atoms of one or more elements. Thus we have a molecule of oxygen (O_2) with two atoms of oxygen, while sodium chloride (NaCl) contains one atom of sodium and one atom of chlorine.

Ion: An electrically charged atom, group or molecule is called an ion. A positively, charged ion is called a **cation,** and a negatively charged one an **anion.** K^+ is an example, of a positive atom and Cl^- is a negative atom; potassium chloride (KCl) is a neutral compound.

Isotopes: Some elements have isotopes, that is they exist in two forms, with two different atomic weights; for example, the atomic weight of carbon is 12, its isotope has an atomic weight of 14 (^{14}C). The ^{14}C isotope of carbon is naturally radioactive.

Acids, Bases, pH: A chemical compound, which when dissolved in water yields hydrogen ions (H^+), is an acid. There are two types of acids, inorganic acids and organic acids. Hydrochloric, sulfuric and phosphoric are inorganic acids. Organic or carboxylic acids contain one or more carboxyl groups (COOH) in their molecule. Fatty acids and amino acids are important organic acids in nutrition.

Hydrogen ion concentration is the amount of hydrogen ion (H^+) per unit volume of an aqueous (water) solution. It is referred to as pH.

Some Chemical Reactions: Some chemical reactions, which occur in biological systems, are listed here.

1. **Salt formation:** When an acid and a base react, salt is one of the products formed.

$$HCl + KOH \rightarrow KCl + H_2O$$
$$\text{acid + base} \rightarrow \text{salt + water}$$

2. **Ester formation:** When an organic acid reacts with an alcohol, an ester is formed. When a fatty acid reacts with glycerol, a fat (an ester) is formed.
3. **Oxidation-reduction:** Oxidation is always accompanied by a reduction, in which electrons are transferred from one atom to another. The atom that gives up the electron is oxidised, the one that receives the electron is reduced. Thus ferric ion is reduced by vitamin C to ferrous form.

$$Fe^{+++} + \text{reduced form of vit. C} \rightarrow$$
$$Fe^{++} + \text{oxidised form of vitamin C}$$

4. **Hydrolysis:** The reaction of water with another compound, with uptake of a molecule of water, is known as hydrolysis. The breakdown of carbohydrates and fats in digestion is an example of hydrolysis.
5. **Phosphorylation:** is a chemical reaction in which a phosphate group is introduced into an organic compound. The formation of ATP from ADP is an example of this reaction.
6. **Synthesis:** When a complex substance is formed from simpler substances by a series of reactions it is known as synthesis. Synthesis of proteins from amino acids is a good example of this reaction.
7. **Degradation:** Complex substances are gradually broken down to simpler ones. The breakdown of glycogen to glucose is an example of degradation reaction.

Use of Food in the Body

The use of food in the body involves three processes — digestion, absorption and utilisation of nutrients in the body.

Digestion is the process, which releases many nutrients in the forms the body can use, by breaking up food in the intestinal tract.

Absorption is the process which carries these nutrients into the circulation system and delivers them to the cell.

Utilisation. Cell is the functional unit of life. Hence a large number of the chemical reactions in the cell utilise the nutrients absorbed to produce materials needed for our existence.

Mechanical processes involved in digestion include chewing of food, swallowing of food, churning action in the stomach and rhythmic contraction of the intestinal tract.

Chewing of food reduces the food particles in size, mixes these with saliva and dilutes it with water, so that it is easy to swallow. The food swallowed is mixed with enzymes and acid by the churning action in the stomach. Further the rhythmic contraction of the intestine, help to break the food into small particles and move the food mass forward through the digestive tract (Figure 2.2).

Chemical reactions in digestion process: The first reaction is *hydrolysis* or splitting with the help of water. Carbohydrates, fats and proteins break up with the addition of water into smaller molecules, which the tissues can use.

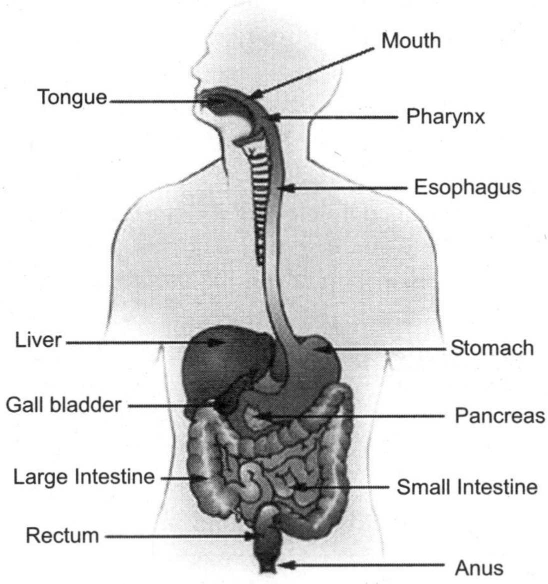

Figure 2.2: The digestive tract.

The chemical reactions are accelerated by enzymes, which are secreted in the mouth, stomach and small intestine. Enzymes are living catalysts, that increase the speed of biological reactions, without being a part of the compound formed. The enzymatic reactions, which take place in the digestion process, are presented in Table 2.1.

As you may know, enzymes are proteins by nature. Their name indicates substance on which they can act, for example, sucrase acts on sucrose. Enzymes are specific in their actions. An enzyme, which hydrolyses protein, will not act on starch. Each enzyme acts optimally at a certain pH, e.g., amylase acts only in alkaline medium.

Some enzymes need another group, known as a coenzyme, to be attached to it to aid their function. For example, B-vitamin serve as coenzymes in the reactions, which release energy from glucose. In enzyme reactions, mineral elements are essential as cofactors. Thus normal body metabolism is dependent on the presence of appropriate enzymes, coenzymes and cofactors specific to each reaction.

The digestive enzymes are only one group of a large number that are essential to regulate body processes. Other enzymes are present in various tissues of the body and help in the utilisation of food that has been absorbed.

Carbohydrates

The digestion process begins with chewing the food in the mouth. The enzyme *ptyalin* (salivary amylase) starts the digestion of starch in the mouth. It hydrolyses starch to dextrins, isomaltose and maltose in neutral or alkaline pH in the mouth. The food tastes sweet due to these products of hydrolysis. The activity of amylase continues in its movement from the mouth to the upper part of the stomach. But as soon as the food mass comes in contact with hydrochloric acid secreted there, this action ceases. Very little digestion of carbohydrate occurs in the stomach as the pH is unfavourable.

The food mixed with gastric juice forms a semi-fluid mass called **chyme.** It takes about three to five hours to form chyme. Small portion of chyme are released through the pyloric sphincter into the duodenum, the first part of the small intestine.

The **small intestine** is so named because of the small diameter of its tube. It is about 20 ft long. Most of the digestive activity takes place in its three compartments namely the duodenum, the jejunum and ileum.

Carbohydrate digestion occurs almost completely in the small intestine, mainly in the duodenum. **Pancreatic amylase** breaks starches into maltose and dextrins. The **maltase** from mucosal cells breaks down maltose to glucose. The brush border, on the surface of the epithelial cells lining the intestines, is the site of this enzyme action.

The enzymes **sucrase, lactase, maltase,** and **isomaltase,** found on the outer cell membranes of the intestines, act on the sugars sucrose, lactose, maltose and isomaltose respectively. The monosaccharides formed—glucose, galactose and fructose—pass through the mucosal cell and via the capillary into the blood stream. These are carried to the liver by the portal vein.

Table 2.1: Enzymatic Reactions in Digestion

Place of Action	*Enzyme*	*Optimum pH*	*Substrate*	*Products of Reaction*
Mouth	Salivary amylase (Ptyalin)	7.0	Cooked starch	Dextrins, maltose
Stomach	Pepsin (protease)	2.0	Proteins	Polypeptides
	Rennin	6.0–6.5	Milk, casein	Calcium caseinate
	Lipase	7.0	Emulsified fats	Fatty acids, glycerol
Small Intestine	**Pancreatic Juice**			
	Trypsin (Protease)	8.0–9.0	Proteins	Polypeptides, some amino-acids
	Lipase	7.0	Fats	Di and mono-glycerides, fatty acids, glycerol
	Amylase	7.1	Starch	Maltose
	Intestinal Juice			
	Peptidases (Erepsin)	8.0	Peptones, Polypeptides	Amino acids
	Sucrase	5.0–7.0	Sucrose	Glucose, fructose
	Maltose	6.7–7.2	Maltose	Glucose (2 molecules)
	Lactase	5.4–6.0	Lactose	Glucose, galactose

1. pH is expressed as the negative logarithm of 'hydrogen ion concentration'. The pH of water is 7; the acids have pH less than 7 and alkalies have pH above 7.

Some glucose is stored in the liver and muscles as glycogen, the rest is transported to tissues to be used for their activities. Fructose and galactose are converted to glucose in the liver.

Cellulose, hemicellulose, lignin and other forms of carbohydrate, which are collectively known as fibre, are not split by human amylases. These are excreted in the faeces.

Proteins

Digestion of proteins starts in the stomach, which serves as a storehouse, where some protein hydrolysis begins. Milk is clotted by a special enzyme rennin and acid is added.

Gastric juice, which is secreted by the stomach, contains hydrochloric acid, pepsin, rennin, mucin and other substances.

Hydrochloric acid has several important functions: (1) it swells the proteins, thus increasing their surface area for enzyme action, (2) it converts the inactive *pepsinogen* to the enzyme pepsin, (3) it provides the acid medium necessary for the action of pepsin, (4) it provides acidic pH for solution of calcium and iron salts, (5) it reduces or destroys the activity of many pathogens (harmful bacteria) present in the food.

Pepsin is the only proteolytic enzyme, which is able to digest collagen, the main protein in connective tissue. Pepsin, a protease in the gastric juice, splits proteins to polypeptides. It also digests the milk curds formed by the enzyme rennin. The contribution of the stomach to the total process of protein digestion is small, as most protein digestion occurs in the duodenum.

As soon as the chyme enters the duodenum, it stimulates the intestinal mucosa to release an enzyme **enterokinase,** which converts inactive **trypsinogen** into active **trypsin.** Trypsin activates other proteolytic enzymes—**chymotrypsin** and carboxypolypeptidases. These enzymes breakdown intact protein and with the help of peptidases continue the breakdown until small polypeptides and amino acids are formed. The last phase of protein digestion also occurs in brush border, in which peptidases hydrolyse di- and tri-peptides into constituent amino acids. But some intact peptides do escape hydrolysis and enter the portal circulation.

The amino acids released are absorbed via distinct active transport systems. Absorbed amino acids and peptides are transported via the portal vein to the liver to be released into the general circulation.

By the time it reaches the jejunum, almost all the protein is absorbed. Only one per cent of digested protein is excreted in the faeces.

Some amino acids, which remain in the epithelial cells, are used in the synthesis of new cells and intestinal enzymes. The endogenous protein released internally (by breaking down of epithelial cells and intestinal secretions) is digested and absorbed from the small intestine along with that ingested in the diet.

Lipids

The stomach lipase does act on emulsified fats in milk, cream, butter and egg yolk, but most of the hydrolysis of fats takes place in the small intestine.

As soon as the food enters the duodenum, the gall bladder releases some bile and the pancreas secrete enzyme-rich juices. These fluids enter the duodenum through a common duct. Bile is a secretion composed of bile acids, bile pigments, cholesterol, lecithin and many other compounds. About a liter of bile is secreted daily due to the stimulus of food in the duodenum.

The bile, which is manufactured by the liver, helps to

- emulsify fat particles, which increases surface area and improves enzyme action.
- neutralise the acid chyme and provide the alkaline pH necessary for the action of the intestinal enzymes.

The pancreatic juices contain trypsin, lipase and amylase, which act upon all components of foods. Thus proteins are broken down by trypsin into amino acids. Large sugar molecules are changed to simple sugars by action of amylase and lipase acts on glycerides and reduces these to fatty acid and glycerol.

The products of fat digestion inhibit the digestion process. The digested meal must be removed from the duodenum over a period of time, to permit digestion to proceed. Hence a fatty meal may remain up to four hours or more in the stomach. Thus there is a feeling of satiation after a fatty meal.

Micelles, a combination of free fatty acids, monoglycerides and bile salts, facilitate the passage of lipids through the aqueous environment of the intestinal lumen to the brush border. The bile salts are then released from the lipid complex and return 3 to 15 times to carry more lipids across the membrane, depending on the amount of food ingested.

The fatty acids and monoglycerides are reassembled into new triglycerides in the mucosal cell. **Chylomicrons** are formed by surrounding a combination of triglycerides, cholesterol, and phospholipids with a beta-lipoprotein coat. Chylomicrons are transported by lymphatic vessels into the blood stream and further on to the liver. The triglycerides are transported to adipose tissue for metabolism and storage.

Cholesterol is hydrolysed by **pancreatic cholesterol esterase** from ester form and absorbed in the same manner as lipids.

The fat soluble vitamins A, D, E and K are also absorbed in a similar fashion. Some forms of the vitamins A, E and K and carotene do not need bile acids for their absorption.

Normally 97 per cent of ingested fat is absorbed into lymph vessels. Fatty acids of 10 carbons or less, due to shorter length and increased solubility, do not need bile salts and micelle formation for their absorption and can be absorbed directly into the mucosal cell. From the mucosal cell these acids go directly via the portal vein to the liver, without esterification.

This is clinically a very useful quality of medium-chain fatty acids. Those patients, who cannot metabolise usual long-chain fatty acids in dietary fat, due to lack of bile salts or some other problem, can be fed triglycerides of medium-chain fatty acids (C_8 and C_{10}). These can be utilised directly.

The digestive process is also aided by friendly bacteria which live in the intestinal tract. They help in hydrolysing food and manufacture some of the nutrients (e.g., vitamin K, folic acid and some B-complex vitamins).

Other Nutrients

Vitamins and water pass unchanged from the small intestine into blood by passive diffusion.

Mineral absorption, which is more complex, occurs in three stages. In the first stage, chemical reactions occur in the stomach and intestines, which are affected by the pH of the mix. In the second stage, these are carried across the membrane into intestinal mucosal cell. In the third stage, minerals are transported into the blood stream or are bound within the cell.

Important interactions occur between minerals in the gastrointestinal tract, which affect the amount that is absorbed.

There is simultaneous absorption of vitamins, minerals and fluids through the intestinal mucosa. About 8 liters of fluids move to and from across the membrane of the gut to keep the nutrients in solution. The current understanding of the sites and routes of absorption of nutrients is depicted in Figure 2.3.

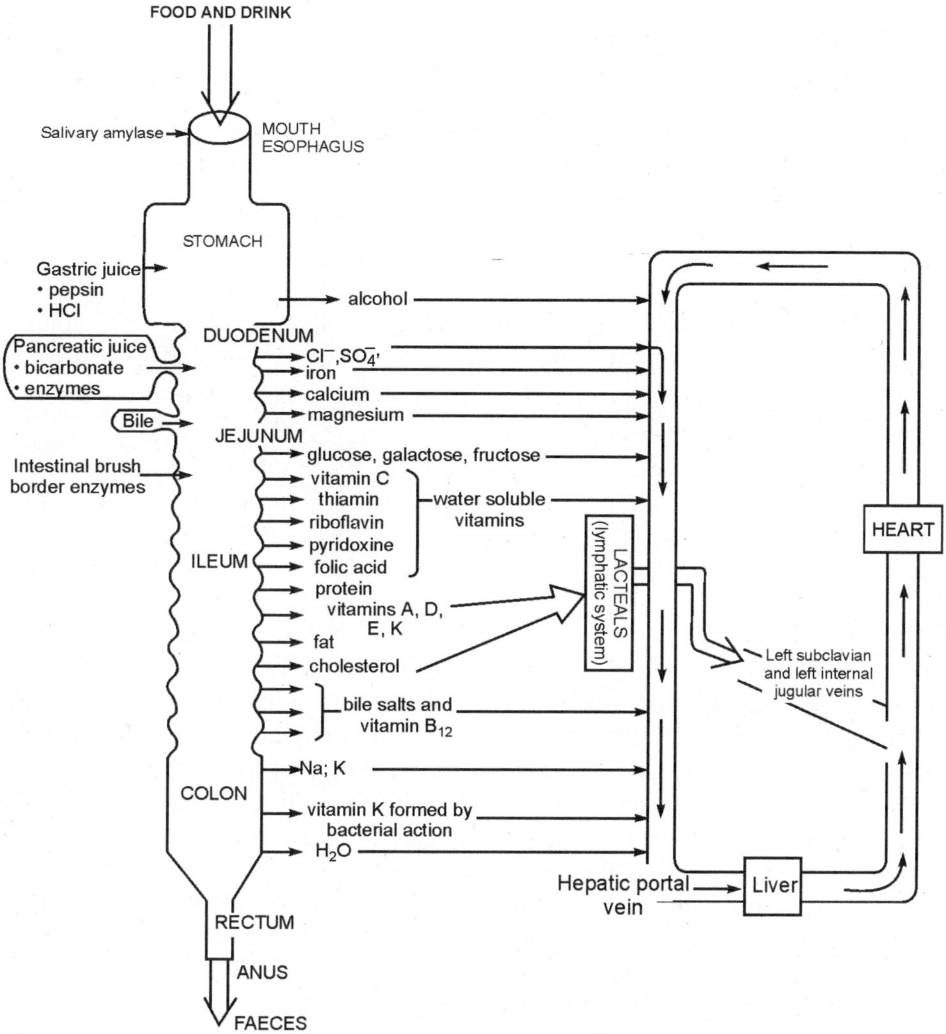

Figure 2.3: Gastrointestinal tract-sites of secretions and absorption.

Factors Affecting Digestion

Several factors affect the digestion process. These include:

1. Psychological factors, which play an important role in food acceptance, ingestion and digestion. If one likes the sight, smell and taste of food, it increases secretions of saliva, stomach juices and motility of gastrointestinal tract. Even the thought of food increases these secretions. On the other hand, if these are not liked, it depresses the secretions.
2. Generally well cooked foods are more digestible than raw foods.
3. Sound teeth to bite, cut and tear food into smaller pieces helps digestion, absence of molars, incisors and/or canine teeth affects the person's ability to grind the food adversely and hence digestion is poor.
4. Sufficient supply of water to dilute the food, permits effective movement through the digestive tract and increases the surface area for efficient enzymatic breakdown.
5. Sufficient bulk (fibre) helps to maintain normal forward movement.

6. Normal secretion of enzymes, bile, hydrochloric acid aids the chemical splitting of food components to small absorbable units.
7. The presence of friendly bacteria in the intestinal tract helps digestion.
8. Relaxation of body permits the processes involved in digestion to occur normally. Any psychological stress, which makes a person tense, interferes with the digestive process by upsetting the occurrence of the normal secretions mentioned above.

Role of Large Intestine

Large intestine consists of cecum, colon, rectum and the canal and is about 5 feet long.

About 500 to 1,000 ml of water in the chyme enters the colon each day. Most of it is absorbed and only 50 to 200 ml is excreted in the faeces. Since the colonic contents move forward very slowly, most of the nutritionally valuable matter is absorbed.

The large amounts of mucus secretion by the mucosa of large intestine protects the intestinal walls from the adverse effects of bacterial and other action. The mucus also helps to hold the faeces together. The neutralisation of acidic products of bacterial action is ensured by the action of bicarbonate ions secreted in exchange for absorbed chloride ions.

Absorption and Transportation

Absorption is the process of sucking up the nutrients in the body. Most of the absorption takes place in the small intestine. Absorption of food from the digestive tract into the blood and lymph takes place after the digested food is moved forward by peristaltic waves (muscular contraction and relaxation) into the small intestine. These peristaltic waves push the food against the absorbing surface of the intestinal wall. The intestinal wall is lined with four to five million tiny finger-like projections called **villi** (see Figure 2.4.). The cells which cover villi permit the absorption of final products of digestion—small molecules of sugars, amino acids and fat products and water, into the vessels that carry away the blood and lymph. The large area of these villi promote efficient absorption of all nutrients. Ordinarily a great deal of time is permitted for the absorptive process because the digested material must traverse the entire length of the intestine a distance of about 20 ft.

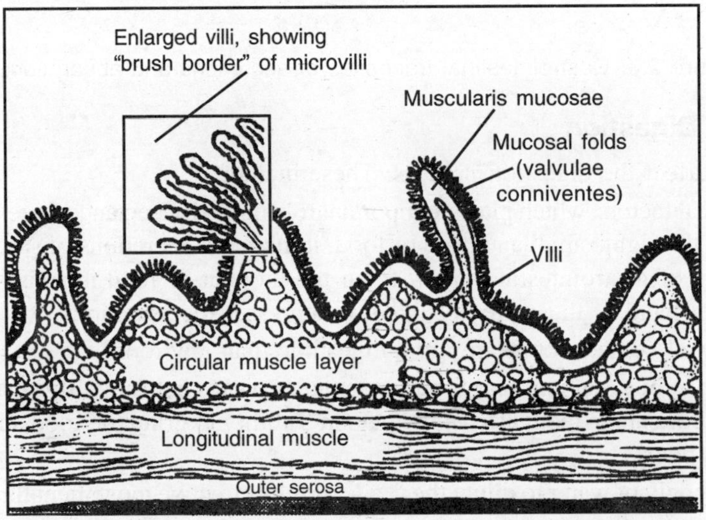

Figure 2.4: Intestinal wall—mucosal folds, villi and microvilli.

Besides the shape and size of intestinal wall, other factors affect absorption of the digested food. For example, bile favours absorption of fats, calcium can be absorbed in the presence of vitamin D and vitamin B_{12} can be absorbed only in the presence of an intrinsic factor in the gastric juice.

The intestine, which is a semipermeable membrane, is highly selective and permits the passage of nutrients only under certain special conditions. Thus absorption is affected by concentrations of the nutrients in the blood. A high concentration in the blood stream may allow less absorption of vitamins and minerals than would be permitted at a time when the blood level of these nutrients is low.

The sugars, amino acids, water-soluble vitamins, minerals salts and possibly some of the fat products are absorbed directly into the blood stream through the intestinal wall and are carried to the liver. The remainder of the end products of fat digestion and the fat soluble vitamins enter into the lymph system.

Individuals in normal health may vary in their capacity to absorb even fully hydrolysed foods. The recommended daily dietary allowances and the daily food guide provide quantities of nutrients generally sufficient to cover the needs of individuals with normal variations in capacities to digest and absorb nutrients.

Utilisation of Nutrients in the Body

Metabolism of all nutrients occurs within the cells of our body. The final oxidation of nutrients into carbon dioxide and water occurs in the mitochondria. About 40 per cent of the energy released is used to synthesise ATP, the remainder is released as heat.

The ATP formed provides energy for the synthetic reactions in the cell. Fatty acid breakdown also occurs in the mitochondria. The individual cells die and are replaced by new cells formed as part of normal life processes.

Glycolysis: Within the tissue cells, the first phase of glucose breakdown occurs in the cytoplasm. This anaerobic stage of carbohydrate breakdown is known as **glycolysis,** in which glycogen or glucose is converted to pyruvic acid. This is schematically presented in Figure 2.5.

Tricarboxylic Acid Cycle (TCA) or Citric Acid Cycle: The intermediate compounds of carbohydrate, fat and protein metabolism are metabolised by a common final oxidative pathway. This pathway is referred to as tricarboxylic acid cycle (TCA) or Citric acid cycle or Krebs cycle. The name tricarboxylic indicates that it involves acids with three carboxyl (—COOH) groups; it is also called Krebs cycle, as Krebs was the first scientist to have worked it out.

In the mitochondria, pyruvic acid is converted to acetyl coenzyme A (CoA) before entering the citric acid cycle.This complex reaction needs five enzymes and four coenzymes, four of which contain four B vitamins (pantothenic acid, thiamin, niacin and riboflavin). The pantothenic acid is a part of coA structure. The two carbon acetic acid combines with four carbon oxaloacetic acid forming citric acid (6–C acid), with release of coenzyme A. This is the starting point of the citric acid cycle, which is depicted in Figure 2.5. In this figure all steps at which hydrogen atoms, carbon dioxide or ATP are formed are shown; a few intermediate substances are omitted.

The cycle moves only clockwise from citric acid to oxaloacetic acid. In each round, one molecule of acetic acid is degraded to carbon dioxide and water with synthesis of ATP. This ATP is the source of energy for many synthetic reactions in the cells.

The **fats** are broken down to fatty acids and glycerol. In the cytoplasm, glycerol is transformed into triose phosphate, which can be oxidised to carbon dioxide and water via TCA cycle or it may be used to form glucose.

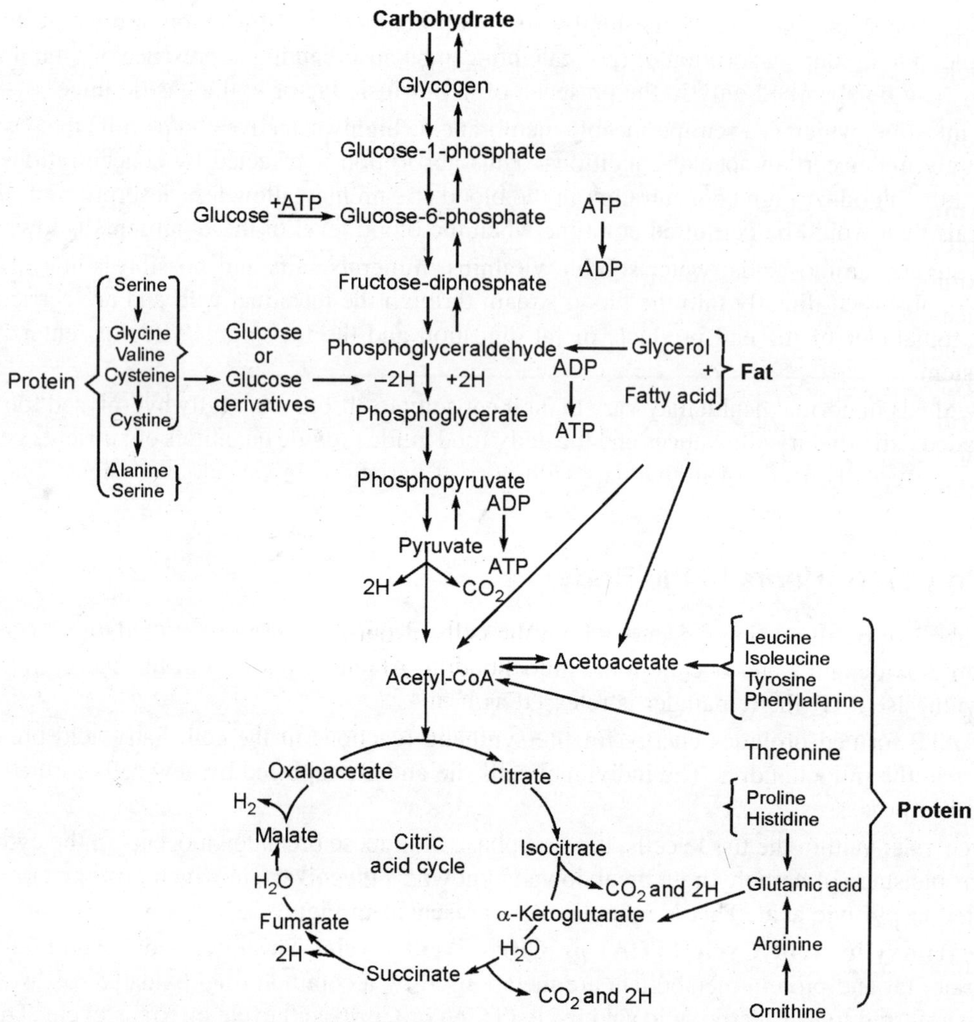

Figure 2.5: Integration of carbohydrate, fat and protein metabolism. The scheme indicates glycolysis, citric acid cycle and their interconnections.

The fatty acids are oxidised to form two carbon units in the form of acetyl coA in a stepwise manner. The acetyl coA enters the citric acid cycle and is metabolised as mentioned above. These reactions occur in the mitochondria.

Beta-oxidation of fatty acids: The fatty acid oxidation is referred to as beta-oxidation, because fatty acid chain loses two carbon atoms at a time, which means the oxidation starts at the beta carbon. When the first two carbons are separated, the new beta-carbon is attacked and so on. This may be represented as follows:

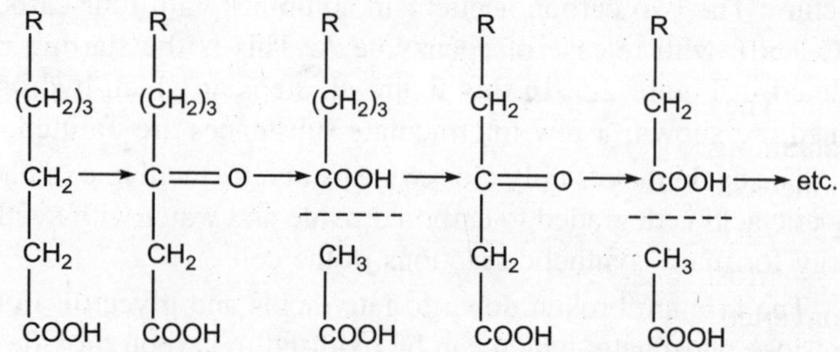

Figure 2.6: Beta-oxidisation of fatty acids.

The two carbon unit combines with coenzyme A and forms acetyl coA which enters the citric acid cycle. The beta oxidation of fatty acids can be shown as given in Figure 2.6. Acetyl coA may be used to synthesise new fatty acids, cholesterol, etc. As noted before, acetyl coA is formed during breakdown of both glucose and amino acids. Thus excess energy intake in any form (fats, carbohydrates, proteins) is deposited as fat in the adipose tissue.

Amino acids, the products of protein digestion are absorbed by the tissues and used to synthesise tissue proteins, antibodies, some hormones and vitamins.

Amino acids are very labile compounds, which can be converted to one another and into other substances. The first step in this process is called **deamination,** the removal of amino group (—NH_2). The amino group may be transferred to a keto-acid to form amino acids, which are normally formed in the body. Hence these amino acids are not essential to be supplied in the diet.

Transamination refers to the transfer of amino groups from one compound to another. Thus L-glutamic acid, loses NH_2 to a keto acid, for example pyruvic acid, to form alanine, an amino acid. Transamination reactions are catalysed by transaminases, which need coenzyme containing vitamin B.

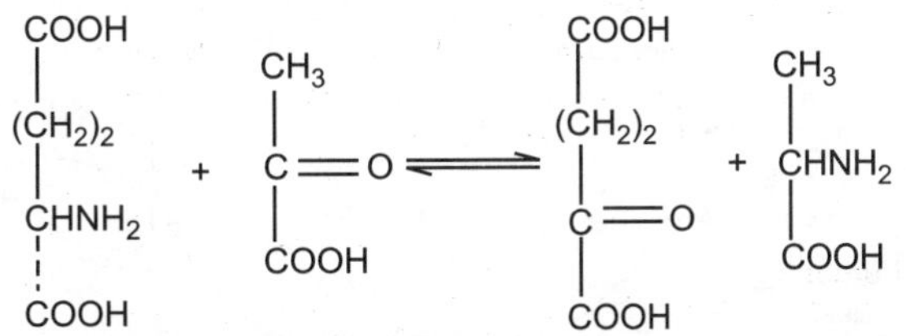

Glutamic acid | Pyruvic acid | Alpha-keto glutaric acid | Alanine

Transaminases are present in all tissues, but heart, muscle, brain; kidney, liver and testes have higher concentrations of the enzyme.

Deamination occurs when the amino group of an amino acid is oxidatively removed by a special dehydrogenase system to form a keto acid and ammonia. Thus glutamic acid is oxidised to form alpha-keto glutaric acid and ammonia as shown below:

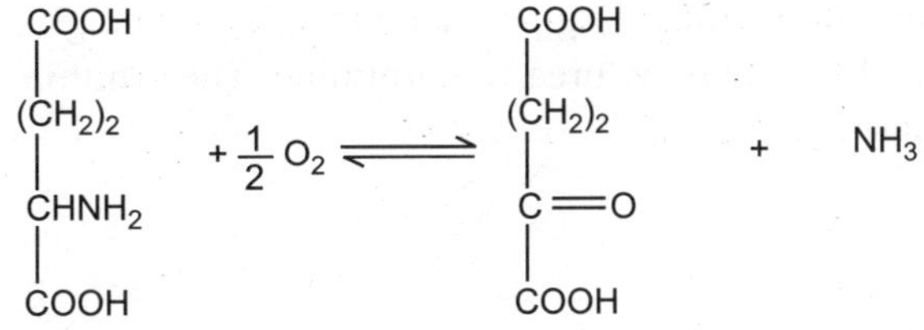

Gllutamic acid | Alpha-keto glutaric acid | Ammonia

The enzyme required for this deamination reaction is amino acid oxidase, which needs a coenzyme containing riboflavin. Liver is the site of most deamination reactions, but if needed, it can occur in the kidneys also. All the deaminated parts of amino acids can enter the citric acid cycle as shown in Figure 2.5.

Most of the nitrogen containing groups, split off from amino acids (80 to 90 per cent), are converted to urea in the liver and excreted in the urine.

Urea Formation: The ammonia formed in deamination is converted in the liver to urea. Urea is the main nitrogenous product of amino acid metabolism. On a normal diet, urea forms 85 to 92 per cent of total nitrogen and it is excreted in the urine. Other nitrogenous constituents of urine are uric acid, ammonia and creatinine, which form a very small fraction of urinary nitrogen.

The schematic formation of urea is given in Figure 2.7.

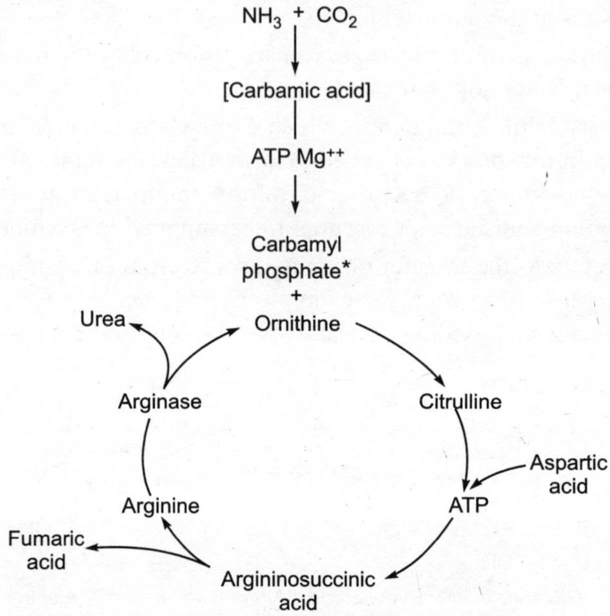

*N-acetyl-L-glutamate is very likely involved in the reactions leading to the formation of Carbamyl phosphate.

Figure 2.7: Formation of urea.

The ammonia formed in deamination of amino acids combines with carbon dioxide yielding compound to form carbamic acid. ATP is required as also Mg^{++} to form carbamyl phosphate, which reacts with ornithine to form citrulline. The enol form of citrulline reacts with aspartic acid in the presence of ATP to form an intermediate (argino-succinic acid) which gives arginine and fumaric acid. The arginine is decomposed by arginase to urea and ornithine. The ornithine is ready to take up CO_2 and NH_3 via carbamyl phosphate again.

Study Questions

1. Explain the following: atom, ion, compound, radioisotope, organic acid and synthesis.
2. List the enzymes involved in the digestion of food and the functions of each enzyme.
3. What are the functions of hydrochloric acid?
4. List the factors which are needed for normal digestion.
5. What are the coenzymes and cofactors needed in the citric acid cycle?

CHAPTER 3

The Recommended Dietary Allowances for Nutrients

Introduction

Each day we need a number of nutrients to enable our body to carry out its activities efficiently. To determine what nutrients we need each day and how much, to keep us in good health, a lot of research has been done. The results of these studies have been used to work out the nutritional requirements of Indian people. Normally, a factor of safety is added to the amount determined in studies of the nutrient requirements. Recommended intakes of nutrients that meet the needs of almost all healthy people of similar age and gender are termed the Recommended Dietary Allowances.

An advisory committee of the Indian Council of Medical Research (ICMR) is responsible for the setting up; review and revision of these RDAs. Let us understand why and how these RDAs were set-up.

Why were the Recommendations Set-up?

In a number of studies, the harmful effects of nutrient deficiencies on the human body and its functions were observed. These were so revealing that the League of Nations thought it necessary to set-up a committee to review available experimental data and recommend daily dietary allowances for each of the nutrients that were known at that time.

During the Second World War (1939–45), the military recruiting officers had to reject a number of young men, who wanted to enlist, because they were underweight. Naturally, the governments in various countries were anxious to rectify this situation. Another related problem was the need to estimate the amount of food to be sent to various army units. This led to the setting up of Recommended Dietary Allowances (RDAs) in number of countries between, 1940 and 1944. India was one of the first countries to set-up Recommended Dietary Allowances in 1944. The desirable dietary intakes of energy, protein, calcium, iron, vitamin A, thiamin, ascorbic acid and vitamin D were suggested in the RDAs set-up in 1944.

On the basis of newer research findings, these recommendations have been revised four times and fifth revision is expected in the near future.

In 1958, the recommendations for energy were revised. In 1968 and again in 1978 allowances of all nutrients except energy were revised. In 1968, additional recommendations were made for four B vitamins, namely riboflavin, nicotinic acid, folic acid and vitamin B_{12}. In 1978, the requirements for a one more B vitamin, pyridoxine (B_6) were included.

In making these recommendations, the ICMR committee was guided by the dietary allowances suggested by Expert group of FAO and WHO and also by the results of studies carried out in India on nutrient requirements.

In the 1978 revision, the unit of energy joule, adopted by International Union of Sciences and IUNS (International Union of Nutritional Sciences) has also been included.

The 1978 revision was entitled Recommended Dietary Intake (RDI), to emphasise the intake of nutrients. The word 'recommended' is used to emphasise that these values need to be revised periodically on the basis of newer research data.

The last revision was made in 1988. The important features of the 1988 revision are:

- the revision of body weight standards for Indians
- complete revision of energy requirements
- definition of quantum and type of fat intakes
- modification of RDAs of vitamin A and D
- inclusion of several nutrients and dietary factors not considered earlier, such as fibre, electrolytes (sodium, potassium), magnesium, phosphorus, vitamin E and K, and
- for the first time a provisional recommendation on trace elements was made.

No substantial changes were made in the RDAs for protein, B-complex vitamins, iron and calcium.

Please note R stands for recommended, not required; D stands for dietary, not daily. It is not necessary to consume RDA for each nutrient everyday; think instead of averaging the RDA for minerals and vitamins over a week.

General Principles of Deriving RDA

A number of general principles are used to arrive at nutritional requirements of an individual or the RDA for a population. These are:

- **Dietary intakes:** This approach has been used to arrive at the energy needs of children. Energy intakes of normally growing children is used as the basis for RDA.
- **Growth:** To define requirements in early infancy, the breast milk intake of healthy infants, or the requirement of any particular nutrient for satisfactory growth has been utilised.

- **Nutrient balance:** As for a number of other nutrients, to arrive at the protein requirements, the minimum intake of nutrient for equilibrium (intake = output) in adults, and nutrient retention consistent with satisfactory growth in children, have been used widely.
- **Obligatory loss of nutrients:** is the minimal loss of the nutrient or its metabolic product through normal routes of elimination (viz., urine, faeces and sweat). It is determined on a diet devoid of or very low in the nutrient. For example, a protein-free diet in case of proteins. This information is used to determine the amount of nutrient to be consumed daily through the diet to replace the obligatory loss. In infants and children, growth requirements are added to the above maintenance requirements.
- **Factorial method:** In this method, the needs for various functions are assessed separately and added up to assess the total daily requirements. This is the method used to arrive at total energy requirements.
- **Nutrient turnover:** Data collected by studying turnover of certain nutrients in healthy persons, using isotopically labelled nutrients has been used to determine their requirements. Vitamin A, vitamin C, iron and vitamin B_{12} requirement have been measured in this manner.
- **Depletion and repletion studies:** These have been used to determine the requirements of water-soluble vitamins. The vitamin status is measured by recording the levels of vitamin or its coenzyme in serum or tissue (e.g., erythrocytes, leucocytes). The requirements of ascorbic acid (vitamin C), thiamin, riboflavin, niacin and pyridoxine have been established using this approach. The subjects are first fed a diet very low in the nutrient being studied until the biochemical parameters reach a low level. After that feeding graded doses of the nutrient is studied. The level at which response increases rapidly indicates the level of requirement of the nutrient.

How is RDA Derived?

RDA is derived on the basis of —

(*a*) A knowledge of the requirement of nutrients for each physiological group.

(*b*) It is based on nutrient requirement determined by one or more of the approaches listed above.

(*c*) The RDA is computed after considering nutrient bioavailability from the diet.

(*d*) It is presumed that the requirement of all other nutrients are met adequately. RDA is applicable only under this condition.

(*e*) RDA is applicable only to a healthy population living under normal conditions.

(*f*) The RDA is computed after considering individual variability.

(*g*) In practice a level of intake corresponding to the Mean +2 standard deviations, which covers the requirements of 97.5 per cent of the population is chosen as RDA. This safe level approach is not used in the case of energy, as excess or inadequate intake is undesirable, only the average requirement of energy is defined as RDA.

For certain nutrients, such as protein, iron, calcium, beta-carotene and vitamin B_{12}, bioavailability from the diet is a critical factor.

For proteins, the essential amino acid mix in the diet, which decides the quality of protein is important. In the normal Indian diet, protein is derived from several sources, such as cereals, *dals* and legumes, milk and milk products and a variety of vegetables. Occasionally fish, eggs and other flesh foods are included according to one's taste and resources. Hence, the quality tends to be satisfactory, due to mutual supplementation of individual proteins.

In case of iron, while the total intake may be satisfactory, absorption from foods is a critical factor. Absorption is affected by the relative presence of both absorption promotors, (acid medium, e.g., ascorbic and other acids) and absorption inhibitors (phytates, tannins, oxalate, etc.). In the diets habitually consumed in India, which are high in inhibitors and low in promotors, iron absorption is only 2 to 5 per cent.

In case of vitamin A, niacin and others, provitamins present in foods, are converted to the respective vitamins in the body. The RDA for vitamin A and niacin are defined after considering these factors.

Reference Body Weights of Indians

The nutrient needs vary with age and weight of an individual. Body weights and heights of children reflect their state of health and growth rate, while adult weight and height represent what can be attained by an individual with normal growth. Anthropometric measurements of Indian children up to 14 years from well-to-do groups have shown that they grow at rates similar to those of children in the developed countries. Desirable heights and weights of both children and adults (not the prevailing ones) are considered in recommending nutrient intakes as the RDA is intended for a healthy and well-nourished population.

In the 1978 revision of RDA, the body weights of well-to-do Indian children and adolescents were used to compute their nutritional needs. But for adults, a reference body weight of 55 kg for men and 45 kg for women have been used since 1944. The weights of adults do not match those of well nourished adolescents. Secondly, with current heights of 163 cm and 151 cm of Indian adult men and women, the corresponding expected body weights would be higher than the reference weights of 55 and 45 kg used so far. Hence, the ICMR committee recommended that the reference weights for Indian man and woman used for RDA be increased to 60 kg and 50 kg respectively.

Table 3.1: Reference Body Weights of Indians of Different Age Groups[1]

	Age (Years)	*Weight (in Kg)*	
		Male	*Female*
Infants	0–0.5	5.4	5.4
	0.5–1.0	8.6	8.6
Children	1–3	12.6	11.8
	4–6	19.2	18.7
	7–9	27.0	26.7
	10–12	35.5	37.9
Adolescents	13–15	47.9	46.7
	16–18	57.3	49.9
Adults	20–50	60.0	50.0

1. RDA for Indians, ICMR, 1990, page 9.

Reference Person

Reference body weights (kg) of Indians of different age groups are given in Table 3.1.
Our nutrient needs vary with the size and age of our body. Therefore an individual of given age and size has been designated as a reference. The reference man and reference woman in the Indian RDA have been defined as–

Reference Woman	Age 20–39 years and weight 50 kg
Reference Man	Age 20–39 years and weight 60 kg

Reference woman is healthy. She may be engaged in 8 hours of moderately active work, in light industry or in general household work. Apart from 8 hours in bed, she spends 4 to 6 hours in light leisure activities and 2 hours in active household work, recreation or walking.

Reference man is healthy, free from disease and fit for work. He is employed in moderately active occupation for 8 hours, spends 8 hours in bed, 4 to 6 hours in leisure activities, sitting and moving about and 2 hours in active recreation, walking or household duties.

Recommended Dietary Allowances for Indians

The recommended dietary allowances for nutrients for an adult reference woman and man are given in Table 3.2. The table contains RDAs for:

Energy and Protein

Minerals—Calcium and Iron

Water-Soluble Vitamins—C and six of the B-group

Fat-Soluble Vitamins—A, E and K

Besides these, there are other nutrients, which are required by our body for normal function. It is reassuring to know that on an average, a diet, which provides a sufficient amount of the above nutrients, will meet the need for these other nutrients also. Please remember that a liberal margin of safety is provided in the recommended dietary intakes to cover differences in needs of healthy persons.

As you can see from Table 3.2, only two nutrients are needed in large amounts—energy and proteins. The RDA for energy is about 40 kcal per kg for a sedentary man and 37 kcal per kg body weight for a sedentary woman. Moderately active man's RDA is 48 kcal per kg and woman's 40 kcal per kg body weight. The RDA of a man engaged in heavy activity is 63 kcal and a woman 58 kcal per kg body weight. Thus knowing your body weight and the type of work you do, you can estimate your energy needs.

The RDA for protein is based on 1 g per kg body weight. It **does not vary** with activity.

The RDA for minerals is much less, calcium is 400 mg per day for both man and woman, while iron is only 28 to 30 milligrammes per day. As you know, a milligramme is one thousandth part of a gramme. An adult woman needs more iron than a man, to make up for the periodic loss of iron in menstruation.

The five water-soluble vitamins, namely thiamin, riboflavin, niacin, pyridoxine and ascorbic acid, are needed in very small amounts and their RDAs are expressed in milligrammes. The remaining two B-vitamins, folic acid and vitamin B_{12} are needed in very minute amounts and hence their RDA are expressed in microgrammes (mcg). A microgramme is one-millionth part of a gramme. The amount of B-Vitamins needed is related to the total energy needs and therefore varies with the RDA for energy. So you notice that an adult man requires slightly higher amounts of these vitamins than an adult woman.

Table 3.2: RDA for Indians (1989)[1]

Group	Particulars	Body Wt kg	Net energy kcal/d	Protein g/d	Fat g/d	Calcium mg/d	Iron mg/d	Vit.A Retinol μg/d	Vit.A β-carotene μg/d	Thiamin mg/d	Riboflavin mg/d	Nicotinic acid mg/d	Pyridoxin mg/d	Ascorbic acid mg/d	Folic acid μg/d	Vit.B_{12} μg/d
Man	Sedentary Work		2425							1.2	1.4	16				
	Moderate Work	60	2875	60	20	400	28	600	2400	1.4	1.6	18	2.0	40	100	1
	Heavy Work		3800							1.6	1.9	21				
Woman	Sedentary Work		1875							0.9	1.1	12				
	Moderate Work	50	2225	50	20	400	30	600	2400	1.1	1.3	14	2.0	40	100	1
	Heavy Work		2925							1.2	1.5	16				
	Pregnant woman	50	+300	+15	30	1000	38	600	2400	+0.2	+0.2	+2	2.5	40	400	1
	Lactation															
	0–6 months		+550	+25	45	1000	30	950	3800	+0.3	+0.3	+4	2.5	80	150	1.5
	6–12 months	50	+400	+18						+0.2	+0.2	+3				
Infants	0–6 months	5.4	118/kg	2.05/kg		500				55 μg/kg	65 μg/kg	710μg/kg	0.1	25	25	0.2
	6–12 monhs	8.6	98/kg	1.65/kg				350	1200	50 μg/kg	60 μg/kg	650 μg/kg	0.4			
Children	1–3 years	12.2	1240	22	25	400	12	400	1600	0.6	0.7	8	0.9	40	30	0.2-1.0
	4–6 years	19.0	1690	30			18	400		0.9	1.0	11			40	
	7–9 years	26.9	1950	41			26	600	2400	1.0	1.2	13	1.6		60	
Boys	10–12 years	35.4	2190	54	22	600	34	600	2400	1.1	1.3	15				
Girls	10–12 years	31.5	1970	57			19			1.0	1.2	13	1.6	40	70	0.2–1.0
Boys	13–15 years	47.8	2450	70	22	600	41	600	2400	1.2	1.5	16	2.0	40	100	0.2–1.0
Girls	13–15 years	46.7	2060	65			28			1.0	1.2	14				
Boys	16–18 years	57.1	2640	78	22	500	50	600	2400	1.3	1.6	17	2.0	40	100	0.2–1.0
Girls	16–18 years	49.9	2060	63			30			1.0	1.2	14				

Narasingha Rao B.S., Y.G. Deosthale and K.C. Pant, *Nutrient Composition of Indian Foods,* p. 94, National Institute of Nutrition, Hyderabad-500007, India, 1989.

The amount of fat-soluble vitamin A, its precursor, beta-carotene and vitamin D required by us is very minute and is expressed in microgrammes (1 microgramme (mcg) = one millionth of a gramme.) The recommendation for vitamin D is given in International Units (IU) and IU = 0.025 mcg.

It is natural that nutrient needs vary with age, activity and physiological status such as pregnancy and lactation. Our physical activity is normally dependent on our occupation or profession. The variation in energy needs with age, physiological status and occupation is illustrated in Figure 3.1.

Use of Recommended Dietary Allowances (RDAs)

The recommended dietary allowances for nutrients have a number of practical uses. These are :

1. To enable government to predict food needs of the population.
2. To provide basis for food distribution quota.
3. To guide agricultural planning policy.
4. To guide policy of food export and import.
5. To guide planning of nutritionally adequate diets for inmates of large catering establishments such as hospitals, hostels, hotels, army canteens, etc.
6. To evaluate the findings of food consumption surveys of population groups.

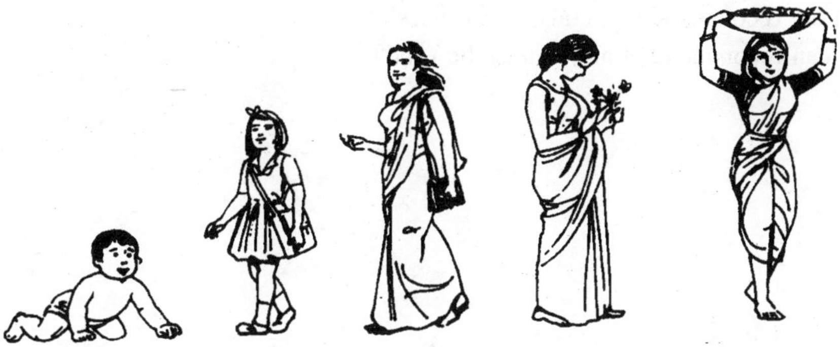

Age – 7-8 months	10 years	25 years	Pregnant	Moderate Activity
Calories – 785	1970	1875	2275	2225
Protein – 11g	57 g	50 g	65 g	50 g
Body Weight – 8 kg	31 kg	50 kg	60 kg	50 kg

Figure 3.1: Energy and protein needs vary with age and occupation.

In practical nutrition classes, the recommended dietary allowances are often used for planning or checking the adequacy of food intake of individuals, or of a given diet plan. You have to be cautious in the use of recommended allowances of nutrients in this manner, because you must consider the body size of the individual, which may differ from that of the reference person.

Secondly a diet that provides the recommended amounts of nutrients may be adequate; a diet which does not meet these may not be a poor one since there is a liberal margin of safety provided in the RDAs. The manner in which you can evaluate the diets of individuals for adequacy will be discussed in a later chapter.

Very often people think that if a little of something is good, a lot must be better. This can lead to trouble, if used in meeting nutritional needs. For example, taking of excess of vitamin A may result in toxic reactions. It is wise to use foods as sources of nutrients and to take nutrient supplements only under medical supervision.

Limitations of RDAs

It is important to note the limitations in the use of RDAs. These are:

(*a*) RDAs are estimates of intakes. of nutrients, which population groups need to consume to meet the physiological needs of all persons in that group.
(*b*) RDAs are not meant to be used to determine nutrient adequacy of an individual's intake.
(*c*) It is implied that intake of nutrients at RDA level will involve very little risk of inadequacy.
(*d*) Individuals, whose intake of nutrients is below that given as RDA are not at risk of deficiency, since many individuals in a population may have requirements well below the RDA.

Study Questions

1. Why are recommended allowances set-up?
2. What are the guiding principles used to derive RDAs?
3. What is a reference man?
4. What are recommended dietary allowances?
5. How can recommended allowances be used?

PART - II

The Nutrients and Energy

CHAPTER 4

Carbohydrates

Introduction

In this chapter we will consider carbohydrates, the primary fuel for our body. Can you imagine a meal without rice, *chapati* or some other cereal preparation? No. Rice, wheat and other grains are an important part of each of our meal everyday. Thus cereals are our staple food. In the Indian dietary, about 65 to 80 per cent energy is provided by carbohydrates.

There are practical reasons for the universal use of carbohydrates in diets. The yield of cereals, the primary source of carbohydrates, is high per unit area. Therefore, they are widely available and are an economic source of energy. They are easily packed and have a long shelf-life in dry storage. They are mild flavoured and combine well with other foods. Carbohydrate foods are easy to prepare.

Let us consider the nature, composition, properties, functions, food sources, utilisation, requirement, and effect of deficiency of carbohydrates.

Nature, Composition and Classification

Carbohydrates are synthesised by all green plants using solar energy, water from the soil and carbon dioxide from the air. This complex process is called **photosynthesis,** the prefix **photo** indicates the importance of sunlight in this process. Plants are thus the primary source of food in the world.

Carbohydrates contain carbon, hydrogen and oxygen. The suffix hydrate indicates that water and oxygen occur in the same proportion as in water.

The members of the simplest class of carbohydrates have a single unit—**monosaccharide (mono** or one, **saccharide** or sugar containing). Glucose is an example of this class. The disaccharides contain two sugars linked together to form a chain. Cane or beet sugar (sucrose), milk sugar (lactose), and maltose (malt sugar) are members of this class. Carbohydrates made up, of long chains of sugars are called **polysaccharides (poly**—many). Among them are starch, dextrins, glycogen, cellulose, hemicelluloses, pectins, plant gums and mucilages. Table 4.1 presents the types and sources of carbohydrates occurring in nature.

Table 4.1: Forms and Sources of Carbohydrates

Carbohydrates	*Main Food Sources*	*Remarks*
Polysaccharides		
Cellulose and hemicelluloses	Stalks and leaves of vegetables	Indigestible
	Outer covering of seeds	Indigestible
Pectins	Fruits	Indigestible
Gums and mucilages	Plant secretions & seed exudates	Indigestible
Starch and dextrins	Grains, legumes & tubers	Digestible
Glycogen	Meats and seafood	Digestible
Disaccharides		
Sucrose	Cane and beet sugar, mollasses	Digestible
Lactose	Milk and milk products	Digestible
Maltose	Malt products, some breakfast cereals	Digestible
Monosaccharides		
Glucose	Fruits, honey, corn syrup	Digestible
Fructose	Fruits, honey	Digestible
Galactose	Milk	Digestible

Simple carbohydrates include mono- and disaccharides. These are small molecules, which dissolve in water and are absorbed very quickly in the body. In contrast, starches and dietary fibres are very large, complex molecules, containing several hundred small sugar units and are absorbed slowly. Therefore polysaccharides are referred to as **complex** carbohydrates. Individual members of each of these classes (starch, pectins, gums, mucilages, cellulose, hemicelluloses, lignin) differ in the type of small units they contain and in the way these units are united in the molecule.

Glucose, the most common monosaccharide, is present in honey, fruits and corn syrup. After absorption of food it is transported through blood and hence is present in blood as an easily available source of energy.

Sucrose is the ordinary sugar available in the grocery store and used in beverages and food preparations as a sweetener. As you can note from the table, it is mainly manufactured from cane sugar in the tropics and sugar beets in the temperate regions. It is also present in molasses, honey, fruits and vegetables. Sucrose is hydrolysed to a mixture of equal amounts of glucose and fructose by action of digestive enzymes or when boiled with acid (such as citric acid from fruits). This mixture of glucose and fructose is called **invert sugar** and it is used in preparation of candies and icings.

Maltose does not occur in free form in nature. It is formed during sprouting of grains or in digestion of starch by action of enzymes. It contains two glucose molecules. Lactose is the sugar in milk. It yields glucose and galactose on hydrolysis by lactase. It is less soluble than sucrose and maltose and less sweet than glucose. Persons, who have lactase insufficiency, cannot utilise lactose and hence have to restrict their intake of milk and milk products. Children, who are born without the liver enzyme lactase, cannot digest milk and have to be fed soya milk instead.

Starch is found in cereal grains, legumes and in tubers. Glycogen is found in meats and seafood. These are digestible polysaccharides.

Cellulose and hemicelluloses, pectins, gums and mucilages are indigestible polysaccharides. Celluloses are found in stalks and leaves of vegetables and outer coverings of seeds. Pectins are present in fruits and gums and mucilages are part of plant exudates and seeds.

Properties

Sugars are soluble in water, are sweet to taste and are hygroscopic (absorb water from the atmosphere). As they are hygroscopic, they need to be stored in air tight containers. Sugars vary in their solubility in water; sucrose is more soluble than glucose. Carbohydrates, can be ranked according to their sweetness. Fructose is the sweetest and the most soluble sugar. It is followed by sucrose, glucose, dextrin and lactose. The relative sweetness of sugars is indicated in Table 4.2.

Table 4.2: Comparative Sweetness of Sugars

Sugar	*Sweetness Value*
Fructose	173
Invert sugar	130
Sucrose	100
Glucose	74
Galactose	32
Maltose	32
Lactose	16

Starches are not sweet, but bland in flavour. Tender corn is sweet, as it matures it becomes less sweet as sugars are converted to starch. Raw fruits contain starch, which changes to sugars during the ripening process with development of sweet taste.

Functions

Carbohydrates have many important functions in the body:

1. The **primary function** of carbohydrates in the body is to supply energy. Each gramme of carbohydrate, as starch or sugar, provides 4 kcal/g. Carbohydrates are a source of readily available energy, which is needed for physical activities as also the work of the body cells. The brain and the central nervous system are dependent on the constant supply of glucose from the blood to meet their energy needs.
2. Carbohydrates act also as **reserve fuel supply** in the form of glycogen, stored in muscles and liver. The total amount of glycogen in the body is over 300g. But it must be maintained by regular intake of carbohydrates at frequent intervals, so that the breakdown of fat and protein tissue is prevented.
3. Carbohydrates serve other special functions in the body. Carbohydrates provide chemical framework, which combine with the nitrogen to synthesise non-essential amino acids in the body.
4. Carbohydrates and their derivatives work as precursors of important metabolic compounds. These include nucleic acids, the matrix of connective tissue and galactosides of nerve tissue.
5. Lactose, the milk sugar, provides galactose needed for brain development. It aids absorption of calcium and phosphorus, thus helping bone growth and maintenance.
6. Lactose forms lactic acid in the intestinal track due to the action of the bacteria (lactobacilli) present there. These lactobacilli synthesise some of the B-complex vitamins. It aids, bacteria (lactobacilli) present to suppress the activities of putrefactive bacteria and protects us from their undesirable effects.
7. Carbohydrates are an important part of some compounds, which increase our resistance to infection (immunopolysaccharides). Ribose, a five carbon sugar, is an essential part of DNA and RNA. Carbohydrates are a part of important compounds, which are components of nervous tissue (galactolipid), heart valve, cartilage, bone and skin (chondroitin sulfate).
8. Carbohydrates are needed for ensuring complete normal metabolism of fats, thus preventing acidosis.
9. Carbohydrates are needed to prevent dehydration. A low carbohydrate diet causes loss of water from tissues as also electrolytes (especially sodium and potassium) in the urine and can lead to involuntary dehydration.
10. Dietary fibre acts like a sponge and absorbs water. It helps smooth movement of food waste through the digestive tract and the soft, bulky stools are comfortably eliminated.

Food Sources

Carbohydrates are synthesised by plants and occur in several forms. Starch is found in plant seeds (cereals and legumes), roots and tubers. These foods are the primary energy sources in the human dietary (Table 4.3).

The intake of complex carbohydrate in the form of cereals, *dals* and legumes, in normal Indian dietary is sufficient. Cereals, which are the staple food in the Indian dietary, contribute major part of the energy and proteins, and some minerals and vitamins. *Dals* and legumes provide significant amounts of proteins, iron and B-vitamins, in addition to energy. Potatoes, yams, jackfruit are good source of starch in the diet. Vegetables and fruits provide dietary fibre, minerals and vitamins. Milk is the only animal food, which is the source of a very important sugar—lactose—in the diet.

Sugars are found in fruits; the percentage is about three in melons, ten in citrus fruits and guava and seventeen in mango. Thus fruits are an excellent snack food as they are a dilute source of quick energy and other nutrients.

Sugars found in plant sap or juice (sugarcane and beetroot) is extracted to give pure 100 per cent sugar. It must be used judiciously, as it provides only energy. The intake of foods high in added sugars, such as soft drinks, syrups and sweets needs to be controlled to avoid obesity.

Tabe 4.3: Carbohydrate Content of Foods

Food	*Carbohydrate*		*Calories/unit*
	g/100g	*g/unit*	
Rice, rice flakes, rawa, vermicelli, etc.	75–78	19	86–88
Wheat flour (*atta*), jowar	69–72	17–18	82–87
Dals,	58–60	15	84–87
Tapioca or cassava	38	19	80
Banana*	27	22	95
potato, colocasia, chiku, peas, yam, jackfruit	16–22	8–11	40–49
Mango	17	9	37
Orange, guava, pear, apple, carrot, onion, clusterbeans	7–13	3–6	24–30
Leafy and other vegetables	1–4	1–2	6–17
Milk	5	7	100
Sugar	100	5	20

* One banana has about 80g edible portion

Utilisation in the Body

Starch is partly hydrolysed by *ptyalin* (salivary amylase) in the mouth to dextrose and maltose. Starch and dextrin are further hydrolysed to maltose by amylase in the small intestine. Maltose, sucrose and lactose are further broken down to glucose, fructose and galactose (simple sugar units) by the enzymes maltase, sucrase and lactase.

The glucose formed by the digestion of the starch and sugar is absorbed mainly into the blood through the walls of the intestine and carried to the liver. The glucose thus absorbed helps to maintain the glucose level in blood and the glycogen stores in the muscle and the liver. Whenever we need energy, the glycogen is broken down to glucose which is oxidised and the energy produced is used by the body. Any excess glycogen is converted to fat.

Regulation of Blood Sugar

Liver glycogen is continually converted to glucose and diffuses into the blood to replace the blood glucose used up by the tissues. Muscle glycogen is used for energy by the muscles. Only when muscle glycogen is oxidised to lactic acid, the lactic acid is carried to liver and converted to glucose and glycogen.

In normal persons, the blood sugar level is maintained at a constant level, which is 70 to 100 mg per 100 ml, under fasting conditions. A number of hormones regulate the reactions, and ensure the maintenance of normal blood sugar level. These hormones are insulin, glucagon, epinephrine, glucocorticoids, thyroxine and growth hormones.

Recommended Dietary Allowance

A minimum of 100g carbohydrates are needed in the diet to ensure the efficient oxidation of fats. Most diets supply more than this amount. If the carbohydrate foods are consumed in excess of the body's need, the excess is converted into fat and is stored as reserve. No daily allowance has been fixed for carbohydrates. As it is the cheapest source of food energy, it supplies up to 80 per cent of the calories in the low cost diets in India. If the proteins supply about 10 per cent of the calories, fat 20 per cent, then carbohydrates must supply the remaining 70 per cent calories.

Clinical Problems

Obesity: It is very easy to take sweets, mithais, candy, soft drinks, etc., in excess of one's needs. Most of these sweets contain a lot of fat also, which is a concentrated source of calories. When the energy intake exceeds expenditure, the excess is deposited as fat. Over a period of time, overweight and obesity can occur. Obesity is known to be a predisposing factor for a number of health problems.

Dental caries: If sugar remains in contact with the teeth, it tends to lead to tooth decay. If it is not checked, it may lead to dental caries. Chewy sweets tend to remain in contact with teeth for long periods, unless children are taught to rinse their mouth thoroughly after eating candy, as also food.

Deficiency

If less than required amount of carbohydrates is consumed the body first burns its own fat and then its tissue proteins for heat and energy. To prevent this, daily diet must supply the required amount of carbohydrates regularly.

Dietary Fibre

Cellulose, hemicellulose and pectins which are components of the skins of fruits, coverings of seeds and the structural parts of edible plants are usually referred to as 'Fibre'. Cellulose is not soluble in hot or cold water. pectins which occur in ripe fruits have the ability to absorb water and to from gels. This property of pectins is made use of in the preparation of jams and jellies.

The structural parts of plants, which are not digested by enzymes in the human intestinal tract are known as dietary fibres.

Classification and Sources: Dietary fibre includes:

(*i*) Structural parts of plant cell walls (cellulose, hemicellulose and lignin), which are not soluble in water, are classed as insoluble fibre. Water insoluble fibres are found in whole wheat, wheat bran, seeds, nuts and vegetables.

(*ii*) Viscous plant fibres are soluble in water. These include pectins, gums and mucilages. Soluble fibres are found in fruits, oat and barley, legumes and beans.

Functions: The human body does not have enzymes capable of breaking down cellulose, hemicellulose and pectins and so fibre is not digested in the body. However, in view of their ability to absorb water, these indigestible substances serve a useful purpose in helping with the elimination of intestinal wastes. They stimulate the peristalitic (rhythmic) movements of the gastrointestinal tract by adding bulk to the intestinal contents.

The insoluble fibre needs chewing and may improve mastication of food. Dietary fibre absorbs water, swells and thus increases surface area of the mass. Thus there is increased contact between the food mass and enzymes and hence digestion improves. There is also a feeling of fullness. The spongelike swollen mass of fibre ensures smooth elimination of faeces.

Fibre reduces transit time and binds some minerals such as calcium, iron, zinc, etc. Soluble fibre binds bile acids and cholesterol and helps carry these out of the body. There is no recommended dietary allowance for fibre. However, nutrition researchers and dieticians suggest that fibre intake be increased to 25 grammes or more per day.

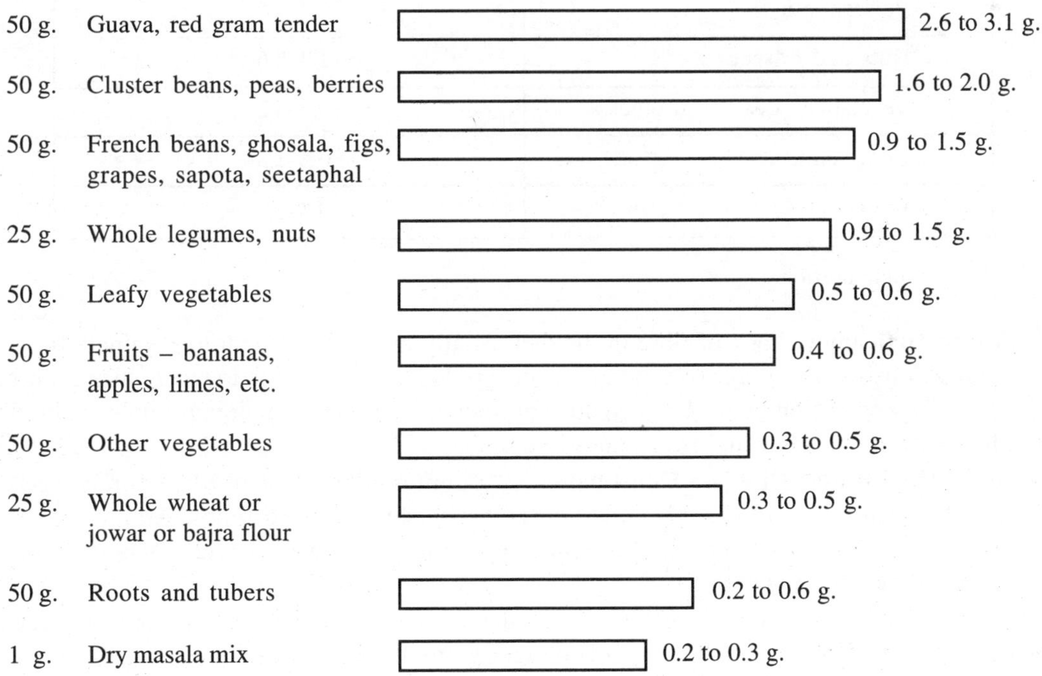

Figure 4.1: Fibre content of foods.

Food Sources: Whole grain cereals, whole wheat flour, fruits such as apples which can be eaten with their skin, bananas, pineapple, vegetables such as cabbage, amaranth are good sources of fibre (Figure 4.1). Unusual sources include agar-agar obtained from sea weed (Table 4.4).

Utilisation in the Body: As has already been described, these groups of substances are not digestible and do not contribute any nutrients to the body. These indigestible substance, however, do serve a useful purpose in facilitating the elimination of intestinal wastes. They stimulate the peristaltic movements of the gastrointestinal tract.

Requirements: The exact amount of fibre needed by the human body cannot be stated. Some experts feel 100 mg fibre per kg or about five to sixs grams per day is sufficient for the adult. An average mixed diet consisting of a raw vegetable, fresh fruit with skins, cooked fruits and vegetables will usually provide sufficient fibre. Fibre content of the diet can be increased by use of some whole grain cereals or whole wheat bread. Chapatis made from whole wheat flour are also a good source of fibre.

Table 4.4: Fibre Content of Foods

Food	*Fibre g/100g EP*[1]
Cereals, whole	1.2–1.9
Cereals, refined	02–0.7
Pulses, whole	3.7–5.3
Pulses, split	0.7–1.5
Nuts and oilseeds	1.3–6.6
Vegetables, Leafy and other	0.5–3.2
Roots and tubers	0.4–1.8
Fruits	0.5–2.7

1. EP-Edible portion.

Effect of Deficiency: Lack of fibre in the diet usually makes it difficult to eliminate food waste from the body. Consistent shortage of fibre in the diet could lead to constipation and other disturbances of the colon. This condition could be corrected by including foods containing whole grain cereals, fruits with skins and vegetable and fruit salads in the diet.

Role in Health and Disease: Constipation is a common problem in large percentage of the population. One of the reasons for this condition is the intake of refined foods. An increase in fibre intake helps to correct this ailment. Eating leafy vegetables, cluster beans, etc., has been found to ensure smooth, regular elimination.

With regular elimination of softer stools, the formation of haemorrhoids is reduced and diverticulosis is prevented or controlled. Pectins and gums bind bile acids and cholesterol and thus reduce their blood levels.

Dietary fibre by increasing bulk and needing more chewing may reduce the food intake. Thus it can help obese persons to reduce total energy intake and lose weight.

The carbohydrate absorption is slowed, which helps to regulate blood sugar and lowers insulin need of diabetics.

Large soft stools may dilute potential carcinogens. Rapid transit of stools may reduce content of carcinogens in colon mucosa and thus reduce risk of colon cancer.

Some problems due to high fibre diets: Dietary fibre is best taken from natural foods and not as fibre supplements. Food sources provide a variety of fibres, vitamins and minerals in combination, whereas fibre supplements do not supply any nutrients. An excessive intake of fibre may result in intestinal obstruction, if it is not accompanied by a liberal intake of water. If fibre intake is increased suddenly, complaints such as cramping, diarrhoea and excessive intestinal gas are common. To minimise these effects, the fibre content of the diet should be gradually increased over a period of several weeks.

Sugar Substitutes

Commercial sugar substitutes or artificial sweeteners are used by people, who wish to reduce their calorie intake. Two of the commonly available sugar substitutes are aspartame and saccharin.

Aspartame is a dipeptide of two amino acids, aspartic acid and phenylalanine. Its trade names are Equal and Nutrasweet. As the dipeptides are unstable to heat, this sweetener cannot be used in cooked or baked foods. Persons, who suffer from phenylketonuria should avoid use of aspartame.

Saccharin is o-sulphobenzimide. It is 300 to 500 times as sweet as sucrose and passes through the body unchanged. It has been used as a sugar substitute for about hundred years without any adverse effects. It is used in beverages and desserts. The only drawback is it leaves a bitter aftertaste, if used in large amount.

Study Questions

1. Why are cereals used as staple food in India?
2. What is photosynthesis?
3. List the properties of sugars.
4. What are the functions of carbohydrates in our body?
5. What is dietary fibre?
6. Why is fibre important in the diet?

CHAPTER

5 Fats and Other Lipids

Introduction

Fats are an essential part of our body, accounting for a sixth of our body weight. The cells and tissues of our body have fat as an integral part. The vital organs (brain, heart, liver) are protected by a sheath of fat and water, which holds them in place and prevents injury. The nerves are also protected by fat. A layer of fat beneath the skin acts as a insulation against cold. The fat around the joints acts as a lubricant and allows us to move these smoothly. Thus fat is a crucial part of the body composition.

Fats are the best known members of a chemical group called, the lipids. They constitute an important part of our Indian dietary and supply 10–30 per cent of the total energy needs. Food fats include solid fats, liquid oils and related compounds such as fat-soluble vitamins and cholesterol.

In the middle of last century, fats were expensive and a meal containing large amounts of fat was called a 'rich meal'. Persons consuming such meals were thought to be healthy. But with the improvement in the methods of production and their availability, there has been an indiscriminate increase in fat intake in some sections of society leading to overweight and obesity. The weight increase discourages movement, increases pressure on the circulation, respiration and skeletal frame. Hence it is recognised as a risk factor for several chronic ailments.

In this chapter, let us consider fats not only as essential body component, nutrient and compact storage fuel, but also as a health hazard. We need to achieve a realistic balance between meeting our needs and avoid health problems due to excessive intake.

Composition

Lipids is an overall group, which includes all fats and related compounds. The word is derived from the Greek word **lipos** which means fat. It is used in combination words to name fat-related health problems, e.g., **hyperlipidemia** refers to elevated level of blood fats.

Like carbohydrates, lipids contain the elements carbon, hydrogen and oxygen, and some contain phosphorus and nitrogen. Lipids have fewer oxygen atoms in their structure than carbohydrates. Therefore more oxygen is needed to oxidise lipids and more energy (about 2.25 times) is released per g of lipid as compared to a g of carbohydrate.

Lipids are an essential part of the body structure. Body fat accounts for 15 to 20 per cent of body weight in healthy non-obese men and 18 to 25 per cent in healthy non-obese women. The fat content of body increases in sedentary individuals and senior citizens if they do noactive leisure activities.

Lipids are widely distributed in nature. They are soluble in organic solvents, namely, ether, chloroform, benzene and other fat solvents. Fatty acids, fats and oils, phospholipids, sterols and lipoproteins are some of the groups of lipid compounds, which are important in the study of nutrition.

Sources

Vegetable oils, used in food preparation, are extracts of oilseeds and nuts. The important sources of vegetable oils are depicted in Figure 5.1. Butter and ghee are animal fats extracted from milk.

Plant oils are hydrogenated to form a almost solid fat known as *vanaspati. Vanaspati* is usually fortified with vitamin A and D, as it is used in place of ghee. The sources of fats in our dietary are listed in Table 5.1. Oils, butter, ghee and *vanaspati* contribute the visible fats in the Indian dietary. The amount of oils and fats in the diet vary with the region. As these are expensive foods, the amount and kind used in the dietary, varies with the socio-economic status of the family.

The animal foods, milk, egg, meat and liver, which contain fat, are sources of hidden fat in the diet. Nuts, oilseeds, milk, eggs and meat supply not only fat but also protein , minerals and vitamins of the B-complex group. Ghee, butter, eggs and liver are good sources of vitamin A. Some refined oils and *vanaspati* are fortified with vitamin A. Use of ghee, butter, fortified refined oil or *vanaspati* helps to meet a part of the day's need for vitamin A.

Table 5.1: Names, Formulae and Melting Points of Some Common Fatty Acids

No. of Carbon Atoms	*Fatty Acids*	*Formulae*	*Melting Point in °C*
Saturated			
4	Butyric	C_3H_7COOH	–7.9
6	Caproic	$C_5H_{11}COOH$	–3.4
10	Capric	$C_9H_{19}COOH$	31.6
16	Palmitic	$C_{15}H_{31}COOH$	62.9
18	Stearic	$C_{17}H_{35}COOH$	69.6
Unsaturated			
18	Oleic	$CH_3(CH_2)_7CH = CH(CH_2)_7COOH$	16.3
18	Linoleic	$CH_3(CH_2)_4CH = CHCH_2CH = CH(CH_2)_7COOH$	– 5.0
18	Linolenic	$CH_3CH_2CH = CHCH_2CH = CHCH_2CH = CH(CH_2)_7COOH$	– 11.0
20	Arachidonic	$CH_3(CH_2)_4(CH = CHCH_2)_4(CH_2)_2COOH$	– 49.5

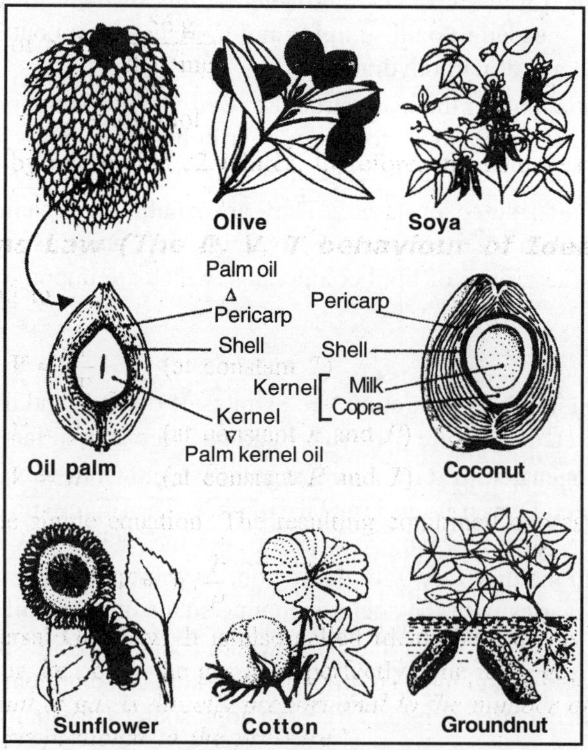

Figure 5.1: Important sources of vegetable oils.

Vegetable oils contain poly-unsaturated fatty acids such as linoleic, linolenic and arachidonic-acid. Linoleic and arachidonic acid are required for growth and maintenance of integrity of the skin. Table 5.2 indicates the sources of fats present in various foods.

It is easier to control visible fats in the diet than that which is hidden. For example, one can monitor use of butter, ghee and oil used directly. Invisible fats include the cream in the milk and *dahi,* nuts used in preparation and as such, egg yolk, oil used in seasoning vegetables, *dal* and salads. Even toned milk contains 3 per cent fat. Invisible fat contributes about 10 or more per cent of total energy in the diet.

Classification

Lipids are classified into three groups on the basis of their chemical structure:

1. Simple lipids, which include fats and oils,
2. Compound lipids, which comprise of phospholipids and lipoproteins, and
3. Derived lipids such as fatty acids and sterols.

Table 5.2: Sources of Fats

Food	*g/100g*	*Calories/100g*
Visible Fats		
Oil, vegetables	100.0	900
Vanaspati	100.0	900
Ghee, cow's	99.5	895
Butter	81.0	729
Invisible Fats		
Oilseeds & nuts	37.0–64.5	537–681
Mutton, muscle	13.3	194
Eggs, hen	13.3	173
Liver, sheep	7.5	150
Milk, cow	4.1	67

Fats, Oils and other Lipids

There is no precise definition of the word 'fat'. The term is applied to foods which are fatty, immiscible in water and greasy in texture.

Every fat molecule has glycerol at its core and three fatty acids attached to it. The nature of the fat/oil depends on the kind of fatty acids linked to the glycerol. The hardness, melting-point and the flavour of the fat is related to the length of the carbon chain and the level of the saturation of the fatty acid. If the substance is a liquid at 20°C it is called an oil, if solid at that temperature, it is known as fat.

Saturated fatty acids are found in solid fats while most of the oils contain unsaturated fatty acids. It may be noted that vegetable oils are a good source of essential fatty acids (Table 5.3).

The unsaturated fatty acids can be converted to saturated ones, thus changing the physical and chemical characteristics of the oil, by a process known as **hydrogenation** in which hydrogen is added on to the oils, in the presence of a catalyst. In the commercial process, hydrogen is added to some (not all) of the double bonds of the unsaturated fatty acids to increase the firmness and the melting point of the product. However, this processing also changes the isomers (shape, configuration) of some of the remaining unsaturated fatty acids. Most unsaturated bonds in nature are in a 'cis' form (folded pattern), but after hydrogenation, many double bonds are in a linear pattern, a 'trans' form. Thus although they are still unsaturated, these 'trans' fatty acids behave like saturated fatty acids.

Table 5.3: Linoleic and Linolenic Acid Content of Edible Oils

S.No.	*Oil*	*Linoleic g/100g*	*Linolenic g/100g*	*Total EFA g/100g*
1.	Safflower (*Kardi*)	74.0	0.5	74.5
2.	Soyabean	52.0	5.0	57.0
3.	Sunflower	52.0	trace	52.0
4.	Maize (corn)	50.0	2.0	52.0
5.	Cottonseed	50.3	0.4	50.7
6.	Sesame (*til*)	40.0	0.5	40.5
7.	Rice bran	33.0	1.6	34.6
8.	Groundnut	28.0	0.3	28.3
9.	Rape/mustard	13.0	9.0	22.0
10.	Palmolein	12.0	0.3	12.3
11.	Olive			
12.	Vanaspati	3.4	–	3.4
13.	Coconut	2.2	–	2.2
14.	Ghee	1.6	0.5	2.1

Fatty Acids

Fatty acids are the main building blocks of fats. Fatty acids have a methyl group (CH_3) at one end and a carboxyl group (COOH) at the other end with a chain of carbon and hydrogen atoms in the middle (formula at the end of the chapter).

About **twenty** fatty acids are found in foods and body tissues. The fatty acids have three important aspects, chain length, saturation and essential fatty acids.

The number of carbon atoms in fatty acid decides the chain length. Thus short chain fatty acids contain 4 to 6 carbon atoms, medium chain 8 to 12 carbon atoms, long chain fatty acids have 14–18 carbon atoms and extra-long-chain fatty acids have more than 20 carbon atoms in the molecule. Milk, fat, vinegar and coconut contain short chain fatty acids, long chain fatty acids are found in most vegetable oils and animal fats. Fish oils contain the extra-long chain fatty acids (Table 5.4).

Saturated fatty acid has a single bond between its carbon atoms, thus the molecule is **saturated** with hydrogen. Stearic acid is an example of a saturated fatty acid.

Unsaturated fatty acids have one or more double bonds in their molecule and are thus **not saturated** with hydrogen.

Further **monounsaturated fatty acids** (MUFA) have only **one** double bond in the molecules. Oleic acid, found in olive oil, is a monounsaturated fatty acid.

Table 5.4: Some Fatty Acids in Foods

Name	*No. of C atoms*	*Chain Length*	*Type*	*Food Source*
Acetic	2	Short	Saturated	Vinegar
Butyric	4	Short	Saturated	Butter
Caproic	6	Short	Saturated	Butter
Caprylic	8	Short	Saturated	Coconut
Myristic	14	Long	Saturated	Nutmeg and Mace
Palmitic	16	Long	Saturated	Palm oil and lard
Stearic	18	Long	Saturated	Beef tallow
Oleic	18	Long	Monounsatd.	Olive oil
Linoleic	18	Long	Polyunsatd.	Groundnut, sesame, corn oil, sunflower
Clupanadonic	22	Extra-long	Polyunsatd.	Fish oils

Polyunsaturated fatty acids (PUFA) have **two or more** double bonds in the molecules. Corn oil contains polyunsaturated fatty acids.

The **methyl end** of the fatty acid molecule is called the **omega** end. If the first double bond in the fatty acid is in the *third carbon atom from the methyl end,* it is called **omega-3** fatty acid; if it is in the sixth carbon from the methyl end, it is called **omega-6-** fatty acid and when it is in the ninth carbon, it is called **omega-9** fatty acid.

Examples of these are:

Oleic acid — Omega-9-fatty acid, which is a MUFA

Linoleic acid, omega-6-fatty acid, which is a PUFA.

Linolenic acid, omega-3-fatty acid, which is also a PUFA.

Fatty acids are found in all simple and compound lipids. Palmitic (16 carbons), stearic (18 C), oleic (18 C) and linoleic (18 C) are some of the common fatty acids.

A small part of free fatty acids are bound to the protein albumin of the blood and are transferred from the adipose cells to the liver, muscles and other sites.

Triglycerides

Fatty acids combine with glycerol to form a glyceride. When only one fatty acid combines with glycerol, it forms a **monoglyceride. Diglycerides** have two fatty acids and **triglycerides** three fatty acids attached to glycerol. Most of the fatty acids in the body as also in foods occur in the form of triglycerides.

Triglyceride molecules contain glycerol — a three carbon alcohol, as a backbone. Three fatty acids are attached to the three hydroxyl groups (–OH) of glycerol and three molecules of water are released in this formation of a **triglyceride.**

The fatty acids which combine with glycerol may vary in the length of the chain (–R) and vary in degrees and type of saturation.

Every time a triglyceride crosses a cell membrane, it must be broken or deesterified and after it enters the cell it is reesterified. In digestion, most triglycerides are hydrolysed to form free fatty acids, monoglycerides and glycerol, which are absorbed into the intestinal cells and the majority of these are rebuilt into triglycerides.

Phospholipids, which are present in every cell, are formed mainly in the liver from fatty acids, glycerol, phosphoric acid and a nitrogenous base. Phospholipids look like triglycerides, but contain a phosphate attached to glycerol in place of one fatty acid. For example, lecithin, a phospholipid contains choline-phosphate attached to one hydroxyl of the glycerol molecule (formula at the end of the chapter).

Lecithin is an important component of all membranes. It takes part in fat digestion. Egg yolk contains lecithin in abundance. Two other phospholipids – sphingomyelins and cerebrosides – are found in the brain. It is not necessary to provide phospholipids in the diet, as our body makes these when and where it needs.

Phospholipids are important as components of active tissues (brain, nervous tissue and liver). They are powerful emulsifying agents and are essential for the digestion and absorption of fats. Phospholipids help to carry lipid particles across the cell membrane in the blood stream.

Sterols are lipids with a multiringed (steroid) structure. Three sterols with functions associated with nutrition are:

Ergosterol a plant sterol

7-dehydrocholesterol an animal sterol and

cholesterol an animal sterol

Ergosterol and 7-dehydrocholesterol are two precursors of vitamin D.

Cholesterol is an important sterol. It is a waxy substance. As you can see (in the formula at the end of the chapter), cholesterol contains a hydroxyl group (–OH), but it does not resemble a triglyceride. Like all other lipids, it dissolves in organic solvents (ether, chloroform, etc.). It is the best known of the sterols and has attracted attention because of the association of elevated blood cholesterol levels with heart ailments.

Triglycerides, phospholipids and sterols share a common background — most parts of these molecules are synthesised from a derivative of acetic acid, which is the smallest fatty acid.

Cholesterol is an essential part of each cell and every type of human cell makes cholesterol. Each day our liver makes about 800 mg of cholesterol, which circulates through the blood stream and is used wherever it is needed.

It is a precursor of vitamin D, hormones and bile acids. The hormones made from cholesterol include corticosteroids, estrogens, testosterone and calcitriol (the active vit. D hormone). **Bile acids** needed for fat digestion, are formed from cholesterol.

The cholesterol content of heart, liver, kidney and egg (embryonic stage of life) is quite high. In infancy and toddler stage, new tissues are formed, especially brain which needs cholesterol. Hence fat should not be restricted in the diet of children up to five years of age.

Lipoproteins are synthesised in the liver. They are composed of three-fourth to two-third lipids and the remainder protein. These serve as the major vehicle for fat transport in the blood stream. The blood is mainly water and fat needs a water soluble cover of protein to permit it to be carried by blood. The lipoproteins contain triglycerides, cholesterol and other substances such as fat soluble vitamins. The density of lipoproteins is dependent on the amounts of fat and protein in it. The higher the fat content, the lower the density.

Four groups of, lipoproteins that have been identified are chylomicrons, low density lipoproteins (LDL), high density lipoproteins (HDL), and very low density lipoproteins (VLDL). The LDLs carry fat and cholesterol to cells. The HDLs carry free cholesterol from body tissues to the liver for breakdown and excretion. Like cholesterol, there is much interest now in these lipoproteins because their concentration in the blood plasma needs to be maintained within certain limits for good health. Their levels in blood plasma are routinely tested to detect lipid disorders, which are related to heart ailments.

Functions

Fat is a major nutrient and it has several functions. Oils and fats are concentrated sources of energy. Each, gramme supplies 9 calories.

Besides providing energy, oils and fats have several functions in the body. Food fats are a source of two groups of essential nutrients — essential fatty acids (EFA) and fat soluble vitamins A, D, E & K and their precursors. Food fats also aid the transport and absorption of fat-soluble vitamins.

Cholesterol is an essential lipid synthesised in the liver. Some important hormones and bile acids are formed from cholesterol. Fat forms the fatty centre of cell walls, helping to carry nutrient materials across cell membranes.

Fats are used to synthesise phospholipids, which are found in all cells.

Fat stored in various parts of the body is known as adipose tissue. The vital organs in the body are supported and protected by a web-like padding of this tissue. Fats act as a cushion for certain vital organs. Nerve fibres are protected by the fat covering and it aids relay of nerve impulses.

Since fat is a poor conductor of heat, a layer of fat beneath the skin helps to conserve body heat and regulate body temperature.

The flavour, palatibility and satiety value of foods is increased by fats. The slower rate of digestion of fat as compared to carbohydrates results in a feeling of satisfaction.

Fats may have other functions, which are not as yet clear.

Essential Fatty Acids (EFAs)

Linoleic acid (omega-6 PUFA) and linolenic acid (omega-3 PUFA) are called essential fatty acids because

1. these are not synthesised in the human body
2. these are required for important functions in the body and
3. these are available only through diet.

The EFAs have several important functions. They are essential for growth in the young and maintenance of normal healthy skin. Their other functions are as components of membranes to ensure their permeability to water and other small molecules. They are precursors of eicosanoids, a group of important metabolites which regulate vascular function, one of these are prostaglandins.

The omega-3 fatty acids, DHA (decosa hexenoic acid) and EPA (eicosa pentenoic acid) have an important role in fetal brain and eye development. These acids also protect against rheumatoid arthritis and cardiovascular diseases.

Certain varieties of fish are the richest food sources of these fatty acids. In some countries 'designer eggs' have been produced with enhanced levels of these omega-3 fatty acids by including DHA-rich algae in the chicken feed.

Common plant oils with the exception of coconut are good sources of linoleic acid.

Green leafy vegetables, cabbage and lettuce are good sources of omega-3-fatty acids. Soyabean and rape seed are also good sources of omega-3-fatty acids. Fatty fish, such as tuna, sardines and salmon are good sources of omega-3-fatty acids and a weekly consumption of any of these fish can help to meet the need.

The U.K. Dept. of Health Publication (1991) recommends that linoleic acid (n-6) should provide at least one per cent and linolenic acid (n-3 at least **0.2** per cent dietary energy for infants, children and adults) to meet their EFA requirements (Table 5.3).

EFAs are used to synthesise certain prostaglandins. **Prostaglandins** prolong bleeding time, reduce the thickness and stickiness of platelets, lower levels of triglycerides and very low density lipoproteins (VLDL) in the blood. Thus artery blockage is reduced. Prostaglandins also reduce inflammation and thus reduce pain in certain ailments (e.g., in rheumatoid arthritis).

Deficiency of EFAs: Deficiency of EFAs results in a flaky skin, development of itchy sores on scalp and retardation of growth. Diarrhoea and other symptoms may also develop. These symptoms of deficiency appear in low-birth weight infants fed fat-free formulas and in adults fed for long periods on intravenous solutions, which contain no lipid.

EFA deficiency results in changes in the fatty acid composition of many tissues, which include biological membranes and mitochondria.

Digestion and Absorption

The digestion of fats starts in the stomach, where a coarse emulsion forms due to churning action. The chemical changes necessary for fat digestion occur in the small intestine. The entry of fat in the duodenum, the first part of the small intestine stimulates secretion of the bile from the gall bladder. The fat gets emulsified by the bile preparing it for digestion.

The fat is broken into small particles, thus increasing the surface area and the surface tension is lowered improving the enzyme action and penetration. **Pancreatic lipase** breaks off one fatty acid at a time from the triglyceride. Thus one fatty acid plus a diglyceride, then another fatty acid plus a monoglyceride and glycerol are produced. Each subsequent step of this process occurs with more difficulty.

The **cholesterol esterase** from pancreatic juice acts on the free cholesterol to form a combination of cholesterol and fatty acids for absorption first into the lymph vessels and finally into the blood stream.

Lecithinase, secreted by the small intestine, acts on lecithin to break into its components for absorption.

The products of digestion are absorbed through the walls of the small intestine and circulated through the lymph. Some of these are used to synthesise important lipid compounds needed for body function. Some fat is used to supply energy. The rest is stored as fat in the adipose tissues for future use.

Fat Intake in India

Diet surveys by National Nutrition Monitoring Bureau (NNMB) of India show that the daily intake of visible fats vary from 3 to 20g/day in rural India and 20 to 42g/day in urban areas. In addition invisible fat intake may vary from 16 to 30 g and 50g/day in some population groups. Thus the total fat intake may contribute 10 to 30 per cent of dietary energy.

The nature of edible oil used in the diet varies from one part of the country to another; it is groundnut oil in west and south India, coconut oil in Kerala, rape/mustard oil from Punjab to West Bengal along the Gangetic plain and safflower in north Karnataka and parts of southern Maharashtra.

While a minimum amount of fat in the diet is essential, excess is harmful. Hence the minimum level and the safe upper limit of fat intake have to be considered.

Recommended Dietary Allowances

The fat requirement is based on two factors, namely to meet energy and the essential fatty acids needs. About 10 per cent of the total energy need is met by invisible fat in the diet. A minimum of 5 per cent of total energy needs to be provided as visible fat in the diet. This works out to about, 12 g of fat per day. A higher, level of intake of 20 g/day is desirable to provide energy density and palatability for normal adults.

It is desirable that an upper limit of 20 g/day of fat intake for adults and 25 g/day for young children be followed, in view of the possible complications resulting from excessive intake of fat. However, in order to meet the essential fatty acid needs, the diet should contain at least 10 g of vegetable oil, which is a good source of linoleic acid.

Diet and Heart Ailments

Fat is essential for our health, but too much of it can lead to ill health. A section of Indians have a high intake of fat, a large part of it is saturated fats (milk sweets, eggs and other flesh foods), and a very sedentary lifestyle. Their energy intake in excess of needs leads to obesity and an unacceptable blood lipid profile. If unchecked, there is deposition of fatty material with formation of plaques in the arteries, which disturbs the movement of oxygen and nutrients. It leads to a variety of heart ailments, such as atherosclerosis, high blood pressure and others.

There are a number of factors associated with susceptibility to heart ailments that can be controlled to a great extent. These include elevation of plasma lipid levels, obesity, physical inactivity and heavy smoking.

The risk factors related to diet will be discussed here.

Effect of Diet on Plasma Lipids

Plasma cholesterol (CHOL): Research conducted at Stanford and other medical centres throughout the world has proved that few heart attacks occur in people, who have total CHOL readings in the 160mg/dl range. The risk of heart disease accelerates as the total CHOL level creeps past the 200 mg/dl mark.

Animal fats, a source of saturated fats in the diet, are also high in CHOL content. The saturated fats are known to increase the total CHOL and LDL production in the liver, leading to increased levels in the blood plasma.

Increased serum CHOL level above 200 mg/dl and low density lipoproteins (LDL) above 130 mg/dl are associated with increased risk of coronary heart disease (CHD). The high-density lipoproteins (HDL) level in the blood is a beneficial factor, as it protects the blood vessel against formation of fatty deposit (atheroma), by moving the fatty material away.

The following changes in lifestyle can help normalise the plasma CHOL and LDL level:

- Reduce in intake of saturated fats (ghee, butter, *vanaspati,* lard, etc.).
- Reduce food cholesterol intake to 300 mg/day or less.
- Increase physical activity to alter cholesterol components in the blood plasma.
- Attain and maintain ideal body weight for your body build and height by controlling your total energy intake.

Plasma triglycerides (TRG): Triglycerides, another blood fat, have been identified as the transporter that moves fat in the bloodstream from one location to another. For instance, it moves it to your liver when it needs it, to your muscles when you are exercising or to your waistline when you are not.

High triglyceride levels are linked to coronary heart disease (CHD), though the connection is still not well understood. When a high LDL and high TRGs (levels over 200 mg/dl) were found together; the risk for subsequent heart attacks, increased. It appears that refined sugar causes TRGs to rise; one of the reasons for controlling excessive sugar intake in a heart-healthy diet.

The level of fat in the diet has been the subject of many studies. In one study, healthy, normal-weight volunteers were placed on either an ultralean 10 per cent fat diet or a rich 40 per cent fat diet. Each volunteer ate the number of calories required to maintain his/her body weight. Each ten days their TRG level in plasma was checked. They found that the volunteers on high-fat diet were manufacturing little or no fat. But those on low-fat diet were producing copious amounts of saturated fat. Sensing that a fat famine was under way, their bodies had cranked up the machinery that converts carbohydrates into fat, one of the built-in mechanisms that permits humans to survive in lean times. In fact, 30 to 57 per cent of the fatty acids in their TRGs was self-made saturated fat. Thus moderate intake of fats may be desirable to maintain normal TRG levels.

Research findings suggest that meal patterns may influence the blood lipid levels. In a college study, it was found that the mean CHOL and TRG values were the lowest in those eating **six** meals a day and highest in those eating **one** meal a day. Thus **frequent,** regular meal times, with appropriate, moderate mix of fat and carbohydrate components, and appropriate calorie restriction, can help to decrease plasma TRGs level and maintain it at normal level.

Physical Activity: Besides diet, physical activity is an important component in the control of obesity, plasma lipid levels and prevention of CHD. Exercise lowers fasting plasma TRG levels even during periods of increased energy intake. It is also known to increase the level of HDL, which protects the health of the blood vessels.

Thus it is possible for us to prevent disabling heart disease and ensure the health of our heart.

Study Questions

1. What are fatty acids? What are the main differences in various fatty acids?
2. Write short notes on triglycerides, phospholipids and cholesterol.
3. What are the functions of fat in the body?
4. What are essential fatty acids? Discuss their functions and effects of their deficiency.
5. What are lipoproteins? What is their significance in the body?
6. Trace the digestion of fat in the gastrointestinal tract.
7. What is the basis of current RDAs for fat?
8. Discuss the relationship between fat and heart ailments. What are the suggested ways to prevent heart ailments?

Structural Formulae

Cholesterol Structure

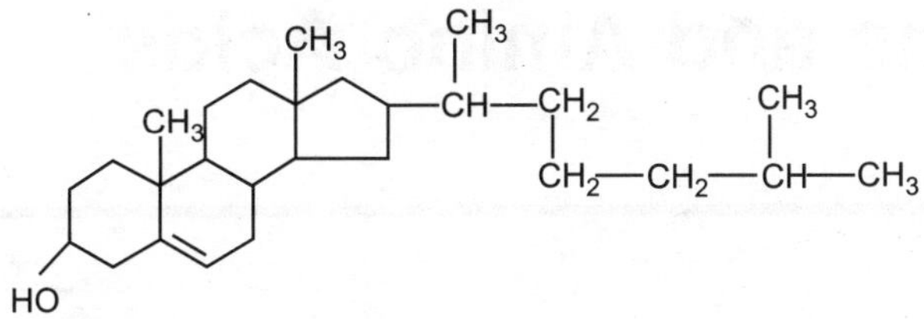

L–α–Lecithin Structure – a phospholipid

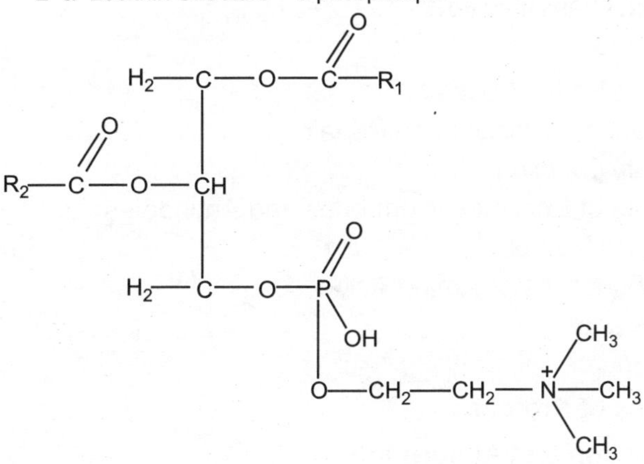

Triglycerides–Structure

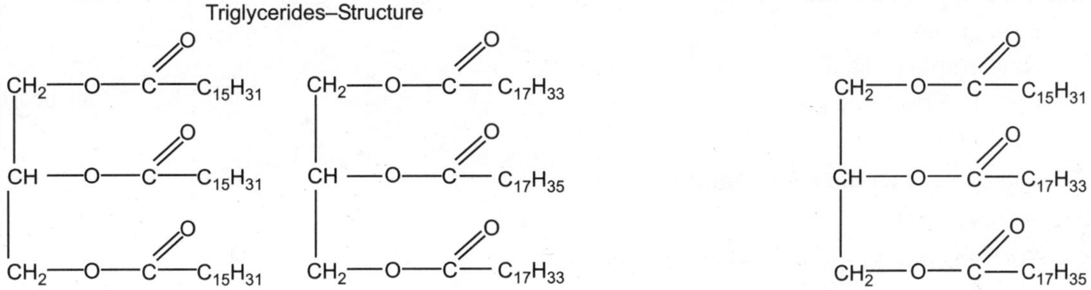

Tripalmitin Stearo-diolein Palmito-oleostearin

CHAPTER

6

Proteins and Amino Acids

Introduction

Next to water, protein is the most abundant component of the body. It accounts for about a sixth of the live body weight and a third of it is found in the muscles, a fifth in the bones and cartilage, a tenth in the skin and the remainder in other tissues and body fluids.

There are thousands of different specific proteins in the body, each having a unique structure and function. For this reason, the word protein implies not one but a large group of complex compounds.

Proteins are present in all living tissues, both plant and animal. They are essential to life because vital parts of the nucleus and protoplasts of every cell are proteins.

Composition

Proteins are very large organic compounds. Proteins, like carbohydrates and fats, contain carbon, hydrogen and oxygen. In addition, proteins contain about 16 per cent nitrogen, which is their unique feature and distinguishes them from carbohydrates and fats. Some proteins also contain sulphur and sometimes phosphorus, iron and cobalt. Proteins are more complex than fats and carbohydrates, as the size of the molecule is large and there is a great variation in the units from which it is formed.

Plants are the primary source of proteins in nature. Proteins are synthesised by the plants from the nitrates and ammonia in the soil. Herbivorous animals use plant proteins to meet their protein needs. Man uses plant foods as also animal foods (milk and meat) to meet his protein needs. Nitrogen is returned to the soil through degradation of products of animal metabolism, excretion of nitrogen compounds in urine and faeces, and decomposition of animal body at death, to complete the natural *nitrogen cycle.*

Structure and Classification

All proteins in our body and food are built from basic units or compounds known as **amino acids.** Amino acids combine to form proteins by means of a **peptide** bond, which joins a carboxylic carbon of one amino acid with nitrogen of another.[1] The resulting peptide has a free carboxyl at one end and a free amino group at the other, permitting addition of other amino acids at either end. The proteins are amphoteric in nature due to the presence of a free acid and a free amino group in their molecule. Polypeptiddes thus formed constitute the **primary structure** of proteins. The **secondary structure** formed by linking several polypeptide chains may be helical, pleated or random coil. More complex proteins have a **tertiary structure** in which the polypeptide chain is wound into a globular form.

Proteins exist in fibrous or globular form. Fibrous proteins appear in structure elements, e.g., collagen of connective tissue, myosin of muscle tissue and keration of hair. Globular proteins are very soluble and occur in tissue fluids; these include casein, egg albumin, albumins and globulins of blood plasma and haemoglobin. In conjugated form, they form most of the intracellular enzymes.

1.The word 'amino' indicates that they contain a — NH_2 group; the word 'acid' indicates that they contain a —COOH (an acid or carbonyl group).

The common structure of an amino acid is $R-CH\langle^{NH_2}_{COOH}$ where, 'R' indicates the remainder of the molecule.

This attachment may be a hydrogen atom or a more complex group; its structure accounts for the difference in various amino acids.[1]

Simple proteins yield only amino acids on hydrolysis. Albumins, globulins, glutelins, prolamins and albuminoids are simple proteins. Albumins and globulins, which are soluble in water and salt solution are present in animal fluids (milk, blood, plasma). Those which are less soluble are present in tissues (muscle, protein, myosin).

Conjugated proteins are combinations of simple proteins with non-protein substances. The combinations result in formations, which are functionally very important to the body. **Conjugated proteins** include:

- Lipoproteins (proteins + lipids) found in blood plasma (HDL, LDL, VLDL, etc.).
- Nucleoproteins (proteins + nucleic acids) found in cells (RDA, DNA).
- Mucoproteins and glycoproteins (proteins + polysaccharides) found in gastric secretion (mucin).
- Phosphoproteins (proteins + phosphoric acid) are found in milk, e.g., casein.
- Metalloproteins (proteins + metals) are found in ferritin, hemosidirin.

Derived proteins are proteoses, peptones and peptides formed in the various stages of protein metabolism.

Functions

The primary function of proteins is tissue building.

Proteins are the main solid matter in the muscles, they are also the major constituents of blood, matrix of bones, teeth, skin, nails and hair. Our body, which consists of about 60 per cent water and 19 per cent fat is held together by only **17 per cent proteins** and 4 per cent minerals.

The principal functions of proteins in the body are discussed below.

Body-Building or Building of New Tissues: Protein is an essential part of every cell. We cannot synthesise (form) protein from simple nitrogen compounds as plants do. Therefore amino acids must be supplied in the diet for building new tissues. Proteins provide the amino acids needed for the formation of new cells. They also provide the material from which nucleic acids are formed, e.g., DNA and RNA, which carry the genetic code.

The amount needed at various stages of life varies with the rate of growth. Infants need more proteins per unit of body weight than adolescents, because the rate of growth is the highest during infancy. More protein is needed in the last part of pregnancy as compared to the first part.

There may be a need to supply extra protein, to rebuild tissues after their loss or destruction. The loss may occur in any one of the following ways;

1. Donation of blood,
2. Excessive menstruation,
3. Haemorrhage after an accident,
4. destruction of tissues due to burns, in wasting diseases such as TB (tuberculosis0, rheumatic fever, etc.

Maintenance of tissues: The need for protein to maintain and repair the old tissues continues throughout life. Proteins in the body tissues are not static; they are constantly being broken down and replaced by new protein synthesised from amino acids from dietary and tissue sources. For example, the lining of the intestinal tract is renewed almost everyday and a half; the protein in the liver and blood plasma is broken down and remade every six days, blood cells have a life span of 120 days and adequate replacement must be supplied to avoid anaemia. In fact, all body proteins are constantly being degraded and synthesised at varying rates. Thus there is a continuous need for protein to provide for the maintenance of tissues already built.

Regulatory Functions: Haemoglobin, a protein and iron complex, ensures the smooth running of respiratory cycle by being the vital oxygen carrier in the red blood cells.

Proteins in fluids such as blood help to regulate body processes. Plasma proteins contribute to osmotic pressure and thus exert an important influence on the exchange of water between tissue cells and the surrounding fluids and on the water balance of the body as a whole.

The amphoteric[1] nature of proteins is useful in maintaining acid-base balance of blood and tissues. Their amphoteric nature further makes them ideal carriers of nutrients across cell membranes. The blood proteins (haemoglobin and oxyhaemoglobin) combine with the carbon dioxide formed in cellular metabolism and excrete it in the expired air. The metabolic products which are acidic or basic combine with protein and are carried through the system without affecting the tissue pH excessively.

Proteins as Precursors of Enzymes, Hormones and Antibodies: A small amount of protein (or of amino acids) is needed for synthesising **enzymes, hormones** and **antibodies.** All enzymes are proteins and are essential catalysts in digestion and metabolic processes in the tissues. Hormones, secreted by various glands are proteins in nature. Hormones regulate and co-ordinate body processes and activities. Hormones are chemical messengers, synthesised in the body. They are responsible for regulating all the activities of the body. Examples of hormones are insulin, thyroxine, growth hormones, steroid hormones, etc. Proteins form antibodies and special white blood cells defend the body against infection and disease and thus participate in the body's immune system.

Transport of Nutrients: Due to their **amphoteric** nature, proteins are ideal carriers of nutrients across cell membranes. Proteins as lipoproteins transport triglycerides, cholesterol, phospholipids and fat soluble vitamins across the cell wall. Specific protein carriers ensure transport of many vitamins and minerals. Albumin carries free fatty acids, bilirubin as also many drugs.

Special Functions of Amino Acids: Almost all amino acids have some unique functions in the body. A few of these are listed here. **Tryptophan** serves as a precursor for the B-vitamin niacin and serotonin, a neuro-transmitter. **Glycine,** a simple ubiquitous amino acid is used in synthesis of porphyrin nucleus of haemoglobin. It is also a constituent of one of the bile acids. It combines with many toxic substances to form harmless products, which are excreted.

Glycine, methionine and **arginine** synthesise creatinine, which with phosphate forms creatine phosphate, an important, form of high energy compound in the cell.

Histidine is used in the synthesis of histamine used as a vasodilator in the circulatory system. **Glutamic acid** is a precursor of a neuro-transmitter. **Phenylalanine** is a precursor of **tyrosine** and together they lead to the formation of thyroxine and epinephrine. Tyrosine is also the precursor of skin and hair pigment. **Methionine,** the sulphur-containing amino acid, is the principal donor of methyl groups in the synthesis of choline and other important compounds.

Milk Formation : Mother's milk is the first food for a young of any mammal. Human milk contains about 1.2 per cent protein. The milk proteins are synthesised in the mammary gland from the available dietary and tissue proteins. A nursing mother needs to take extra protein in her diet to meet the demands of protein for milk formation.

Energy Supply: A small part of the body's need for energy (about 6 to 12 per cent) is supplied by products of protein metabolism. Each gramme of food protein yields four calories to the body.

---

1. Amphoteric: capable of acting both as a base and an acid.

Food Sources of Protein

Plants are the primary source of protein, because they can synthesise protein by combining nitrogen and water from the soil and carbon dioxide from the air. Animals depend on plants to fulfill their protein requirement.

The food sources of protein are listed in Table 6.1. It may be observed that pulses, whole and split, nuts and oilseeds, milk, eggs, fish, poultry and meat are good sources of protein in the diet. Cereals and their products are a major source of protein in the Indian dietary (Figure 6.1).

Cereals and pulses, when cooked in water, supply only one-third or less of the protein present in the raw foods, as these foods absorb at least two times their weight of water. There is no increase in weight of milk, eggs, meat and fish during cooking. Therefore, there is likely to be very little decrease in the amount of protein supplied by these foods when cooked.

Another aspect of evaluating the foods as sources of protein is the quantity of food that is normally consumed and the frequency of the use of the food. In India, cereals are consumed in large quantities and are included in almost all the meals. Therefore, these contribute a large part of the day's need for protein in the Indian dietary. Secondly, pulses are included in most of the meals, along with the cereals, which results in a high quality protein in the diet. Proteins from leafy vegetables are an excellent supplement to the cereal diet.

Milk is one animal food, which is accepted and included in menus for feast as well as fast. The quantity of milk included depends on the availability and cost. Thus cereals, pulses, milk and milk products contribute most of the protein in the Indian dietary.

Dry, salted or smoked fish and meat are inexpensive concentrated sources of protein. These contribute valuable protein in the diet of people from coastal regions.

Table 6.1: Sources of Protein

Food	*Units recommended for adults*	*Protein*	
		g per unit[1]	*g in units recommended*[2]
Cereals—rice, wheat, millets and their products	10	2–3	20–30
Dals, pulses	2	6	10–12
Milk, Curds, etc.[3]	1–2	5	5–10
Eggs[3]	1	6	6
Meat, Fish, Poultry[3]	0–1	5–6	5–6
Vegetables			
Leafy green	1	1–2	1–2
Beans and Peas	1	2–4	2–4
Roots, Tubers and Others	1	1	1
Fruits (vitamin C-rich)	1	1	1

1. Amount of food per unit is indicated in, Chapter 14, Table 14.1.
2. Units as recommended in the food guide in Chapter 14.
3. Units of animal foods included in the diet, vary with dietary pattern and cost.

Eggs are included in one meal of the day by those who accept them. Normally fish, meat and/or poultry are included one or two times a week. Please remember that the importance of any food as a source of protein depends on how often and how much of it is consumed.

It may be observed that the concentration of protein in most vegetables and fruits is small. Therefore, these may not be counted to supply more than 10 per cent of the day's intake. Though the quantity supplied may be small, these proteins do enhance the quality of protein in the diet.

It is known that if the kinds and amounts of amino acids in the food proteins in a meal are in keeping with the body's need, the protein mix is efficiently utilised. Thus when cereals and pulses are included in the same meal, the essential amino acid content of the two together is more in keeping with the body's needs than that of each of these taken singly.

Any additional foods such as curd (buttermilk) and vegetables or fish/meat, which may be included in the meal may help improve the quality of the protein by virtue of the essential amino acids they supply. Thus including two or more sources of protein in the menu for each meal helps to improve the quality of protein and its utilisation. Some of the regional dietary patterns are based on this principle.

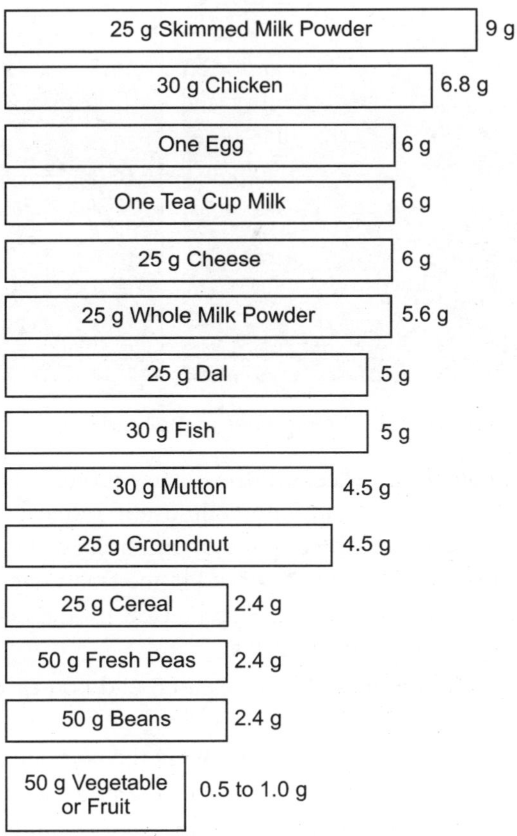

Figure 6.1: Food Sources of Protein.

Protein Digestion and Absorption

Protein digestion starts only in the stomach as there are no protein splitting enzymes in the saliva. In the stomach, protein is hydrolysed by the enzymes with the help of hydrochloric acid into peptides or amino acids. This process continues in both the duodenum and the small intestine, where the pancreatic and intestinal enzymes complete the hydrolysis by converting almost all the protein into amino acids.

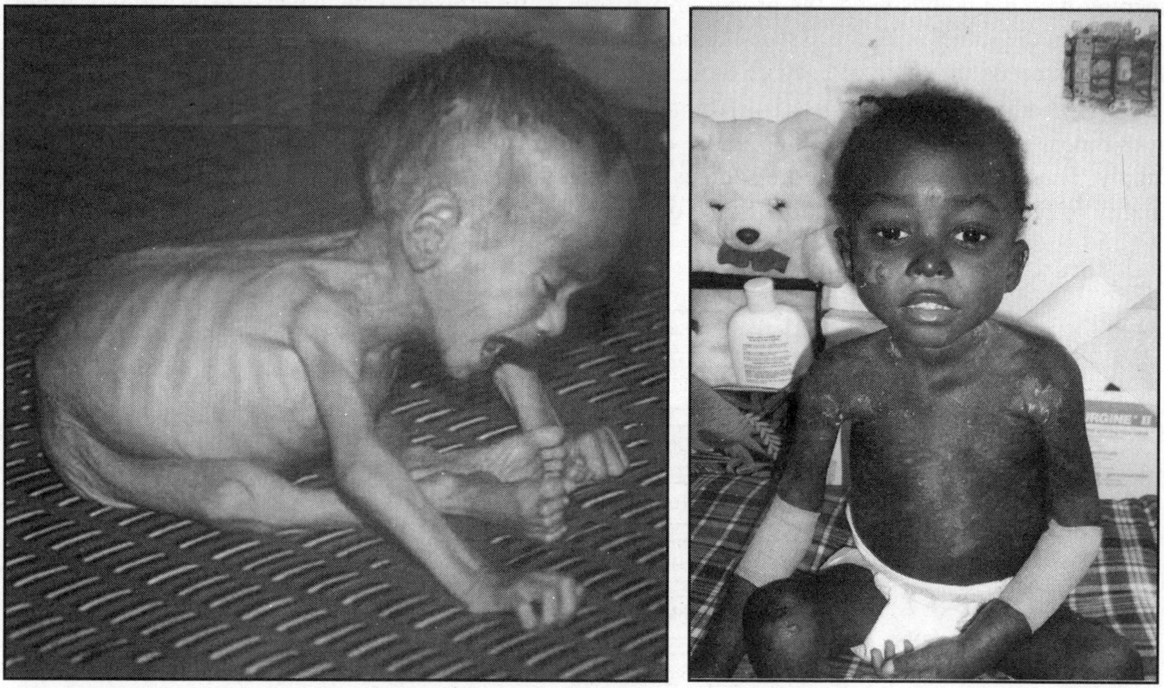

Figure 6.2: Protein-energy malnutrition.

It is reported that approximately 92 per cent of the dietary protein is digested from a mixed diet. Proteins of plant origin, especially those bound with cellulose are digested less than those of animal origin. The amino acids thus formed are absorbed either by the stomach wall, the intestinal walls or by the colon. Most of the amino acids are, however, absorbed in the small intestine. After passing through the walls of the digestive tract, the amino acids are picked up by the circulating blood stream and transported to the liver and to the various body tissues.

For the synthesis of proteins in the body, both essential and non-essential amino acids must be available in adequate amounts.

Non-essential amino acids can be formed in the body by the combination of essential amino acid groups with metabolic products of carbohydrates and fats by a process known as transamination.

Some of the amino acids are split off by a process known as deamination. The nitrogenous by-products, if not utilised, are excreted in urine as urea, uric acid and creatinine.

Essential Amino Acids

There are 22 (or more) amino acids, all of which are vital to human life and health. The body is able to synthesise 13 of these but is unable to make 9 others. These nine amino acids have to be provided in the diet in sufficient amounts and are called **essential amino acids.**[3]

Arginine is called **semiessential,** because it may not be synthesised in sufficient amounts to meet the rapid growth of infants, especially premature ones and may need to be supplied in the diet.

Non-essential amino acids: The word non-essential is misleading for these are necessary in the body for tissue building, repair and other metabolic functions. These are so important that the body synthesises these itself. The only reason these are termed non-essential is because these **need not be provided in the diet.** The formulae of amino acids are given at the end of the chapter.

Protein Quality

The food proteins vary greatly in their amino acid composition. Protein quality depends on the kinds and amounts of the essential amino acids present in the food proteins. It is reported that certain food proteins lack one or more essential amino acids. For example, cereals are low in lysine, most of the pulses contain a small amount of methionine. Most of the animal proteins such as milk, eggs, poultry, fish and meat contain all essential amino acids.

However, as cereals and pulses are normally consumed together with other foods such as vegetables, curd, etc., the lack in one food is supplemented by the other foods. In other words, various foods when eaten together in a meal, complement each other and improve the quality of protein supplied to the body.

Measurement of Protein Quality

There are several methods to determine the quality of protein in the diet. These are biological value (BV), net protein utilisation (NPU), protein efficiency ratio (PER) and chemical score.

Biological Value: Biological value is the percentage of the absorbed nitrogen (N) retained by the body. The nitrogen content of the food eaten by an animal and the nitrogen content of the urine and faeces are determined. The biological value (BV) is calculated by using the formula:

$$\text{BV} = \frac{N \text{ retained by the body (dietary } N \text{ - (urinary } N + \text{faecal } N) \times 100}{N \text{ absorbed (dietary } N \text{ - faecal } N)}$$

The quality of protein is directly related to its BV. The BV increases with increase in the percentage of nitrogen absorbed being retained.

The BV of milk is 84, brown rice 73 and whole wheat 65.

Due to complementary effect of food mixtures, the BV of mixed diets is higher than the arithmetical average of the component of food proteins.

Net Protein Utilisation (NPU): Net protein utilisation is digestibility of protein multiplied by its BV.

Protein Efficiency Ratio (PER): Protein efficiency ratio is not based on intake and output of food protein residues. Therefore it is less accurate than BV and NPU. But the technique is easy and it is also easy to use. In this method, a known amount of test protein in an adequate diet is fed to young rats for four weeks under standardised conditions and the weight gain is determined. The PER is obtained by dividing the weight gain by grams of protein fed.

3. Eight amino acids needed by adults are isoleucine (I), leucine (L), lysine (L), methionine (M), phenylalanine (P), threonine (T), tryptophan (T) and valine (V). One needed by growing children is histidine (H).

$$\text{PER} = \frac{\text{weight gain in g}}{\text{protein fed in g}}$$

The PER of milk is reported to be 3 and polished rice 2.2.

Chemical Score: Chemical score is based on the comparison of amino acid composition of the food protein with the amino acid of a reference protein such as milk, egg or FAO reference protein (1973). The amino acid score is the concentration of the limiting amino acid per gram in the food/food mixture as a percentage of the same amino acids per gram in the acid of the reference protein.

The formula used is:

$$\frac{\text{mg of limiting amino acid / g of test protein} \times 100}{\text{mg of the same amino acid / g of reference protein}}$$

Recommended Dietary Allowance

The requirement of the body for protein as determined by nitrogen balance studies is between 0.5 to 0.6g/kg of body weight in adults, when the source of protein supplies the amino acids in the proportion needed by the body. In practice, the amino acids of the food combination may not be so well proportioned; therefore the recommended daily allowance for protein is set to 1.0 g/kg of body weight for adults.

During infancy, pregnancy and lactation there is an increased need of protein for growth. Persons suffering from burns or wasting diseases such as tuberculosis and rheumatic fever, also need additional protein for regeneration of wasted tissues. Similarly if there is loss of blood due to excessive menstruation, haemorrhages or blood donation, more protein is needed in the diet.

The recommended dietary intake of proteins are presented in Table 6.2.

Table 6.2: Recommended Dietary Intakes of Proteins.[1]

Particulars of the Individual	*Protein g/day*
Man (60 kg)	60
Woman (50 kg)	50
Woman, pregnant (latter half of pregnancy)	65
Woman, nursing mother (0–6 months of lactation)	75
Infants, 0–6 months	2.05 g/kg/day
Infants, 7–12 months	1.65 g/kg/day
Children, 1–3 years	22
Children, 4–6 years	30
Children, 7–9 years	41
Boys 10–12 years	54
Girls 10–12 years	57
Girls 13–15 years	70
Boys, 13–15 years	65
Boys, 16–18 years	78
Girls, 16–18 years	63

1. Recommended Dietary Intakes for Indians, ICMR, 1990.

Vegetarian Diets

A large number of Indian people (10 to 15 per cent of the population) are vegetarians, due to their religion and belief in the principles of non-violence. A large section of non-vegetarians (about 80 per cent) restrict their consumption of animal foods to one or two days of the week. Thus they are vegetarians for 5 to 6 days each week. One important feature of the Indian diet is that milk and milk products are accepted universally in the vegetarian diet. Thus they are lactovegetarians. It is easy to plan a nutritionally adequate lactovegetarian diet. Indian vegetarians, therefore, do not face the problems encountered by vegans and fruitarian in meeting their nutritional needs.

Protein Sources in the Indian Vegetarian Diet: The protein sources in the Indian vegetarian diet are cereals, *dals* and legumes, milk and milk products, immature beans and peas, vegetables and fruits. Over six varieties of cereals and millets and sixteen types of *dals* and legumes are used in Indian diet. Being a tropical country there are over 150 varieties of leafy and 250 other vegetables to choose from, resulting in nutritionally rich combinations.

In the normal Indian diet, cereals are the staple food and *dals* or legume, milk and vegetable preparations are served with cereal preparations. Naturally the quality of the protein combination is excellent.

Clinical Problems

Protein Excess: Though protein is a vital need of the body, intake of excess creates stress on the body function. The liver has to deaminise the extra amino acids and synthesise urea. The loss of calcium in the urine is increased with high protein intake. High protein from animal foods carries undesirable saturated fats also along with it.

As protein foods are expensive, their increased intake may lead to lesser intake of nutrient rich, foods and thus reduce the quality of the diet. Adequate protein is good; but excess intake is not desirable.

Deficiency of Proteins

Latent stage: The deficiency of proteins accompanied by that of energy is one of the most common nutritional deficiencies in India. In the early stages, it may not be noticed. Research reports indicate that animals on low protein diets tend to be small, but their functioning is not affected. Children tend to have retarded growth but this may not be noticed, if all children from the neighbourhood are of small stature due to protein deficient dietary. Further it may also result in thin, lanky bodies in teens.

Protein deficiency during pregnancy may result in stress, which could give rise to complications such as vomitting, swelling of feet, etc. If these symptoms are commonly prevalent, they are accepted as a normal part of pregnancy. Some think it is a hereditary condition. Thus due to ignorance, protein deficiency in pregnancy may not be detected and thus there will be no improvement in the diet. This condition may not be restricted to low socio-economic groups. It may adversely affect the growth of the foetus and foetal stores for future. Thus the infant's survival and health are affected by maternal nutrition. In children, lack of protein in the diet results in stunted growth and low weight.

Severe Deficiency: If there is severe deficiency of protein in the first two years of life, it could affect mental development, learning ability and behaviour.

In India and other tropical developing countries, protein-energy malnutrition (PEM) is a common disorder during childhood. When the child is weaned, the diet often does not contain an adequate quantity and quality of protein which results in deficiency diseases. When an infant is fed high carbohydrate low protein foods such as ogi (corn starch porridge) as in West Africa, **kwashiorkor**, a typical protein deficiency condition occurs. When both protein and calorie are very low in the diet, **nutritional marasmus** could occur. In other words, kwashiorkor is a deficiency disease due to severe lack of protein but nutritional marasmus is due to sheer starvation (Figure 6.2).

The education of prospective parents about childcare and nutrition can ensure good nutrition of infants and young children and prevent protein-calorie malnutrition. Greater attention is needed to appropriate supplementary nutrition for children in the 0–2 age group, the most critical period in terms of brain and body growth.

Study Questions and Activities

1. List the functions of proteins and discuss these.
2. What are essential amino acids?
3. Write short notes on: protein quality, biological value, special functions of amino acids, deamination, urea cycle, vegetarian diet.
4. Prepare dishes which supply 5–6 g of proteins. Record the cost of each preparation.
5. Prepare *khichdi, idli, thalipeeth* using 100 g of the major ingredients. Record the number of servings obtained from the preparation. Calculate the protein and energy obtained from a portion of each preparation.

Essential Amino Acids

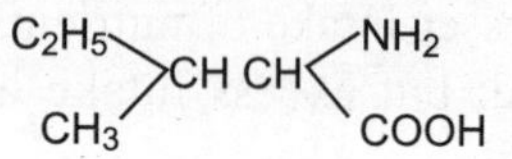

Isoleucine

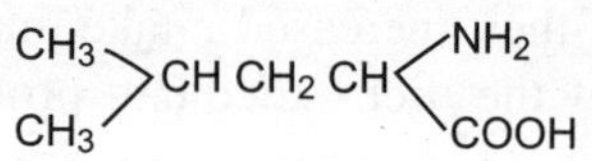

Leucine

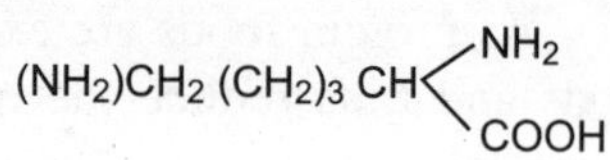

Lysine

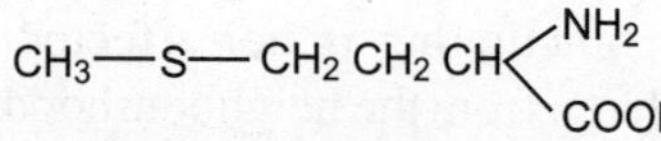

Methionine

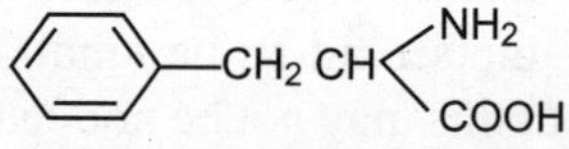

Phenylalanine

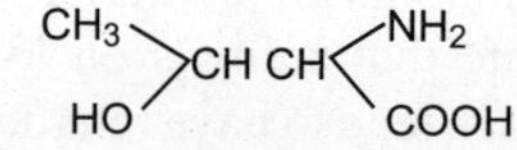

Threonine

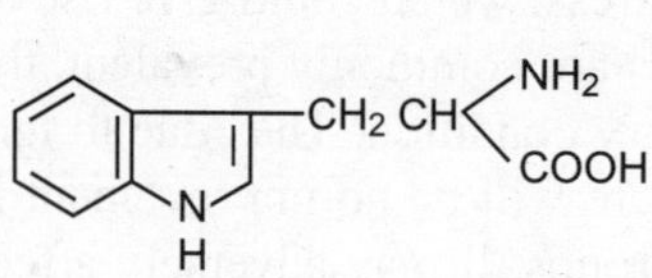

Tryptophan

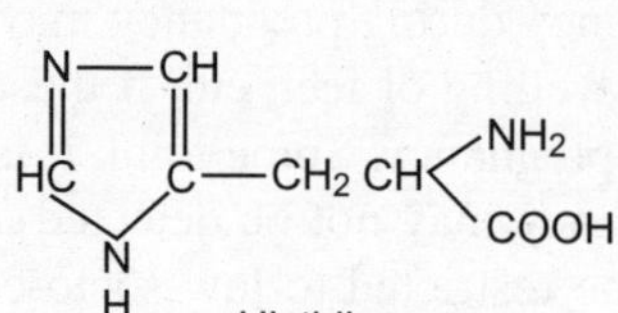

Histidine

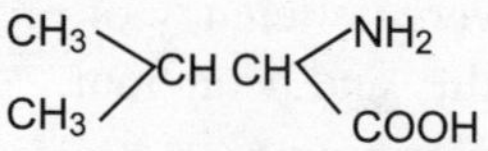

Valine

Semi-essential Amino Acids

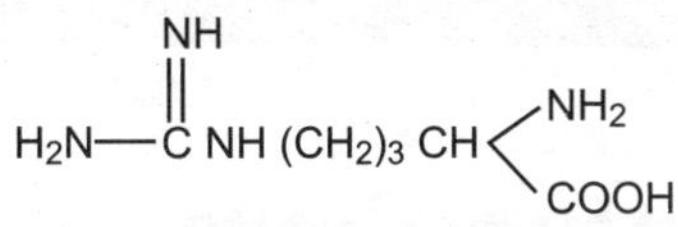

Arginine

Non-essential Amino Acids

Amino acids, which are synthesised in the body, therefore *non-essential* in the diet.

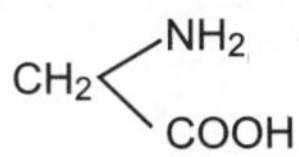

Glycine

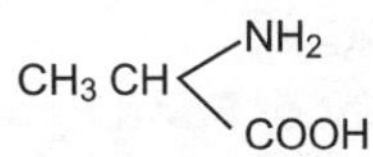

Alanine

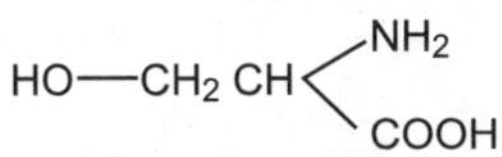

Serine

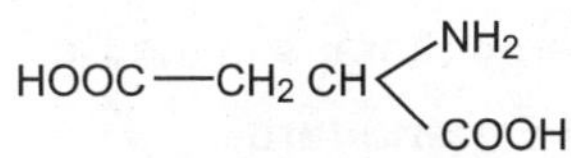

Aspartic acid

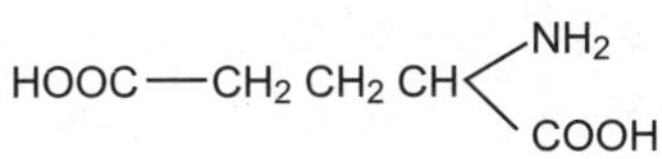

Glutamic acid

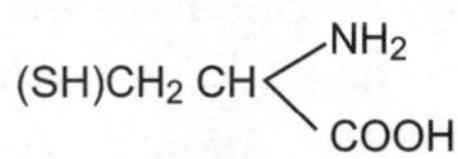

Cysteine

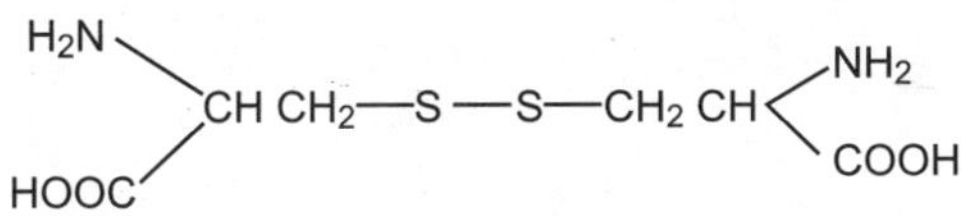

Cystine

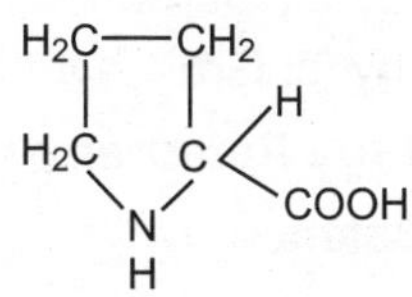

Proline

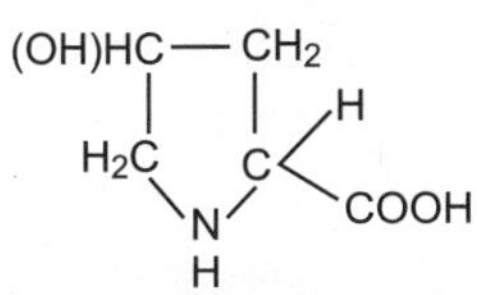

Hydroxyproline

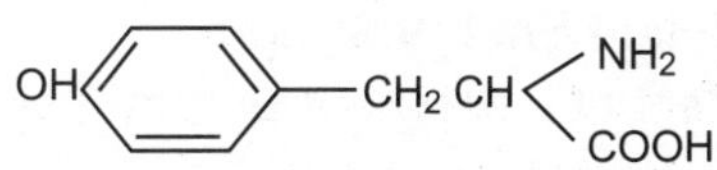

Tyrosine

CHAPTER 7

Energy Metabolism

Introduction

Our body needs three inputs to ensure its normal function.

Air (oxygen), Water and Food

Food supplies the energy components (carbohydrates, fats, proteins), as also nutrients (minerals and vitamins), which ensure their use in the body.

In this chapter, we will consider energy, its definition, measurement and balance.

What is Energy?

Energy is the capacity to do work. Energy exists in a number of forms. It may occur as heat generated by chemical, mechanical or electrical means. Examples are:

1. Heat produced by chemical means, e.g., when lime and water are mixed.
2. Heat produced mechanically in the grinding stone when cereals are ground.
3. Heat generated by electric current for boiling water in a tea kettle.

One form of energy can be converted to another form.

In physiology and nutrition, energy is defined as the capacity of a body to do work. Just as a machine needs fuel to keep it operating, the body needs food to provide the energy to perform its various tasks.

The energy released in the body from food is measured as a unit of heat the kilocalorie (kcal). By definition, one kilocalorie is the amount of heat required to raise the temperature of one kilogramme of water through one degree Celsius (*i.e.*, from 14.5° to 15.5.°C).

Some efforts have been made to introduce the joule (J)[1] as a unit of energy. One joule is equal to the energy expended when one kilogramme is moved through one meter by a force of one newton (N). But joule cannot be used in practical nutrition, until food composition tables are prepared giving the energy value of foods in joules, and RDA are set in joules.

It must be remembered that the human body uses energy in many forms hence the unit used in measurement is only an indirect indication of the energy available to the body in various forms (chemical, thermal, mechanical, electrical, etc.).

Food supplies the energy we need for everything we do. Two components of food, carbohydrates and fats, supply 85 to 92 per cent of the total energy in the Indian dietary, the rest is provided by proteins.

Measurement of Food Energy

The energy value of foods is determined in the laboratories by the use of special equipment called the bomb calorimeter. In the bomb calorimeter, the heat given off by a food in direct combustion or burning, is measured under controlled conditions.

Energy value of a food can also be measured indirectly by measuring the oxygen used in burning a known amount of food.

---

1. 1 kilocalorie = 4.184 kilojoules (kJ)
   1000 joules = 1 kilojoule (kJ)
   1000 kilojoules – 1 megajoule (mJ).

The average fuel values of the energy giving components of foods have been found to be:

Carbohydrates	4.10 kcals/gramme
Fats	9.45 kcals/gramme and
Proteins	5.65 kcals/gramme

The energy available from food in the body, called the physiological fuel value, is less than its fuel value given above because:

- Some partially oxidised products are excreted.
- Some food is excreted in undigested form.

The carbohydrates and fats (after digestion) are completely oxidised in the body, but some partially oxidised end products of proteins are excreted in the urine. The energy value of these end products on an average is equivalent to 1.25 kcals/gramme of protein consumed. This figure is derived from a normal American diet about sixty years back. This correction is made in calculating energy available from proteins in the body.

The averages of coefficients of digestibility[1] for the components of a typical dietary were:

Carbohydrates	98%
Fats	95%
Proteins	92%

The physiological fuel value (*i.e.*, the energy available to the body) was calculated as follows:

$$\text{Carbohydrates} = (4.10) \times 98\% = 4.01 \text{ kcal/g}$$

$$\text{Fats} = (9.45) \times 95\% = 8.98 \text{ kcal/g}$$

$$\text{Proteins} = (5.65 - 1.25) \times 92\% = 4.05 \text{ kcal/g}$$

For practical use these physiological fuel values were rounded off to the nearest whole number to get the kcalorie values we use in practical nutrition.

Table 7.1: Calorie Content of Dal

Components	*Dal* *a*	*Calories per g* *b*	*a × b*
Carbohydrates	57.6	4	230.4
Fats	1.7	9	15.3
Proteins	22.3	4	89.2
Moisture	13.4	0	0
Minerals	3.5	0	0
Fibre	1.5	0	0
Calories per 100.0 g of Dal			= 334.9

1. The coefficient of digestibility is a measure of digestion and is calculated as follows

$$\text{Coefficient of digestibility} = \frac{(\text{Nutrient intake - Nutrient in faeces}) \times 100}{\text{Nutrient intake}}$$

Carbohydrates	4 kcals / g
Fats	9 kcals / g
Proteins	4 kcals / g

Please remember that these fuel values refer to the edible portion of the food. Thus firstly, the energy content of the food is related to the food composition. Table 7.1 illustrates how to calculate the fuel value of food on the basis of composition.

Secondly, energy value of food is affected by water or moisture content of food, as it is given in the food composition tables. As you may note from Table 7.2, water or moisture does not provide any energy. Therefore foods, which have a large percentage of water, have a low calorie content.

Thirdly, energy content of foods varies with their fat content. As we learnt earlier, fat provides 9 kcals per gramme, therefore foods with high fat content, have a high energy value (Table 7.2).

Fourthly, the energy value of foods is affected by preparation or processing. As rice absorbs water, while cooking, cooked rice has about one-third the number of calories as an equal weight of raw rice. The reverse is the case when foods are dried. Dried fruits are concentrated source of energy as compared to fresh fruits. Seasoning with oil increases the energy content of salads, vegetables and *dals.* Frying foods such as *papad, shev,* wafers, invariably increases their energy content. Examples of effect of preparation on energy content of foods is presented in Table 7.3.

Thus any change in the composition during processing or preparation affects the calorie content of the food product. It is important to take these changes into account, while calculating the energy content of food preparations, used in the dietary.

Table 7.2: Moisture, Fat and Caloric Content of Foods

Food	*Moisture %*	*Fat %*	*Calories per 100 g*
Cucumber	96	0.1	13
Tomato	94	0.2	20
French beans	91	0.1	26
Orange, Carrot	88	0.2	48
Milk, cow's	87	4.1	67
Grapes	79	0.3	71
Potato	75	0.1	97
Egg	73	13.3	173
Mutton, muscle	71	13.3	194
Wheat	13	1.5	346
Groundnut (Peanuts)	3	40.1	567
Butter	19	81.0	729
Oil, Ghee or *Vanaspati*	0	100.0	900

Table 7.3: Change in Calorie Content with Preparation & Processing

Food	*Moisture %*	*Fat %*	*Calories per 100 g*
Rice, raw	13	0.5	345
Rice, cooked	71	0.2	115
Grapes	79	0.3	71
Raisins (dry grapes)	20	0.3	308
Methi leaves, fresh	86	0.9	49
Methi leaves *bhaji*	80	8.0	113
Papad, roasted	20	0.3	228
Papad, fried	3	26.0	512
Bengal gram *dal* flour	10	5.6	372
Shev (made from besan)	3	38.0	568

Calorie Density

The word density is derived from dense, which refers to the concentration of a material in a particular substance. Thus calorie density indicates the concentration of energy (calorie) in a food. Fat or foods containing fat have a higher calorie density than those containing carbohydrate or proteins. If you refer to Table 7.3, you will observe that fried *papad* is calorie dense as compared to roasted *papad.*

Energy Intake

The main source of energy for all the body activities is food, along with the energy store in body tissues as reserve.

Our body needs fuel to carry out its work on a continual basis. This need starts at birth and continues as long as one lives.

Energy is the primary need of the body and takes precedence over all other needs. The metabolic products formed by digestion of carbohydrates and fats, which are simple sugars, glycerol and fatty acids, provide most of the energy needs of the body. One can summarise the energy production from foods as:

$$\text{Glucose, fatty acids, glycerol or amino acids + oxygen} \rightarrow$$
$$\rightarrow \text{energy + carbon dioxide + water}$$

The actual process involves a series of complex reactions, which lead to the common pathway known as Kreb's cycle or the tricarboxylic acid cycle, its end products being energy, carbon dioxide and water. The energy released is trapped in energy-rich compounds (ATP), from which it is released as required.

Food Energy Intake: You can calculate your own energy intake by keeping an accurate record of a day's actual food consumption. A sample form given in Table 7.4, can be used and energy value of foods eaten can be calculated by referring to food composition table in the appendix (Appendix F).

Energy Storage in the Body

While we may eat two, three or four meals a day, which supply energy to the body at intervals, our body activities (voluntary and involuntary) go on throughout the day, even while we sleep. The body draws on its stores of energy to meet its continuous need for energy.

Glycogen: Glycogen stored in the muscles and liver (about 300–350 g), acts as an energy reserve. Glycogen stores maintain blood glucose at normal levels for use of body functions during hours of sleep. Thus our first meal of the day, which breaks the night long fast, is very important for replenishing glycogen stores.

Table 7.4: Record of Food Energy Intake

List all meals and snacks for 1 day:

Food (description and amount)	*Carbohydrates (g)*	*Fat (g)*	*Protein (g)*	*K calories*
Breakfast				
Lunch				
Snacks				
Dinner				
Snacks				
TOTAL				

Adipose tissue: Food energy in excess of body's needs is stored efficiently in the adipose tissues. This store is larger than glycogen stores. The amount thus stored varies from person to person. A well balanced amount needs to be maintained as an added reserve energy source.

Muscle mass: In the muscle mass, a limited amount of energy is stored as protein. This lean muscle mass needs to be maintained for good health. The body draws on these tissues for energy, only when it is under stress due to long periods of fast or starvation.

Energy Expenditure

Our body spends the energy from food and body reserves to carry out its functions related to maintenance of life and to carry out physical activities. The energy expenditure of adults is decided by three types of needs for energy: basal metabolism, physical activity and use of food in the body.

Measurement of Energy Expenditure

Energy expended by the human body at rest or in activity can be measured directly by measuring the heat evolved. This is known as *direct calorimetry,* which is easy in principle, but very cumbersome in practice. It needs a small insulated chamber in which the human subject is kept and all the heat produced is accurately measured. There may be less than ten such equipments in research laboratories in the world. Atwater and Ross about hundred years back, studied human energy metabolism, using such a chamber. They were able to demonstrate that in man.

1. The fundamental physical law of Conservation of Energy is obeyed. Thus total energy expenditure (heat produced + activity done) is equal to the net energy provided by the food consumed (total chemical energy in the food – the energy lost in faeces and urine), when the person is in energy balance.
2. Total energy expenditure is quantitatively related to the oxygen consumption in man.

Total energy spent is quantitatively related to the oxygen used in the body. The oxygen consumed when an organic substance is completely used (oxidised) in the body is proportional to the energy released as heat. Hence the measurement of oxygen consumption by the body can be used to determine energy spent by the body at rest (BMR) or in various activities. This is an indirect way to determine energy expenditure and is therefore, known as *indirect calorimetry.*

The oxidation of glucose proceeds quantitatively as follows:

$$C_6H_{12}O_6 + 6O_2 \longrightarrow 6CO_2 + 6H_2O + \text{Heat}$$

The ratio of carbon dioxide produced to the oxygen used is known as respiratory quotient (RQ). The RQ for oxidation of glucose is 1.0. Similarly the RQ for protein is 0.8 and for fat 0.7, indicating that more oxygen is needed to oxidise proteins and fats than that needed to oxidise carbohydrates.

Energy for Basal Metabolism

Energy needs of the body at rest is called basal metabolism. It can also be aptly be called the cost of living. A number of processes go on to ensure the continuance of life without any conscious effort. These include the beating of heart, the circulation of the blood, breathing, the regulation of body temperature, glandular activities, etc. These processes are known as the basal metabolic processes.

Basal energy expenditure (BEE) or resting energy expenditure (REE) is the energy used by the body at rest. The energy used is measured as the basal metabolic rate (BMR) or resting metabolic rate (RMR). The terms are used interchangeably.

The basal energy needs account for, about 60 per cent of the total energy requirement for most people. The highly active tissues (liver, brain, heart, kidney and gastrointestinal tract), which form less than 5 per cent of the body weight, use about 60 to 70 per cent of the basal metabolic energy. The rest of the tissues, which account for most of the body weight, need much less energy to maintain their basal function.

Measurement of Basal Metabolic Rate (BMR)

The BMR is normally measured early in the morning, after the subject awakens and is in a post-absorptive state (10 to 12 hours after the last meal).

In clinical cases, the normal exchange of oxygen and carbon dioxide in regular breathing used to be measured with a calorimeter to determine the BMR. The amount of energy used to be calculated from the oxygen used. This test is used only in research now.

A number of new efficient tests are used in clinical practice currently. These tests measure the activity of the thyroid gland. There are several ways of measuring the activity of thyroid gland, which produces the hormone thyroxine. The blood levels of thyroxine, the hormone which controls the BMR, can be measured. Iodine is used in the synthesis of the thyroid hormone. Hence serum levels of protein-bound iodine (PBI) and radioactive iodine uptake tests are also used to determine BMR.

Basal energy needs can be estimated using a general formula 1 kcal/kg body weight per hour for men and 0.9 kcal/kg body weight per hour for women.

The classic Harris-Benedict equations are also used to estimate the basal or resting energy needs of adult hospitalised patients.

Female REE = $655 + (9.56 \times W) + (1.85 \times H) - (4.68 \times A)$

Male REE = $66.5 + (13.8 \times W) + (5.0 \times H) - (6.76 \times A)$

Where W = weight in Kilogrammes (kg), H = height in centimeters (cm) an A = age in years

Factors affecting the BMR: Body size and composition, age and growth, sleep, state of nutrition, climate and certain ailments affect the basal requirement.

Body Size and Composition: The heat loss from the body is related to body size; energy needed to maintain lean muscle mass at rest is related to body composition.

Original work on energy measurement was based on body surface area. Recent studies have demonstrated that the metabolic rate is primarily dependent on lean body mass (LBM). LBM can be accurately determined by under water weighing or total count of body potassium.

Athletes, who have developed muscles due to exercise, have 5 per cent increase in BMR as compared to non-athletes. Women have 5 to 10 per cent lower metabolic rate as compared to men of same weight and height, because they have more fat and less muscle in their body than men do. If BMR is calculated on the basis of lean body mass, there is no difference between men and women.

Age: There is a decrease in metabolic energy expenditure of 2 to 3 per cent per decade after early adulthood, due to the shift in the proportion of muscle to fat in the body. The basal metabolic rate gradually decreases after reaching adulthood; the decrease is about 30 per cent between 30 to 75 years.

Growth and Repair: The metabolic rate is highest in the stages of rapid growth, namely the first and second years of life. There is a lesser peak in metabolic rate in the years of puberty and adolescence in both sexes. Infants may store 12 to 15 per cent of their energy intake in the form of new tissue. The metabolic rate increases in pregnancy due to growth of the foetus and related increased growth activity.

Sleep: The metabolic rate falls by about 10 per cent while sleeping as compared to the resting rate when awake. This is due to relaxation of muscles and reduced activity of the nervous system during sleep.

State of Health: The metabolism is decreased due to malnutrition; the decrease in basal metabolism is proportional to the degree of malnutrition. It is mainly due to decrease in the amount of active tissue and a decrease in the metabolic rate.

When one suffers from fever, the increase in temperature of the body increases metabolism. The increase is about 7 per cent per each degree Fahrenheit above normal (98.6°F or 37°C).

Hormonal Control: A hormone known as thyroxine, controls the speed of our involuntary activity. The thyroid gland, situated in our neck, synthesises this hormone.

If too much thyroxine is released, the rate of energy expenditure is increased; if too little is released, the energy expenditure is reduced. The basal metabolism may decrease by 30 to 40 per cent when the synthesis of thyroxine is inadequate. On the other hand, the BMR may almost double due to a hyperactive thyroid gland. These conditions need prompt medical treatment.

Luckily for most of us such abnormalities are not very common. Most of us have a normally functioning thyroid gland and hence a normal basal metabolic rate.

Climate: Extreme environmental temperatures affect the metabolic energy needs. The metabolic rate of persons in the tropics is 5 to 20 per cent higher than those in temperate regions.

In hot climate (if the temperature is greater than 86°F), the metabolic rate increases by about 50 per cent due to increased activity of sweat glands. The increase in metabolic rate due to cold depends on the body fat insulation and use of warm clothes.

Table 7.5: Energy Cost of Some Common Activities in Terms of BMR Units.[1]

Activity	*Energy cost of activities in BMR units*	
	Indian data	*International data*
Sitting quietly	1.20	1.25
Standing quietly	1.40	1.33
Sitting at desk	1.30	1.36
Standing and doing lab work	2.0	1.95
Harvesting	3.6	3.5
Hand saw	7.4	7.5
Typing (sitting)	1.58	1.69
Walking 3 MPH	3.71	3.77

1. BMR of man = 1.05 kcal/hr/kg and woman = 0.975 kcal/hr/kg.

Energy for Physical Activity

Physical activity is that activity, which we choose to do; so it is also known as voluntary activity. It includes;

- the work related to one's occupation, profession or job.
- activities related to personal necessities, such as bathing, brushing teeth, dressing, eating, washing clothes and utensils, commuting to work, market, etc.
- leisure activities such as reading, watching television, playing games (badminton, tennis), gardening, playing with children, walking, etc.

The energy cost of some common activities in terms of BMR units is given in Table 7.5.

Please remember that energy spent in these activities is in addition to that used for basal metabolism. The total energy needed for physical activities includes that spent in personal necessities, professional work, housework and leisure activities.

The additional energy output due to voluntary physical activity varies from as little as 10 per cent for a bed-ridden patient to as high as 50 per cent for an athlete. Factors, which affect energy need for activities, are body size, the efficiency in activity and level of fitness of the person.

Mental work or study does not need extra energy. Similarly, anxiety or any other emotional state does not increase energy needs, but any agitated movements, muscle tension or restlessness may require extra energy.

Typical disposal of food energy is presented in Figure 7.0.

Energy for Utilisation of Food

Some energy is used to take food into the body, digest it and carry the nutrients to the tissues and eliminate the waste products produced in the process. This is known as the specific dynamic action of foods or the energy for utilisation of food.

The energy required for the utilisation of mixed diets in Western countries is reported to be 6 to 10 per cent of the total energy need. The energy needed for the utilisation of the carbohydrate-based Indian diet may be lower than that percentage.

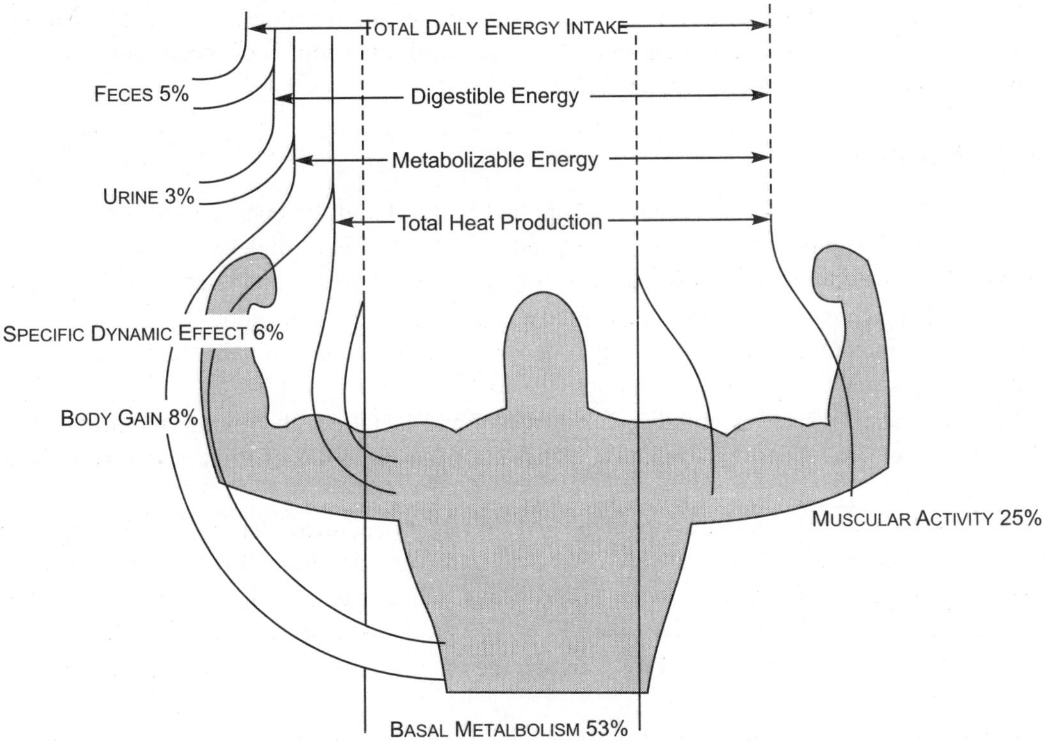

Figure 7.0: Typical disposal of food energy

Energy for Growth and Repair: Extra energy is needed during periods of rapid growth for the building of new tissues. These stages of life include pregnancy, early childhood and adolescence.

The total energy need of one pregnancy is estimated to be about 40,000 kilocalories. In the lactation stage, the secretion of milk for the infant increases the mother's need for energy, the additional need is in the range 700 to 1000 kilocalories per day.

Infants, whose growth rate is the highest in the entire life-cycle, have been observed to store 12 to 15 per cent of their total energy intake. Adolescent growth spurt results in extra need for energy; it may be as high as 25 to 30 per cent more than the adult needs.

Persons, recovering from wasting diseases, from burns, from blood loss, etc., need additional energy for replacing the tissue damaged or lost with new tissues.

Total Energy Requirements

The number of calories we need each day is decided by the involuntary as well as the voluntary activities of our body. The total energy needed for our body daily is the sum total of the energy for

1. Basal metabolic processes, which are involuntary
2. Muscular (physical) activity, which is voluntary
3. Utilisation of food or specific dynamic action of foods and
4. Energy for growth and repair.

To maintain daily energy balance, food energy intake must be equal to body's energy expenditure in a healthy adult.

Loss of weight excessively, as in anorexia nervosa, results from deficient intake of food energy over a long period of time. Treatment consists of counselling about food needs for health, gradual increase in food intake as also moderate activity and rest.

Energy Balance

In an adult, a balance between energy supplied by food and the energy used by the body for its activities, ensures maintenance of ideal weight and good health. Thus underweight and overweight are states, which indicate the extent of imbalance in body's energy needs and energy intake.

Energy balance is the level of energy intake of an individual from food that will balance energy expenditure and maintain body weight, when he/she is healthy and maintains body weight and has a body size, body composition and level of activity consistent with good health.

In growth stages, such as childhood, pregnancy and lactation, the energy requirement includes energy needed for growth or the formation of tissue or the secretion of milk at rates consistent with good health.

The ICMR expert committee adopted the FAO/WHO procedure of using BMR factors for arriving at the energy requirements of Indian reference man and woman. These BMR factors for Indian men and women engaged in sedentary, moderate and heavy activity are 1.6, 1.9 and 2.5 respectively. The energy requirement of Reference Indian man and woman as given in RDA 1990 is presented in Table 7.6.

For individuals with different body weights, the energy needs can be computed from the above figures arithmetically.

Energy requirement decreases with age beyond 30 years, due to gradual decrease in basal metabolic rate. By 75 years of age, the decrease is about 30 per cent.

Table 7.6: Energy Requirement of Reference Indian

Sex	*Activity*	*Body weight (kg)*	*Energy (kcal)*
Man	Sedentary	60	2425
	Moderate	60	2875
	Heavy	60	3800
Woman	Sedentary	50	1875
	Moderate	50	2225
	Heavy	50	2925

Cut-off Point for Assessing Energy Inadequacy

During famine and drought situations, scarcity of food and work exists. An individual's energy intake can go below the cut-off point. It is important to set-up a cut-off point for energy for determining the extent of energy inadequacy. The cut-off point derived from weighted average of daily energy requirement for entire population on the basis of present RDA will be 2,200 kcal. The same cut-off point can be used to determine the extent of poverty and energy inadequacy in our population.

Recommended Dietary Allowance (RDA)

The recommended dietary allowances for energy are given in Table 7.7. It may be observed that in adults the energy intake is related to the physical activity (Figure 7.1). The energy need for pregnancy

Table 7.7: Recommended Daily Allowances for Energy

Particulars	*kcal/day*	*Particulars*	*kcal/day*
Man (60 kg)		**Infants**	
Sedentary work	2425	0–6 months (5.4 kg)	108/kg
Moderate work	2875	6–12 months (8.6 kg)	98/kg
Heavy work	3800	**Children**	
Woman (50 kg)		1–3 years (12.2 kg)	1240
Sedentary work	1875	4–6 years (19.0 kg)	1690
Moderate work	2225	7–9 years (26.9 kg)	1950
Heavy work	2925	Boys 10–12 years (35.4 kg)	2190
Pregnant woman	+300	Girls 10–12 years (31.5 kg)	1970
Lactation		Boys 13–15 years (47.8 kg)	2450
0–6 months	+550	Girls 13–15 years (46.7 kg)	2060
7–12 months	+400	Boys 16–18 years (57.1 kg)	2640
		Girls 16–18 years (49.9 kg)	2060

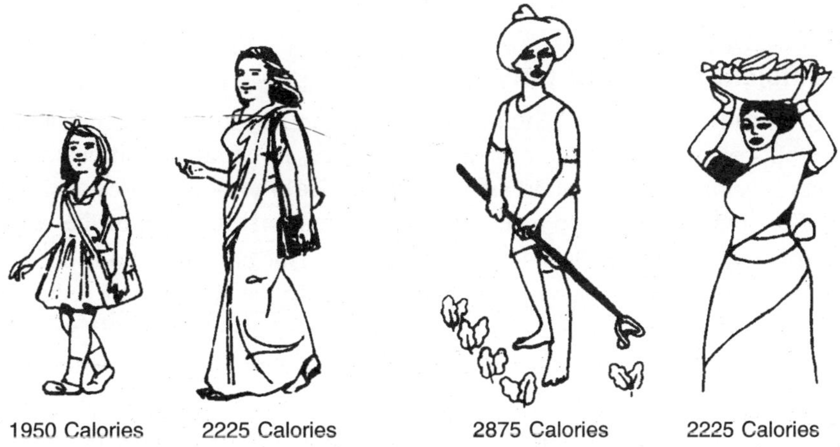

Figure 7.1: Energy needs vary with activity.

is increased in the latter half when the growth is rapid and some storage occurs to be utilised during the early part of the lactation for the secretion of milk. The extra energy needs for pregnancy and lactation are indicated below, as also the energy needs during various stages of growth. In the first year of life as the growth is very rapid and individual variation in weight is great, the recommendation is made in terms of energy per unit weight (kcal/kg). The growth rate slows from the second year of life and so also the energy need per day. The variation in energy needs with occupation and physiological state is depicted in Figure 7.2.

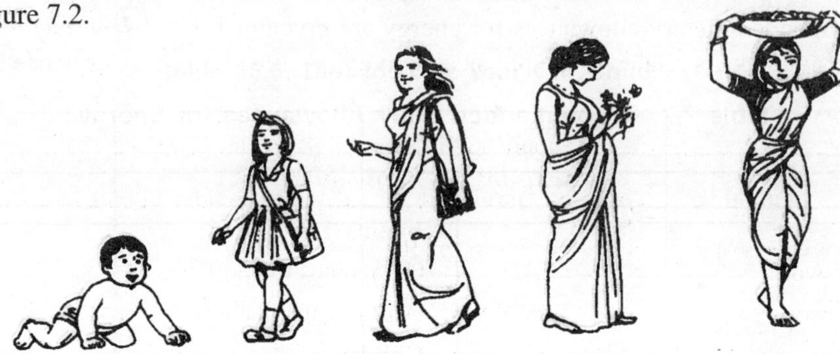

Age – 7-8 months	9 years	25 years Sedentary	Pregnant	Moderate Activity
Calories – 845	1950	1875	2175	2225
Body Weight – 8.6 kg	26.9 kg	50 kg	60 kg	50 kg

Figure 7.2: Energy needs vary with age, occupation and physiological state.

Insufficient Energy Supply

The effects of insufficient energy supply throughout life may result in low life expectancy. For a large section of the rural population, who do not get sufficient food, the cause may be traced to too many persons per unit of family land; poor yields or poor harvests; the landless labour may have no work during part of the year. In the cities the causes may be full or partial unemployment or too many dependents per earning member in the lower socio-economic groups. A small section of the population may have insufficient intake due to faulty food habits. These may include missed meals, poor schedules, neglect or poor health practices.

Effects of Insufficient Energy Supply

The effects of insufficient energy supply vary with the age group affected and the extent of insufficiency. In adults, it may affect their capacity for work, in children it affects their growth and activity. If the energy supply is very short of what is needed, the body stores of fat may be used, followed by use of the muscle tissues to meet the need for minimal function of the body.

Working Capacity: The energy needs for work are next to the basal metabolic needs in magnitude. When there is an insufficient energy supply, the body adjusts to the shortage by reducing activity.

In children, this may result in reduced movement or play, depending on the age of the child and may pass unnoticed. In adults, it results in reduced activity, slow deliberate movement and avoidance of continuous effort.

In a number of studies, dramatic losses in working efficiency have been reported, during periods of food shortage. In Germany, steel output fell from 120 tons to 80 tons per man per month, when energy supply for work was reduced from 1900 to 1150 calories per day.

In India, where about 65 to 70 per cent of the population is engaged in agriculture, it will affect the agricultural production adversely.

Wasting of Tissue: When adults have to do strenuous manual work with meagre food intake, the extra energy needed is mobilised by burning body tissues. This has been euphemistically called 'wasting of tissue'. This is what happens to many farm workers who have very little food reserves. When the planting season comes, and they have to go through the whole cycle of strenuous operations involved in producing the crop, with meagre food intakes.

The wasting of tissues is observed in adults in pre-harvest periods in many farming communities. This population goes through the cycle of want annually. What it means in terms of loss of potential human resources and human misery is hard to estimate.

The women folk in these communities, who have the additional burden of child-bearing, are subjected to greater stress and it is bound to affect the health of the mother and the child adversely.

Stunted Growth: It has been observed that underfed mothers tend to have smaller babies, who have very little reserves of nutrients at birth. Inadequate food during infancy results in stunted growth.

Unfortunately, as most children in such communities suffer from a similar problem, the retarded growth may not be noticed by the parents. Thus the subnormal may pass for normal growth. This is not a malady in itself, but insufficient food intake is not only deficient in energy, but in other nutrients, making the child vulnerable to diseases.

Any childhood infection such as diarrhoea, dysentery, measles, chicken pox creates a stress and the body tissues are used up to meet the extra demands imposed by the infection. The child may not survive, if it suffers from repeated attacks of such infections, in the absence of improved quantity and quality of food intake.

Aged persons, in such families may also suffer from tissue wastage, as they are dependent on their relatives, who are unable to provide food for them.

Maintenance of Body Weight

Weight is one of the gross parameters of our health. The life insurance companies collected data about weights for heights of healthy individuals to set-up norms (of weights for heights) to be used as guides in the medical examination of their clients. The clients, who were overweight or underweight were found to be greater risks, and therefore had to pay higher premiums. Thus overweight can be a financial liability.

A healthy normal person reaches the desirable weight for his/her height by 25 years of age. It is advisable for a person to maintain that weight throughout life. This is the reason why all tables indicate desirable weight for height for men and women at 25 years (Tables 7.8 and 7.9).

When energy intake is equal to body needs, body weight is maintained at a fairly constant level, in a healthy adult. Thus constant body weight is an index of energy balance in healthy adults.

Consistent intake of inadequate food, which is unable to meet the body's need for energy, leads to use of body fat to make up the deficit and there is loss of weight. An underweight person has reduced capacity for work, vitality and decreased resistance to disease.

On the contrary, continuous intake of energy in excess of one's needs, results in deposition of fat. If this practice is continued, the gain in weight may be unsightly. Overweight is associated with ailments of heart, circulatory system, kidneys and diabetes. Please remember that there is no reason for a person to weigh more when he is 40 than what he weighed at 25 years of age. The same is true of later years.

Table 7.8: Males (25 yrs.) Weight for Height for Males and Overweight-Underweight Limits

Height (*cm*)	*Weights*[1.2] (*kg*)	*Overweight limit*[3] (*kg*) (+20%)	*Underweight limit*[3] (*kg*) (–20%)
148	47.5	57.0	38.0
152	49.0	59.0	39.0
156	51.5	62.0	41.0
160	53.5	64.0	43.0
164	56.0	67.0	45.0
168	59.0	71.0	47.0
172	62.0	74.5	49.5
176	65.5	78.5	52.4
180	68.5	82.0	55.0
184	72.0	86.5	57.5
188	75.5	90.5	60.5
190	77.5	93.0	62.0

1. Derived from Life Insurance Corporation, Agent's Manual.
2. Weights have been rounded off to the nearest half kilogram.
3. Overweight and underweight limits are calculated from weight in column 2, by adding or subtracting 20%.

Table 7.9: Females (25 yrs.) Weight for Height and Overweight-Underweight Limits

Height (*cm*)	*Weights*[1.2] (*kg*)	*Overweight limit*[3] (*kg*) (+20%)	*Underweight limit*[3] (*kg*) (–20%)
148	46.5	56.0	37.0
152	48.5	58.0	39.0
156	50.5	60.5	40.5
160	52.5	63.0	42.0
164	55.0	66.0	44.0
168	58.0	69.5	46.5
172	60.5	72.5	48.5
176	64.0	77.0	51.0
180	67.0	80.5	53.5
184	70.5	84.5	56.5
188	74.0	89.0	59.0

1. Derived from Life Insurance Corporation Agent's Manual.
2. Weights have been rounded off to the nearest half kilogram.
3. Overweight and underweight limits have been calculated from weight in column 2, by adding or subtracting 20 per cent.

Excess Energy Intake

Continued increase in weight in a healthy adult after the age of 25, indicates intake of energy in excess of body needs. The body has no mechanism to rid itself of this extra energy and therefore stores it in the form of fat.

The excess intake does not have to be large. It can be as little as 50 extra calories a day, which when taken regularly, will result in 2 kilogram gain in weight in a year. This gain is not serious in the short run, but over a decade it adds up to 20 kilogram, which is when it becomes noticeable.

Most people add weight after the age of 35 or 40 years, because they continue the energy intakes that they needed at the age of 25 years. But their need for energy decreases with age, due to the lowering of the basal metabolic rate and perhaps change in the activities from more active ones to less active ones.

Most women are less active at this age, as the children are of school-going age and do not need the kind of care they needed as babies. Both men and women may be more efficient in whatever jobs they do and may have given up active exercise or sport for sedentary entertainment like playing bridge or watching television. This is also a stage where people can afford the luxuries of life such as eating rich and expensive foods. Thus, there is an intake of excess food energy which is not utilised, and is deposited as fat.

It is necessary to reduce energy intake to a level lower than one's needs, to use up the deposited fat. Exercise in the form of outdoor games, walking and indoor fitness exercise help in weight reduction. But it must be accompanied by consistent, regular, carefully planned reduction of energy intake.

Study Questions and Activities

1. List the nutrients, which supply energy. Discuss the factors which affect the energy needs of the body.
2. List the amounts, kinds and cost of foods which you include in your daily meals:
   (a) Compare the cost of 100 calories from foods such as rice, wheat, *dal,* bread, milk, oil, butter.
   (b) Calculate your energy intake per day.
   (c) Calculate the percentage of calories supplied by foods from various groups.
   (d) What happens if the energy need of a person is not met?

CHAPTER 8

Fat-soluble Vitamins

Introduction

A number of deficiency diseases plagued people, whose diets were restricted. Thus half the sailors, in the fifteenth to seventeenth century voyages, died of scurvy, due to lack of fresh vegetables and fruits in their diets. In Asia, beriberi plagued rice-eating people. Pellagra claimed many lives of corn-eating population in Southern United States in the beginning of last century.

Today we rarely see these deadly diseases in the sections of society, who have varied diets of ordinary natural foods. But in over 70 developing countries, crores of children still lose their sight due to lack of vitamin A.

It was thought that a diet containing proteins, carbohydrates, fats, minerals and water was adequate to maintain life, until the beginning of last century. But research conducted in the early part of the last century proved that some vital factor was missing from the diet. This vital factor was given the name vitamin. Later it was found that there was more than one factor involved.

Now we know that vitamins are one of the six classes of nutrients supplied by food. They are required for normal growth and maintenance of all animal life. Vitamins are important for their regulatory and protective functions. Unlike most other nutrients they are required in very small amounts. But it is necessary to provide these in the diet because many of them cannot be manufactured by the body. The lack of vitamins results in definite deficiency disorders, which are specific for each particular vitamin.

Vitamins have captured public interest in the last sixty years. This may be because they have been synthesised and marketed by a large pharmaceutical industry. Their efforts have been supported by medical practitioners and health conscious public. Some people have often been misled into thinking 'if little is good, more may be better'.

Surely vitamins are essential nutrients. We need to understand what they do, how much we need them and where we can get them. Can we get enough of these in foods or do we need pills to meet our needs of some vitamins? Most important, can mega-doses of vitamins hurt us? We need sound answers to these questions.

Definition

A substance can be classified as a vitamin if it satisfies the two criteria:

1. It must be a vital, organic dietary substance, which is neither a carbohydrate, fat, protein, or mineral and is necessary in only very small amounts to perform a specific metabolic function or to prevent an associated deficiency disease, and
2. It cannot be manufactured by the body, and, therefore, must be supplied by the diet.

Nature of Vitamins

Vitamins are organic substances, which occur in small amounts in foods. They are necessary for life and growth. Chemical structure of each vitamin is specific; some like vitamin C have a simple structure, while others such as vitamin D have a complex structure.

Vitamins do not provide calories, but are essential in the metabolic reactions, which release energy from carbohydrates, fats and proteins. Vitamins are essential co-factors in hundreds of metabolic reactions in the body. They may act singly or in co-ordination with each other. Each vitamin has specific functions and so one vitamin cannot substitute for another in the body.

Vitamins may occur in preformed or its active form in the food, or as a precursor compound which can be changed into active form in the body.

Vitamins are conveniently classified into two groups on the basis of their solubility into **fat-soluble** and **water-soluble** vitamins. Fat-soluble vitamins include A, D, E and K. Water-soluble vitamins include the B-group and vitamin C.

Foods differ greatly in the amount and kinds of the vitamins they supply. Selection and intake of foods according to the food guide (chapter 14) can help to meet one's need of the various vitamins.

Fat-Soluble Vitamins

Fat-soluble vitamins can only be absorbed in the presence of fat. Therefore, the presence of some fat in the diet is essential for their absorption. Fat-soluble vitamins can be stored in the body and hence occasional intake of very high sources may help the body tide over periods of low intake. The requirement for fat-soluble vitamins may be met by intake of a precursor or the vitamin itself. Not much of fat-soluble vitamins are lost in normal cooking procedures.

Vitamin A

This was the first fat-soluble vitamin to be discovered. It has a number of important functions in the body. Vitamin A is found only in animal foods, mainly as retinol. Plants provide a source of vitamin A for animals in the form of orange-yellow pigments called the carotenoids. The chief source in human nutrition is beta-carotene, which the body converts to vitamin A in the intestinal mucosa during absorption. The conversion is partial and varies from 25 to 50 per cent.

Vitamin A activity in foods used to be expressed in International Units (I.U.), with the following equivalencies:

1 IU = 0.3 mcg retinol
1 IU = 0.6 mcg beta-carotene
1 IU = 1.2 mcg other provitamin A carotenoids

Now it is expressed as microgram (mcg) of retinol or beta-carotene or retinol equivalent (RE) as indicated in Table 8.1.

As, you may have noted, the amount of vitamin ester and carotenoids provided decreases with increasing weight of the vitamin A compound. About 6 to 12 times weight of carotenoids are needed to provide one unit RE, depending on the form present.

Table 8.1: Retinol Equivalents (RE)[1] of Vitamin A Compound and Carotenoids

Compound	*mcg*	*IU/mcg*	*mcg/RE*
All-trans retinol[2]	0.300	3.33	1.00
All-trans retinyl acetate	0.344	2.91	1.15
All-trans retinyl palmitate	0.549	1.82	1.83
All-trans beta-carotene[3]	1.800	0.56	6.00
Mixed carotenoids[4]	3.600	0.28	12.00

1. Sight and Life Manual on Vitamin A Deficiency Disorders (VADD), 2nd ed., 2001, p. 11.
2. Molecular wt. = 286.44; 3 mg = 10.000 IU.
3. Molecular wt. = 536.85.
4. Provitamin A carotenoids other than beta-carotene.

Functions

Vitamin A has a number of different functions in the body. In recent years, knowledge of the functions of vitamin A has increased greatly. The Sight and Life Manual on Vitamin A Deficiency Disorders has updated the information about the major functions of vitamin A.

It is necessary for normal growth and development. If the intake of vitamin A is not sufficient for normal growth, the bones will stop growing, before the soft tissues are affected. This may result in overcrowding of the brain and nervous system, cranial pressure and consequent brain and nerve injury. In some instances the pressure on the optic nerve may result in blindness. Vitamin A deficiency may sometimes cause degeneration of nervous tissue without causing bone malformation.

Function in Vision: Vitamin A occurs in the retina of the eye and is required in the process of vision to adjust to light of varying intensity (dark adaptation). It occurs in the light receptor cells in the retina in combination with protein. This substance is known as visual purple (rhodopsin). It is bleached in the presence of light, which enables a person to see. Some vitamin A is used up in the process. If more vitamin A is not available, ability to adjust to changes in intensity of light is impaired. Night blindness occurs in severe vitamin A deficiency; it indicates the inability of a person to see at night, when the amount of light is far too little to permit adequate vision.

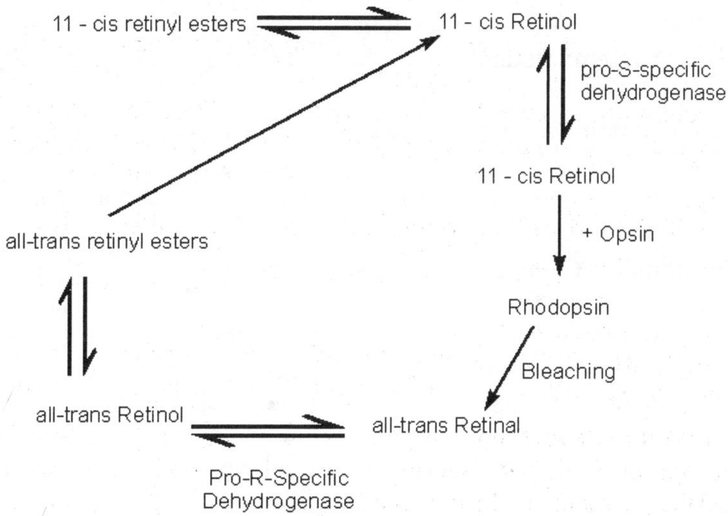

Figure 8.1: Current model of the visual cycle (Ranalo 1994).
(Sight & Life Manual of VADD, p. 32, 2001)

The current model of the visual cycle is given in Figure 8.1.

Health of Epithelial Tissues: These tissues cover the outer surface of the body, line the major cavities and all the tubular systems in the body. These are specialised tissues, of which the outer covering is resistant; protective epidermis and the internal tissue is a secretory mucous membrane. Inadequate supplies of vitamin A results in suppression of the normal secretions and produces a keratinised (dry, horny) type of epithelium. The skin may become excessively dry and mucous membrane may fail to secrete normally and hence be prone to bacterial invasion.

In vitamin A deficiency keratin-producing cells replace mucus-secreting cells in many epithelial tissues of the body. This is the basis of the pathological process termed xerosis that leads to the drying of the conjunctiva and cornea of the eye. The process can be reversed by vitamin A. It has become clear recently that vitamin A mainly in the form of retinoic acid plays a key hormone-like role in cell differentiation throughout the tissue and organs of the body. Hence the formation of retinoic acid must be regulated precisely.

Immune Response: Many of the epithelial tissues are important barriers to infection. Vitamin A deficiency impairs this function in a non-specific way. In addition, vitamin A in a more specific way helps to maintain the lymphocyte pool. Vitamin A also functions in T-cell-mediated responses. Some aspects of the immune response, such as immunoglobulin production, are now known to be affected by retinoids.

Haemopoesis: Vitamin A deficiency in man and experimental animals is consistently associated with an iron deficiency type of anaemia. In these conditions, vitamin A is required in addition to iron for a full response.

Growth: Retinoic acid is known to play its hormone-like function in control of growth and development of tissues in the musculo-skeletal system, just as it does elsewhere.

Other Functions

Energy Balance: It has been recently shown that an enzyme in mitochondria, which controls the local production of energy as heat is under the transcriptional regulation of retinoic acid.

Central Nervous System: Retinoic acid plays a major role in the development of the foetal central nervous system.

Gap Junctional Communication: Gap junctions are narrow, hydrophilic pores connecting the cytosol of two adjacent cells. The gap junctions are reported to be involved in regulation of morphogenesis, cell differentiation, secretion of hormones and growth. Retinoic acid and its analogues act as ligands of nuclear receptors.

Activity of Carotenoids: Carotenoids carry out several important functions in animals and plants. Some carotenoids are only precursors of vitamin A and its derivatives. They act as accessory pigments in energy transfer in photosynthesis. Carotenoids have a photoprotective role in man and bacteria. They are also involved in phototropism in simple and higher plant forms and in plant growth regulation. Carotenoids act in the trapping or tying up of single oxygen. They are used as colouration of food for mankind.

Food Sources

Vitamin A is present in animal foods only. Liver is the richest source of vitamin A. Other sources include butter, ghee, milk, curds and egg yolk. Refined oils and vanaspati are good sources of vitamin A if these are fortified with vitamin A. These may be fortified with vitamin A to the extent of 750 mcg (2500 IU) per 100 g. Table 8.2 lists the important food sources of vitamin A (Figure 8.2).

Vitamin A is not present in vegetable foods, but these foods contain the pigment, beta-carotene, which is the precursor of vitamin A and is therefore also known as 'provitamin A'. On the basis of its chemical structure one molecule of beta-carotene should be able to yield two molecules of vitamin A. In the body, however, the absorption and conversion of beta-carotene is not that perfect and may range from 25 to 50 per cent (Please refer to formulae at the end of the chapter)

Leafy vegetables such as spinach, amaranth, coriander, and drumstick leaves as well as ripe fruits such as mango, papaya, and yellow pumpkin are good sources of beta-carotene. Generally, dark green leafy vegetables contain greater amounts of carotene than those which are light in colour (Table 8.2).

Lycopene, a carotenoid from tomatoes, is an antioxidant. It has the ability to protect against vascular degeneration, the leading cause of adult blindness. Algal carotenoids lutin and zeaxanthin have the same ability and are used as food additives. Lycopene is known to inhibit carcinogenesis in specific animal systems and is expected to have similar protective effects in humans. Lycopene supplementation can reduce prostrate cancer risk by approximately 45 per cent.

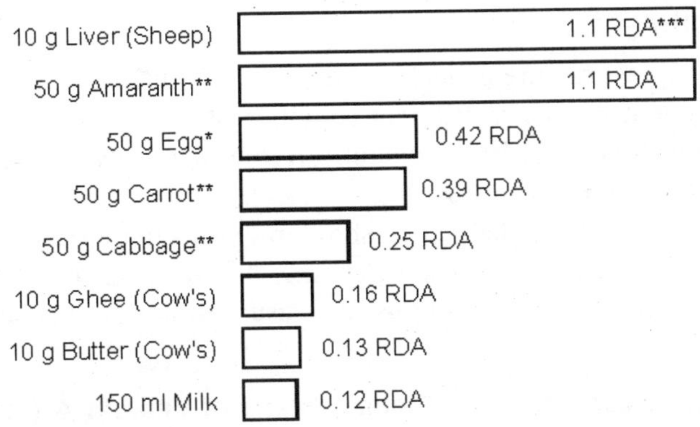

Figure 8.2: Food sources of vitamin A.

* includes beta-carotene

** Only beta-carotene present

*** RDA: Recommended Daily Allowances (of vit. A)

Large intake of vitamin A in times of plenty are stored in the liver and help the body to tide over periods of shortage. Similarly an occasional intake of a concentrated source also helps to meet the requirements for this vitamin.

Table 8.2: Sources of Vitamin A

Food	*Vitamin A value*	
	Vitamin A mcg/100 g	*Carotene mcg/100 g*
Liver, sheep	6,690	–
Eggs	360	600
Butter, ghee (cow's)	600–960	–
Milk	48–52	6
Leaves:		
Dark green, e.g., amaranth, radish, spinach	–	5000 or more
Light green-cabbage, lettuce	–	750–2000
Yellow or orange, vegetables and fruits, e.g., carrots, mango, papaya, orange	–	665–2740
Immature beans and peas, capsicum, tomato	–	80–595

Liver oils of shark, halibut, cod and saw fish are some of the richest known sources[1] of vitamin A. However fish liver oils do not form part of the diet and have to be taken as a supplement.

1. Fish liver oils contain preformed vitamin A, the contents per one gramme being 200 to 700 mcg in cod liver oil, about 700 mcg in shark liver oil and 10,000 mcg in halibut liver oil.

Human Requirements

It is customary to express requirements for vitamin A for humans in terms of Retinol Equivalents (RE/day) taking into account the many different activities of retinol and the provitamin carotenoids. Table 8.3 gives RDIs for vitamin A from several different agencies. These were meant to prevent deficiency and provide a margin of safety.

However recent evidence has emerged to show the protective effects of increased amounts of antioxidant nutrients such as carotenoids against chronic diseases. Since these beneficial effects were not thought of in forming the recommendations, it is usual to advise increase in the intake of fresh vegetables and fruits.

Table 8.3: Recommended Dietary Intake of Vitamin A (mcg/day)*

*ASG***	*FAO/WHO*	*USA*	*UK*
0–1	350	375	350
1–3	400	400	400
4–6	400	500	500
7–12 years	400	700	500
10–12 years	500	700	500
12–15 years	600	700	600
M 15–18 + years	600	1000	700
F 15–18 + years	500	800	600
Pregnancy	600	800	+100
Lactation	850	(I half) 1300 (II half) 1200	+350

* McLaren, D.S. & M. Frigg. Sight & Life Manual on Vit. A Deficiency Disorders. 2nd ed., 2001, p. 36.
** ASG = Age-Sex-Grouping for FAO/WHO, USA & UK.

Table 8.4: Recommended Dietary Allowances of Vitamin A (mcg/day)*

*ASG***	*Retinol*	*Beta-carotene*
Infants (6–12 months)	350	1400
1–6 years	400	1600
7–12 years	600	2400
13–18 years	600	2400
Adult Man and Woman	600	2400
Pregnant Woman	600	2400
Lactating Woman	950	3800

* Recommended Dietary Allowances for Indians, ICMR, 2000, p.53.
** ASG = Age-Sex-Grouping.

Recommended Daily Allowances

The daily requirement of an adult for vitamin A is of the order of 600 mcg of retinol or 2400 mcg of beta-carotene per day derived from foods of either animal or vegetable origin (Table 8.4). The allowance for infants is 350 mcg (about 1400 mcg of beta carotene). The need increases gradually as the child grows to adolescence. No increased allowance during pregnancy is recommended but the allowance is increased to 950 mcg or 3800 mcg of beta-carotene during lactation. This is in conformity with the FAO/WHO recommendations.

Effect of Deficiency

The deficiency may result from dietary lack of vitamin A, the provitamin, or poor absorption of these. The deficiency results in growth failure, affects the vision, the skin and the immune function adversely.

The earliest symptom is impaired ability to see in dim light (dark adaptation); the next stage is inability to see normally in dim light which is known as night blindness or **nyctalopia.**

The next symptom is usually dryness of lining of eyelids and eyeball (conjunctiva). A later and more severe stage of deficiency is xerosis (dryness) of the cornea. The cornea becomes dry and loses its transparency (xerophthalmia). In the last stage of the disease, keratomalacia, the cornea becomes soft and results in permanent blindness.

In early stages, treatment with vitamin A will restore full vision; however, if advanced changes have taken place, blindness is inevitable. The term xerophthalmia refers to clinical manifestation of vitamin A deficiency. The skin changes include dryness, wrinkling, slate gray discolouration and thickening of the outer layer (hyperkeratosis). The hair may lose lustre.

There is a noticeable shrinking, hardening and progressive degeneration of epithelial cells, which increases susceptibility to severe infections of the eye, the nasal passages, the sinuses, middle ear, lungs and genitourinary tract.

Overdosage

An overdosage of vitamin A may cause serious injury to health. Self-administration of highly potent concentrates is likely to cause a serious condition from which recovery is slow. Some of the symptoms of overdosage are irritability, headache, nausea and vomiting. Symptoms subside gradually on stoppage of intake of vitamin A.

Vitamin D

Pure vitamin D was isolated in crystalline form in 1930 and was called calciferol. Vitamin D is now considered a pro-hormone than a vitamin. Vitamin D is sometimes called the 'sunshine vitamin' because the body is able to convert a precursor 7-dehydrocholesterol, a sterol present in the skin, to vitamin D in the presence of sunlight. It can be synthesised in the body in adequate amounts by simple exposure to sunlight even for five minutes per day.

Vitamin D activity is shown by a group of chemical substances called sterols, which are wax like substances. These compounds are insoluble in water, but are soluble in fats. They are stable to heat, acids, alkalies and oxidation.

Functions

Vitamin D performs several important functions in the body. These include:

- Absorption of calcium and phosphorus: calcitriol, a hormone, is an activated form of vitamin D. It acts with two other hormones (the parathyroid hormone and the thyroid hormone calcitonin) and stimulates the absorption of calcium and phosphorus in the small intestine. Without the presence of vitamin D formation of strong and rigid bones is not possible.
- Bone mineralisation: The bone tissue formation from calcium and phosphorus and other materials is regulated by calcitriol. It regulates the rate of deposit and resorption of these mainerals in bone. This balancing process helps to build and maintain bone tissue. Vitamin D hormone can be used to treat rickets in children and osteoporosis (bone loss) in older women.

Food Sources

Irradiation of the skin with sunlight is the main source of vitamin D. The mid-day sun is rich in ultra-violet light and helps in synthesising this vitamin.

Foods are not a good source of vitamin D. It is found in small quantities in liver, egg yolk, milk and milk fat (butter and ghee), obtained form animals fed on pastures exposed to sunlight.

The richest source known is fish liver oils, such as halibut, cod, shark and sawfish. Fish liver oils do not form part of the diet and have to be taken as a supplement.

Vanaspati may be fortified with 180 International units of vitamin D per 100 g. The per capita consumption of *vanaspati* is quite low in India and so the impact of this fortification is limited.

Recommended Dietary Allowance

It is difficult to set requirements for this nutrient due to its unique hormonelike nature, its synthesis in the skin by sun's irradiation of the 7-dehydrocholesterol there and its limited food sources. As the extent of synthesis of this vitamin and dietary intake is not easy to determine, exact data on vitamin D requirement is not available. Only a range of values is usually given. About 5 mcg or 200 International Units[1] are stated to be the daily requirement of a child. The requirements for adults may be less but are not known with any degree of certainty. However, during pregnancy, adequate supply of vitamin D is essential for the healthy development of the foetus.

As already said, exposure to sunlight results in the conversion of a compound present in the skin to vitamin D. Thus a specific recommendation of a daily supplement of 10 mcg or 400 IU per day is made for only people who work at night, those whose habits or style of dress shield them from sunlight and for invalids who stay indoors.

Effect of Deficiency

When adequate quantities of vitamin D are not available, strong and rigid bones are not formed. This leads to a condition in children known as 'rickets' which is characterised by poor growth and bone deformation such as bowed legs, beaded ribs, enlarged joints and skull deformation. The teeth of children may fail to develop normally because of poor calcification and may have pits and cracks which render them prone to decay. In young girls, improper formation of the bones of the pelvis may result in difficult deliveries of babies, later on in their life.

Osteomalacia—a condition similar to rickets may develop in adult women due to lack of vitamin D. This deficiency disease is common in north India and Pakistan especially among women who have had many pregnancies and have nursed their children for long periods. The bones may become so weak that they may not bear the weight of their bodies and may bend or break.

---

1. One International unit (I.U.) = 0.025 mcg of vitamin D.

Overdosage

Intake of excessive amounts of vitamin D is toxic to the body and causes irritability, nausea, vomitting and constipation. Even a dose of 1000 International Units (25 mcg), when administered over long periods of time, has been found to cause toxic side effects in children.

Vitamin E

Vitamin E or alpha-tocopherol is a fat-soluble vitamin.

No definite proof of vitamin E deficiency in human beings has been established.

Functions

The main function of vitamin E, tocopherol, is its ability to prevent tissue breakdown, by virtue of its antioxidant nature.

Vitamin E acts as nature's most powerful fat-soluble antioxidant. In the lipid membranes of body tissues, the polyunsaturated fatty acids present are easy targets for oxygen to break down. Vitamin E protects the cell membrane fatty acids from damage by interrupting this oxidation process. It is believed to prevent the oxidation of vitamin A and carotene in the digestive tract and to regulate the rate of oxidation of foods inside the body.

Selenium is a trace mineral that works as a partner with vitamin E as an anti-oxidant.

There is a paucity of Indian data both on the vitamin E (tocopherol) content of foods and on vitamin E status. Limited information suggests that Indians have blood levels of 0.5 mg/kg/ml which is considered as satisfactory.

Food Sources

The richest sources of vitamin E are the vegetable oils. Vegetable oils are also the richest sources of polyunsaturated fatty acids, which vitamin E protects. This is nature's unique arrangement to package the two together. Other food sources include cereals, leafy vegetables, milk, eggs, muscle meats and fish.

Vitamin E is widely distributed in foods. Even the cheapest kind of cereal diet contains sufficient intake of the vitamin.

Vitamin E requirement is linked to that of essential fatty acids (linoleic and linolenic acids). The requirement of vitamin E suggested is 0.8 mg/g of essential fatty acids.

Vitamin K: Phylloquinone is the major form of vitamin K found in plants. It is also the form found in our dietary.

The basic function of vitamin K is in the blood-clotting process. It is essential for the formation of prothrombin by the liver. Prothrombin is a normal constituent of the blood and helps clotting of blood on contact with air.

Green leafy vegetables are the principal dietary source of vitamin K. Deficiency of vitamin K prolongs clotting time and may result in excessive bleeding after an injury. Human babies do not have reserves of vitamin K at birth and in many hospital it is, therefore, routine practice to give vitamin K to the expectant mother to prevent excessive bleeding at child birth.

The normal formation of vitamin in the intestinal tract is disturbed by the use of sulfa drugs. Patients, who are treated with antibiotics, after surgery, are likely to suffer from vitamin K deficiency, due to killing of intestinal bacteria, which synthesise the vitamin. Thus there may be blood loss due to non-clotting and poor wound healing.

The Indian RDA committee considered that no recommendation need be made for vitamin K, since Vitamin K deficiency is seen in India only occasionally in premature newborn infants. It is suggested that a dose of 0.5–1.0 mg of vitamin K be administered by the intramuscular route to such infants.

Study Questions

1. List the fat soluble vitamins and their precursors. What are their main sources?
2. Explain the role played by
   (a) Vitamin A in vision.
   (b) Sunlight in synthesis of Vitamin D.
   (c) Vitamin K in the blood clotting process.
3. Why should a overdosages of vitamins A and D be avoided?
4. Explain what happens when there is a deficiency of vitamin A in the diet.

Structure of FAT-Soluble Vitamins

Vitamin A (represented by retinol)

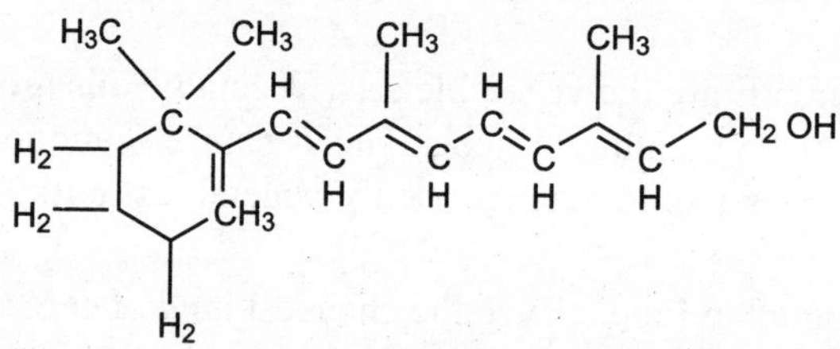

Vitamin D (represented by cholecalciferol, vitamin D_3

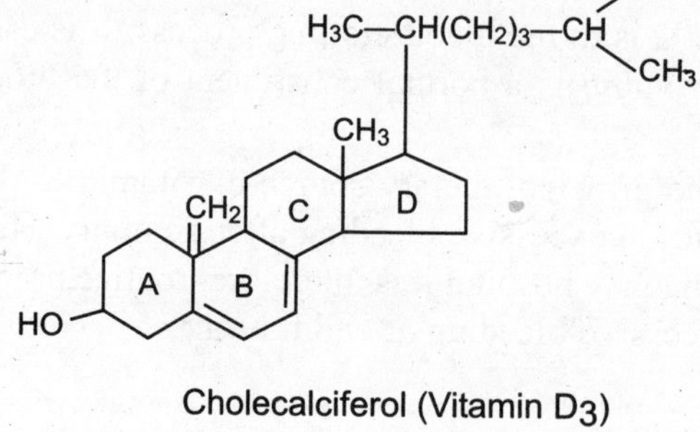

Cholecalciferol (Vitamin D_3)

Vitamin E (represented by alpha tocopherol)

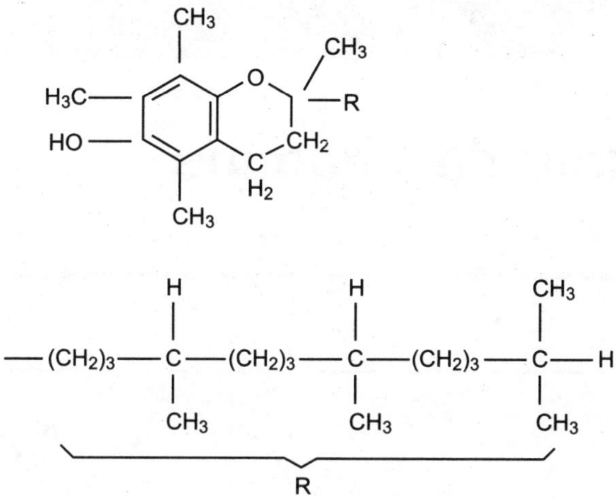

Vitamin K represented by phytylmonoquinone vitamin K_1

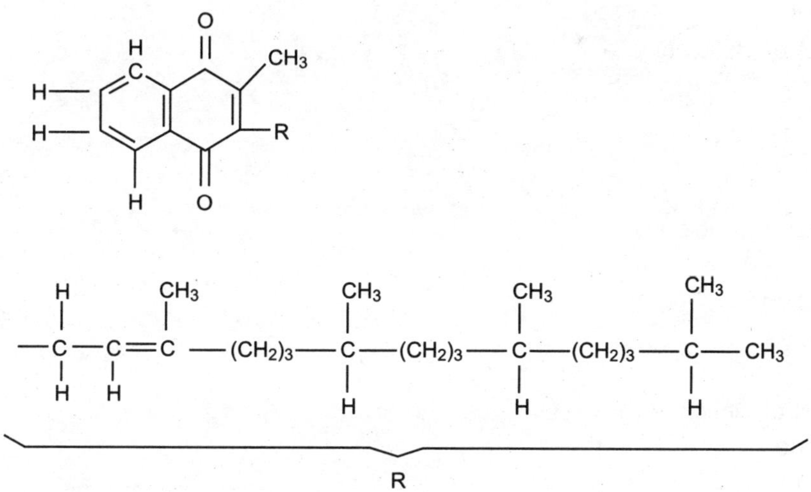

CHAPTER

9

Water-soluble Vitamins

Introduction

WATER-SOLUBLE vitamins consist of a large number of substances. These include ascorbic acid and the B-complex vitamins. The water-soluble vitamins are absorbed quickly in the body and the amounts not utilised are excreted in the urine. Adequate amounts should, therefore, be supplied in the daily diet. Some of the water-soluble vitamins are partly lost in cooking procedures. This factor has to be kept in mind while meeting their requirements.

Vitamin B-Complex

A number of substances have been identified and grouped together under this heading. It must be noted that each of the B vitamins is a separate vitamin in name, structure and function.

Six members of this group, namely, thiamin, riboflavin, niacin, pyridoxine, folic acid and vitamin B_{12} are included in the RDA, because definite requirements of these vitamins have been established through research. A diet, which provides adequate amount of these six vitamins, also, carries enough of the other members of this group. All these vitamins are essential for human nutrition. The structural formulae of the B-complex vitamins and vitamin C are given at the end of the chapter.

Thiamin

Thiamin (also known as vitamin B_1 and aneurin) was first isolated in 1926 from rice polishings by Jansen and Donath. They isolated 100 mg of crystals from 100 kg of rice polishings. Subsequently, it was synthesised in 1936 by R.R. Williams and is now available in the market in the form of thiamin hydrochloride.

The name thiamin is derived from its chemical ringlike structure. Thiamin consists of substituted pyrimidine and thiazole rings linked by a methylene bridge. It exists mainly in various inter-convertible phosphorylated forms, chiefly thiamin pyrophosphate (TPP). It is very soluble in water and is readily broken down by heat in neutral or alkaline solutions.

Functions: The basic function of thiamin as a coenzyme is related to release of energy from glucose and its storage as fat, thus it makes energy available for normal growth and function of the body. Thiamin pyrophosphate, the coenzyme form of thiamin, is necessary for catalysing the oxidation of carbohydrates in the body. This reaction releases energy in the system.

Thiamin is needed to maintain normal function of three systems in the body, gastrointestinal, nervous and cardiovascular system.

Gastrointestinal System: Thiamin helps to produce energy needed for the cells of smooth muscles and secretory glands. In its lack, there is lack of muscle tone and deficient gastric secretions; as a result there is poor appetite, indigestion, constipation and poor stomach function.

Nervous System: The central nervous system needs glucose as energy source for its function. When there is a lack of thiamin, the energy is not released and nerves are unable to work, with loss of response and alertness. The result is apathy, fatigue and irritability. If the deficit continues, nerve tissues may be damaged causing pain and finally paralysis.

Cardiovascular System: If energy supply is not continuous, due to lack of thiamin, the heart muscle weakens and may lead to heart failure. The blood vessel walls become weak, the vessels may dilate and fluid may accumulate in the lower part of legs.

Thus insufficient thiamin supply affects the body systems adversely and body function is disturbed.

Food Sources: Nearly all foods, except sugars, fats and oils, contain some thiamin. Plant sources include pulses, nuts, oilseeds and whole grain cereals. Parboiled rice and fresh peas are good sources of thiamin. Leafy green vegetables and animal foods such as milk, eggs, fish and meat are fair sources.

Most foods, however, contain **only small quantities** and it is necessary to consume a variety of foods to fulfil the daily thiamin needs. Table 9.1 gives the thiamin content of some common foods (Figure 9.1).

The main source of thiamin in the Indian dietary is cereals but refining of cereals reduces thiamin content with most of the thiamin being lost in the polishing. *Chapatis* made form whole wheat flour, when eaten as a staple, provide 50 per cent of the day's thiamin needs. The *dal* eaten with it, provides 25 per cent of the thiamin needed. Seventy-five per cent of the thiamin is lost when wheat flour is refined to manufacture *maida.* Parboiling of rice helps to conserve thiamin. Thiamin being water-soluble is also lost, when water in which cereals or pulses are cooked is discarded. Long cooking also destroys some thiamin.

Under ordinary conditions of cooking, most of the thiamin losses occur due to solution and not because of heat-inactivation. If cooking water is not discarded, most of the thiamin (85–95 per cent) is retained.

Recommended Daily Allowance

As thiamin is directly involved in energy and carbohydrate metabolism, the thiamin requirement is expressed in terms of energy intake. Hence the recommended thiamin allowance is 0.5 mg per 1000 calories for all age groups.

Table 9.1: Sources of Thiamin

Food	*Thiamin*	
	mg/100	*mg/unit**
Pulses, oilseeds and nuts (except coconut)	0.24–1.00	0.06–0.25
Cereals		
Whole	0.20–0.98	0.05–0.24
Refined	0.06–0.12	0.01–0.03
Flesh Foods		
Pork	0.54	0.27
Liver, sheep	0.36	0.18
Other flesh foods, fish, eggs	0.03–0.18	0.01–0.09
Vegetables and Fruits		
Fresh peas, beans, capsicum and seetaphal	0.25–0.55	0.12–0.27
All other vegetables and fruits	0.01–0.25	0.01–0.12
Milk	0.05	0.07

* One unit: Amount as indicated in the Daily Food Guide (Table 14.1).

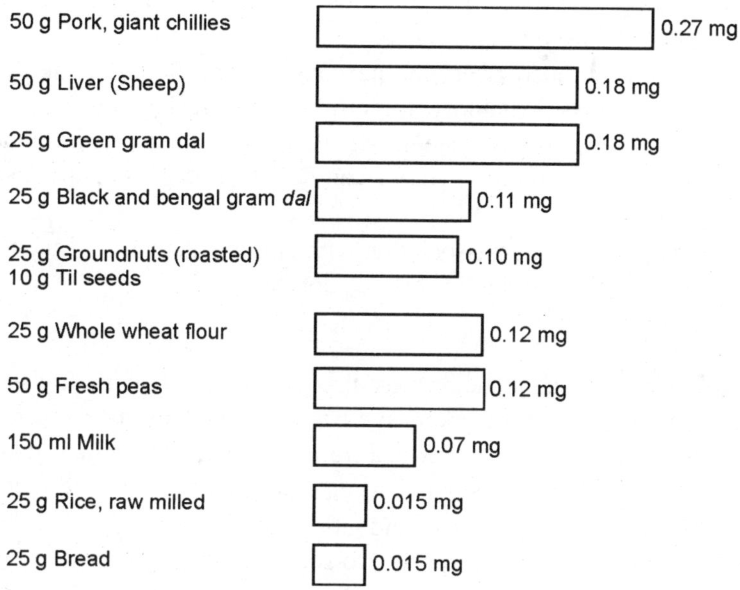

Figure 9.1: Food sources of thiamin.

Table 9.2: RDAs of Thiamin, Riboflavin & Nicotinic Acid*

Thiamin	0.5 mg/1000 kcal
Riboflavin	0.6 mg/1000 kcal
Nicotinic acid (Niacin equivalents)**	6.6 mg/1000 kcal

* Nutrient Requirements & RDAs for Indians, ICMR, 1990.

** $\text{Niacin equivalents} = \text{Niacin mg} + \dfrac{\text{Tryptophan mg}}{60}$

There are very few studies of thiamin requirements of pregnant and nursing mothers and none on the requirement of children. Hence RDA is fixed at 0.5 mg per 1000 kcal and the total intake is related to their energy allowance.

The method used to determine the RDA for thiamin combines erythrocyte transketolase activity, urinary excretion and other findings. The RDA for thiamin is given in Table 9.2.

Stability: Most of the thiamin is in the aleurone layer of the cereal grain. Using whole grain flours to make *chapatis, rotis,* ensures retention of thiamin. Thiamin is water soluble and cooking water should be retained in the recipe made to prevent loss. It is fairly stable, but is destroyed by alkalis and prolonged heat. Cooking the food to just done stage and avoiding use of soda in preparation, helps to retain most of the thiamin in the preparation.

Effect of Deficiency **:** When thiamin intake is deficient, the digestive system is disturbed resulting in loss of appetite (anorexia), poorly toned muscles and constipation. Loss of appetite may be accompanied by nausea and vomitting.

Thiamin deficiency can also affect the nervous system. Some of the symptoms observed are mental depression, moodinesss, irritability, forgetfulness, confusion and fear. Severe deficiency leads to beri-beri, a disease of the nervous system, which has been known since antiquity. The name 'beri beri' is a Singhalese word meaning 'I can't I can't', which describes the disease, as the person is always too ill to do anything.

Thiamin deficiency is found in association with chronic alcoholism, due to very low food intake and increased demand. Intake of thiamin restores normalcy.

Riboflavin

Riboflavin, a more heat-stable factor, was discovered after thiamin. It was isolated from yeast by Warburg and Christian. Kuhn and coworkers synthesised it in 1935. It was formerly known as vitamin B_2 or vitamin G. The name riboflavin is derived from its chemical structure. It is a yellow-green (Latin word 'flavus' means yellow) fluorescent pigment containing the sugar 'ribose', hence the name riboflavin.

It is less soluble in water than thiamin and more stable to heat, especially in acid solutions. When in solution, riboflavin is destroyed on exposure to sunlight.

For example, prolonged exposure of milk to direct sunlight may decrease the riboflavin content of milk considerably.

Functions: The primary form of riboflavin is as an integral part of the coenzymes flavin mononucleotide (FMN) and flavin-adenine dinucleotide (FAD). Riboflavin functions as a vital part of coenzymes in both energy production and tissue protein building.

It is thus essential for tissue health and growth of all animal and plant life (including microorganisms). It plays an important role in maintaining the integrity of mucocutaneous structures.

Food Sources: Milk is a rich source of riboflavin. So also are products derived from milk such as yoghurt (curds), butter milk, milk powder and concentrated milk (Table 9.3). There is no riboflavin in butter and ghee because the vitamin is water-soluble and remains in the water extract during the removal of butter from milk or curds.

Liver and kidney of animals and birds are also good sources of riboflavin. Pulses, green leafy vegetables, eggs, and meat contain a fair amount (Figure 9.2). Cereals, roots and fruits are poor sources of riboflavin.

Recommended Daily Allowance

The requirements of riboflavin have been determined by recording urinary excretion and the concentration of the vitamin in blood cells. In addition, riboflavin requirement is indicated by the intakes of riboflavin necessary to maintain saturated levels of the enzyme glutathione reductase in erythrocytes (EGR) (riboflavin is a co-factor of this enzyme).

Riboflavin requirement is related to total energy requirements. For practical purposes the general RDA standard is based on 0.60 mg of riboflavin per 1000 kcal for all ages. Thus the recommended allowance varies from 0.7mg for an infant to 1.7 mg for an adolescent.

The need for riboflavin increases during pregnancy and lactation and also with increased activity and caloric intake. The disease conditions, in which increased riboflavin in the diet is called for include, recovery from wasting diseases, convalescence (for rebuilding of tissues), diarrhoea and vomitting (to make up for poor absorption).

Table 9.3: Sources of Riboflavin

Food	*Riboflavin*	
	mg/100 g	*mg/unit**
Bael fruit	1.19	0.60
Liver, sheep	1.70	0.85
Dark green leafy vegetables	0.30–0.47	0.15–0.23
Milk	0.10–0.19	0.15–0.30
Pulses, whole and split	0.15–0.39	0.04–0.10
Nuts	0.19–0.97	0.05–0.24
Other flesh foods and eggs	0.09–0.44	0.04–0.22
Cereals and their products	0.03–0.29	<0.01–0.07

* One Unit: Amount as indicated in the Daily Food Guide (Table 14.1).

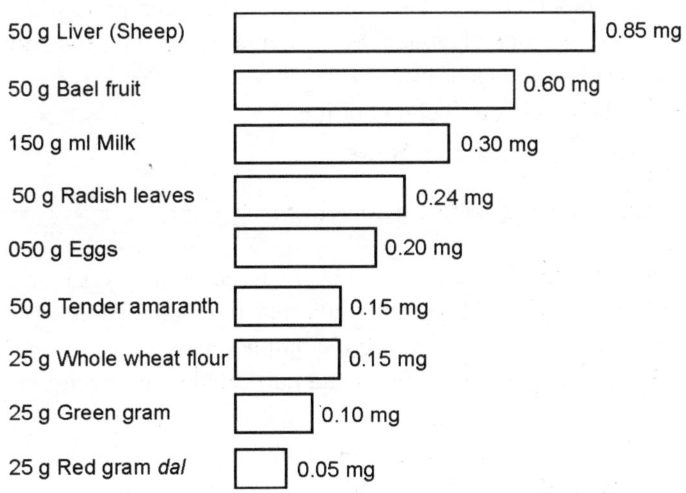

Figure 9.2: Food sources of riboflavin.

***Effect of Deficiency*:** Lack of riboflavin affects the eyes, skin and nerves. The eyelids become rough and the eye becomes sensitive to bright sunlight. This condition is called photophobia (fear of light). The skin changes are found around the area of the mouth, on the lips, tongue and nose. The lips become inflamed, cracks are observed at the corners of the mouth and the tongue is swollen, red and sore. These are clinically known as **cheilosis, angular stomatitis, naso-labial dyssebacia** and **scrotal dermititis.** The deficiency symptoms can be corrected by administering riboflavin.

Niacin

Goldberger in 1915 observed the existence of a pellagra-preventing factor, which he related to B vitamins. He found that the same factor cured black tongue in dogs. In 1937 Elvehjem and coworkers discovered that nicotinic acid was effective in curing black tongue in dogs. Smith and others found that nicotinic acid cured pellagra in humans. Thus a known substance (nicotinic acid) was identified as a vitamin. Cowgill suggested that the term 'niacin' be used for nicotinic acid to avoid association with the nicotine of tobacco.

Niacin, the term which includes both nicotinic acid and nicotinamide, is another vitamin of the B-complex group. The amide is very soluble in water and is the one preferred therapeutically because it has no side reactions. Both products are stable and are not affected by heat, acid or alkali.

***Functions*:** Niacin functions in the body as a component of two important co-enzymes NAD and NADP. The full name is nicotinamide adenine dinucleotide and its phosphate derivative respectively. These coenzymes are involved in tissue respiration and synthesis and the breakdown of glucose to produce energy. Niacin works in close association with riboflavin and thiamin in the cell metabolism system that produces energy. It is necessary for growth.

Requirements: All the factors, which affect energy needs, influence niacin requirement. Since one of the amino acids, tryptophan has been shown to be a precursor of niacin in the body, the total niacin requirement is stated in terms of 'niacin equivalents' to account for both sources. About 60 mg of tryptophan can give rise to one mg of niacin.

Table 9.4 indicates the niacin equivalents in foods.

Niacin equivalents are calculated as follows:

$$\text{Niacin equivalents mg} = \text{Niacin content in mg} + \frac{\text{Tryptophan content in mg}}{60}$$

***Sources*:** In plant foods, groundnuts are the best source of niacin. Liver, an organ meat, is a rich source of niacin (Table 9.5). But both groundnuts and liver are included in the diet occasionally. Therefore cereals, which are used as staples, are the major source of niacin in the Indian diet, and they are supplemented by pulses and meat. Unrefined and parboiled cereals retain more niacin than refined ones.

Milk, eggs, vegetables and fruits contain very small amounts of niacin. Brewer's yeast is a very concentrated source of niacin. It is sometimes added to recipes to increase niacin content of the diet. Figure 9.3 depicts the food sources of niacin.

Table 9.4: Niacin Equivalents in Foods[1,2] in 100 g Edible Portion

Food	*Niacin (a) (mg)*	*Tryptophan (b) (mg)*	*Niacin equivalents (in mg)*
Cereals			
Rice, raw, milled	1.9	87	3.3
Rico, parboiled, milled	3.8	71	5.0
Wheat, whole, flour	4.3	133	6.5
Bajra	2.3	204	5.7
Jowar (sorghum. vulgare)	3.1	116	5.0
Pulses			
Arhar or tur *dal*	2.9	143	5.3
Blackgram	2.0	269	6.5
Green gram whole	2.1	230	5.9
Lentil	2.6	241	6.6
Bengal gram, whole	2.9	137	5.2
Groundnuts	19.9	243	23.9
Vegetables			
Amaranth, tender	0.4	45	1.1
Potato	1.2	26	1.6
Milk	0.1	62	1.1
Egg	0.1	192	3.3
Pomfrets	2.6	196	5.8

1. Gopalan, C. *et al., Nutritive Value of Indian Foods,* National Institute of Nutrition/ICMR Publication, 1990.
2. Niacin equivalents are calculated as follows:

$$a+\frac{b}{60} = \text{(mg of niacin)} + \frac{\text{mg of tryptophan}}{60} = \text{mg of niacin equivalents.}$$

Table 9.5: Sources of Niacin

Food	*Niacin*	
	mg/100g	*mg/unit**
Liver, sheep	18	9
Groundnuts	20	5
Flesh foods**	3–7	<2–3
Cereals	2–5	1–2
Pulses	1–3	<1
Brewer's yeast	40	–

* One Unit: Amount as indicated in Daily Food Guide (Table 14.1)

** Includes pork, beef, mutton.

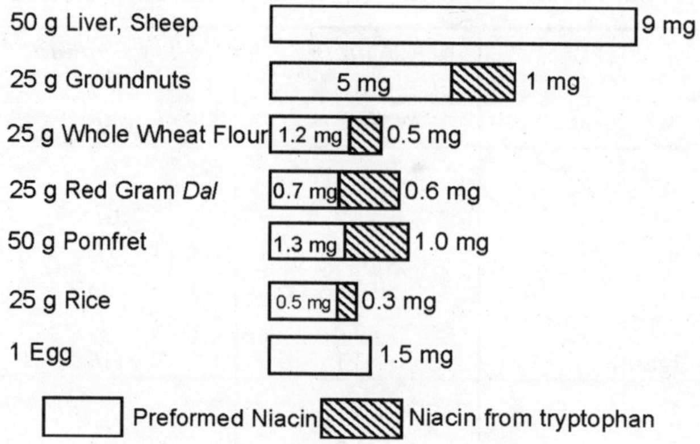

Figure 9.3: Food sources of niacin.

Recommended Dietary Allowance

Since niacin is involved in the utilisation of carbohydrates, the requirement of niacin is related to the total calories in the diet. The figure recommended is 6.6 mg per 1000 calories. The total niacin equivalent required daily on the basis of calorie requirement could range from 8 mg to 26 mg depending on the age and occupation of the individual (Table 9.2).

***Effect of Deficiency*:** Lack of niacin affects the skin, gastrointestinal tract and nervous system. The skin, especially the part exposed to the sun, itches and burns. Lack of appetite in early stages is followed by diarrhoea in later states. Nervous changes include dizziness, insomnia, irritability, fear, depression and forgetfulness; later on there may be dementia. The deficiency disease is known as **pellagra** which is seen in endemic form in some parts of India, where *jowar* (sorghum) is the staple food. Deficiency symptoms can be corrected by administering niacin.

Pyridoxine

Three naturally occurring pyridine derivatives (pyridoxine, pyridoxal and pyridoxamine) are known as vitamin B_6.

Functions: Vitamin B_6 is a co-factor for several enzymes connected with the metabolism of amino acids. It is also believed to have a role in the formation of antibodies.

Sources: Data on the vitamin B_6 contents of foods are limited. However, pulses, wheat and meat are known to be rich sources, while other cereals are fair sources. Vegetables and fruits are relatively poor sources.

Requirements: There is some evidence that the pyridoxine requirements may be related to protein intake. The average requirement for adults would appear to be about 1.5 mg per day. Cooking losses in normal Indian diets are negligible; hence no allowances for losses need be made.

The suggested daily intake varies from 0.4 mg for infants to 2.0 mg for adults and 2.5 mg for expectant and nursing mothers (Table 9.6).

Deficiency: The symptoms of vitamin B_6 deficiency—such as peripheral neuritis, anaemia, glossitis, cheilosis and seborrhic dermatitis are similar to those of other B vitamins. Hence the extent of pyridoxine deficiency in India is not known.

Table 9.6: Suggested Daily Intake of Pyridoxine, Folate, Vitamin B_{12} and Ascorbic Acid

		Pyridoxine mg	*Folate* µg	*Vitamin B_{12}* µg	*Ascorbic acid mg*
Adult man and woman		2.0	100	1	40
Pregnant woman		2.5	400	1	40
Lactating woman		2.5	150	1.5	80
Infant:	0–6 months	0.3	25	0.2	25
	6–12 months	0.4			
Preschool children	1–3 years	0.9	40	0.2 to 1.0	40
	4–6 years		50		
School children	7–9 years	1.6	60		
	10–12 years		70		
Adolescents	13–15 years	2.0	100		
	16–18 years		100		

Folic Acid

Folic acid and related compounds, which is one of the B vitamins, was discovered in 1941, as a growth factor for bacteria. It was found to be essential for all vertebrates including man. Its name was derived from the Latin word *folium,* which means leaf, because it was first isolated from spinach leaves and is widely distributed in green, leafy plants.

Folic acid is pteroyl-mono-glutamic acid. It is quite soluble in slightly alkaline or acid solution; but is reasonably stable in neutral or alkaline solutions, especially in the absence of air.

Functions: The primary function of folic acid is related to the transfer of single carbon in the synthesis of a number of metabolites in the body. It is also involved in the synthesis of nucleic acid along with vitamin B_{12}. Folic acid undergoes a series of metabolic conversions to its various coenzyme forms after it is absorbed.

Sources: It is widely distributed in foods. Green leafy vegetables, liver, legumes and yeast are rich sources of folic acid. It is a relatively stable vitamin but storage and cooking losses can be as high as 50 per cent, especially if cooking water is discarded.

Suggested Daily Intake: The safe level of folate intake would be 100 mcg per day for adults and adolescents with 25 mcg in infancy increasing to 40 mcg at pre-school stage, gradually increasing with age to 100 mcg of folates at adolescence (Table 9.6).

It was observed in one study that the birth weights of infants, born to mothers who had taken 300 mcg folate per day during pregnancy, were higher than those born to mothers who had received 100 or 200 mcg daily. Hence the ICMR suggested intake in pregnancy is 300 mcg of additional folic acid daily. The additional needs may be met through folate supplements, as it may be difficult to provide it in the diet. Nursing mothers need additional 50 mcg of folic acid.

Deficiency: Prolonged and severe folic acid deficiency leads to abnormal formation of red blood cells resulting in megaloblastic anaemia. It responds to administration of folic acid.

Vitamin B_{12}

Vitamin B_{12} or cyanocobalamin was the last member of the B vitamins discovered in 1948. It contains cobalt and phosphorus and is red in colour. It is found only in animal foods and higher plants are unable to synthesise it.

Cyanocobalamin is considered the most potent vitamin and is one of the last true vitamins that has been classified. It was discovered through studies of pernicious anaemia, a condition that begins with a megaloblastic anaemia and leads to an irreversible degeneration of the central nervous system. It was found that the condition could be reversed by feeding afflicted patients large amounts of raw liver. The active material in the liver was found to be vitamin B_{12}, which is present only in very small amount. Suggested intakes are given in Table 9.6.

Cyanocobalamin contains a tetrapyrrole ring system, which is chemically very similar to the porphyrin ring system of the haeme compounds.

Functions: It promotes normal growth and development. It helps with certain types of nerve damage, and treats pernicious anaemia. It is an essential component of several coenzymes, which are needed in the synthesis of nucleic acids. Its metabolism and use in the body is closely related to folic acid. It is essential for the normal functioning of all cells, especially those of bone marrow, the nervous system and the gastrointestinal tract.

Sources: The richest sources are liver, and organ meats. Milk, eggs, muscle meat and fish are good sources. Plant foods do not contain vitamin B_{12}. It is not stable to heat and light; hence processed foods are not good sources. For example, there is 10 per cent loss in pasteurisation and 40 to 90 per cent loss in evaporation of milk.

Deficiency: Uncomplicated deficiency is characterised by symptoms such as sore tongue, weakness, loss of weight, tingling of extremities, apathy, mental and other nervous abnormalities. When there is a lack of intrinsic factor, essential for the absorption for the vitamin, pernicious anaemia results, in which there is degeneration of the spinal cord. There is a low level of vitamin B_{12} in the blood and an inability of new RBCs to develop normally resulting in megaloblastic anaemia. The condition can be cured by injecting vitamin B_{12}-intramuscularly.

Ascorbic Acid (Vitamin C)

Ascorbic acid (vitamin C) was isolated and its chemical structure elucidated in 1932 by C.G. King. Its lack in human diet has long been known to cause a disease called scurvy. In olden days, sailors to whom fresh fruits and vegetables were not available for many days during long voyages at sea developed this disease. It is reported that 100 out of the 180 men who sailed with Vasco da Gama, died of scurvy before they reached India in 1498.

Ascorbic acid closely resembles glucose in structure. The vitamin is a white, crystalline, odourless compound readily soluble in water. It is a strong reducing agent. It is comparatively stable in an acid medium but is destroyed by the action of heat, oxygen and catalysts such as copper.

It is now made synthetically and the synthetic product is relatively inexpensive.

Functions: Ascorbic acid performs a number of important functions in the body. It is a part of the cementing material which hold the body cells firmly in place. Thus it plays an important role to build and maintain strong tissues in general, especially connective tissues (bone, cartilage, dentin, collagen, etc). Blood vessel tissue depends on vitamin C to form strong capillary walls.

Vitamin C is an important partner of protein for tissue synthesis. Naturally it is needed in growth stages of life. High concentrations of vitamin C are found in metabolically active tissues in the body, indicating its importance in their function. These include brain, liver, kidney, pancreas, adrenal glands, thymus and spleen.

It helps the body to build resistance to infection. It helps in the absorption of calcium and ensures the health of bones. By aiding absorption of iron, it makes it available for haemoglobin synthesis. It is needed in wound healing, infections and fever to help recovery.

Being a strong reducing agent, it helps to tie up free radicals and thus protects the body from their deleterious effects.

Sources: Amla (nellikai, also called Indian gooseberry) is one of the richest sources of ascorbic acid, which contains 600 mg/100 g of the fruit. Guavas and cashew apples contain 200 to 300 mg/ 100 g. Citrus fruits such as oranges, sweet lime, grape-fruit and pomelo are also excellent sources of ascorbic acid. Drumsticks also have a high ascorbic acid content (Table 9.7).

Leafy vegetables such as drumstick leaves, amaranth, cabbage, which are more frequently available, are excellent sources of vitamin C (Figs. 9.4 & 9.5).

Sprouted pulses such as Bengal gram and green gram are good sources and have proved to be of value during drought and famine conditions when other sources of ascorbic acid, such as fresh fruits and vegetables are not available.

Stability: Vitamin C is a labile nutrient. It oxidises easily on exposure to air and heat. It is stable in acid medium, so acid fruits (citrus) and vegetables (e.g., tomato) retain their vitamin C content. It is soluble in water and hence cooking water must be utilised to prevent loss. It is not stable in alkaline pH, so soda should not be added in food preparation to prevent loss.

Table 9.7: Sources of Vitamin C

Fruits	*Vit. C mg/100g*	*Vegetables*	*Vit.C mg/100 g*
Amla	600	Drumstick leaves	220
Guava	210–310	Capsicum	137
Cashew fruit	180–210	Drumstick	120
Orange juice	64	Bitter gourd	88
Limes	63	Knol-khol	85
Papaya	57	Radish leaves	81
Mausambi	50	Cabbage	55
Lemon, sweet	45	Methi leaves	52
Pineapple	39	Cluster beans	49
Plantain	20	Tomato, ripe	27
Mango	16	Potato	17
Bananas, Sapota	7	Other beans	25
Apples, Grapes	1		

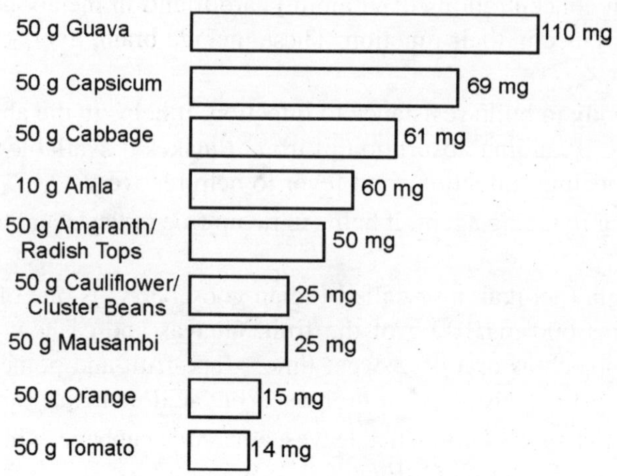

Figure 9.4: Food sources of vitamin C.

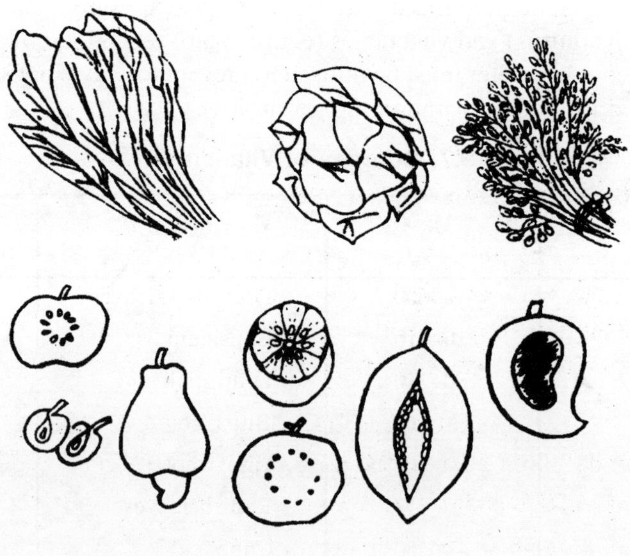

Figure 9.5: Fruit and vegetable sources of vit. C.

***Recommended Dietary Allowance*:** Ascorbic acid cannot be stored in the body. The requirement has to be supplied daily. Even if excess is ingested, it is excreted in the urine. The recommended daily allowance increases with age from 20 to 40 mg for children and is 40 mg per day for adult. An intake of 80 mg per day is recommended for a nursing mother. The amount recommended is liberal, as ascorbic acid is a very labile nutrient (Table 9.6).

***Deficiency*:** If ascorbic acid is not present in sufficient quantity, the cementing material is not formed in adequate amounts. Tiny breaks occur in the walls of very small blood vessels and haemorrhages result. The tissues of the gums become tender and often bleed. In severe cases, soft tissues around the joints become swollen and are painful. There is general weakness, lack of appetite and thickened and scaly skin. Spongy gums and haemorrhages in body tissues are other symptoms of scurvy; these can be reversed by including ascorbic acid rich foods in the diet.

Study Questions

1. List the requirements of the following nutrients:
   (*i*) Thiamin
   (*ii*) Riboflavin
   (*iii*) Niacin.
   Do these vary with age? Why?
2. List the main sources of
   (*a*) Thiamin
   (*b*) Riboflavin
   (*c*) Niacin.
3. Describe the symptoms of deficiency of
   (*a*) Thiamin
   (*b*) Riboflavin
   (*c*) Niacin.
4. Discuss the functions of pyridoxine, folic acid and cyanocobalamin in the body.
5. Discuss the functions of vitamin C.
6. What are the sources of vitamin C?
7. Describe the symptoms of vitamin C deficiency.

Structures of Water-Soluble Vitamins

Ascorbic Acid (Vit C)

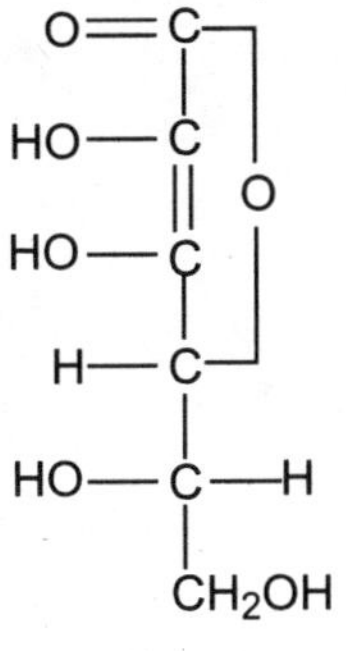

Riboflavin

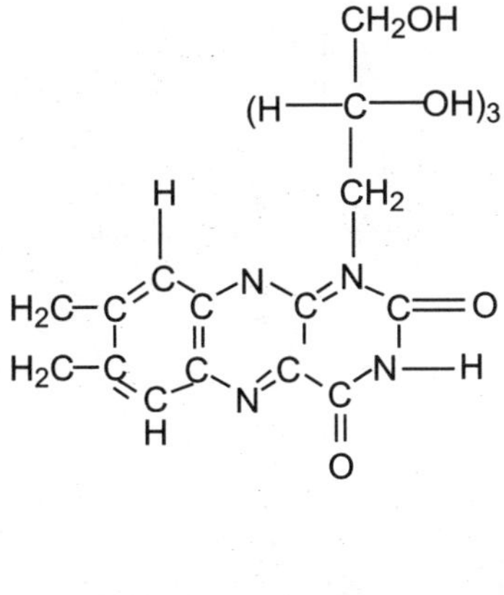

Thiamin Vitamin B_1

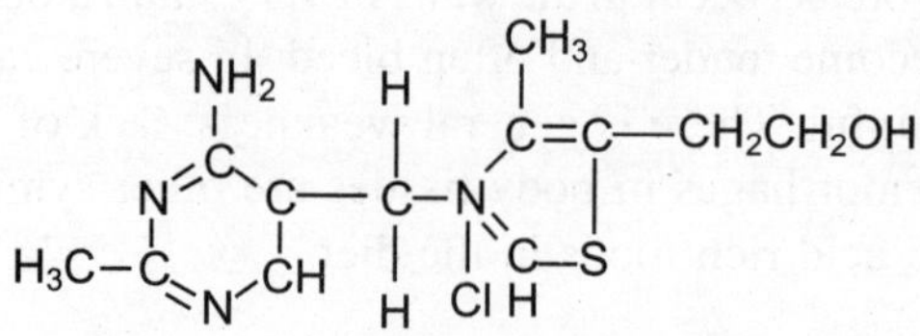

Niacin Group

Nicotinic Acid

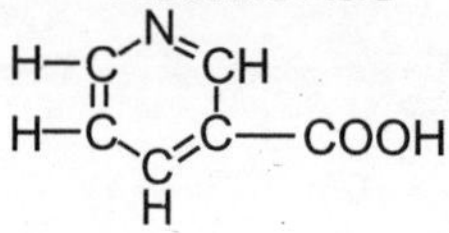

Nicotinamide

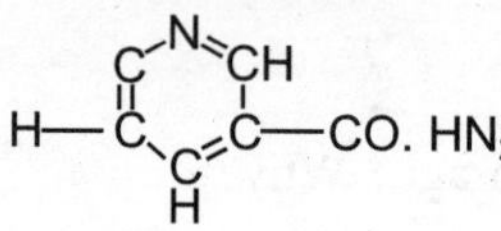

Vit B_6 Group

Pyridoxine

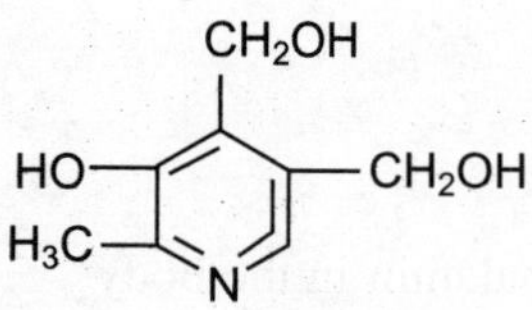

Pyridoxal

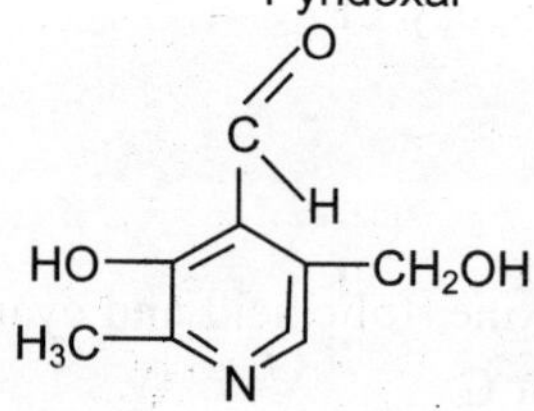

Pyridoxamine

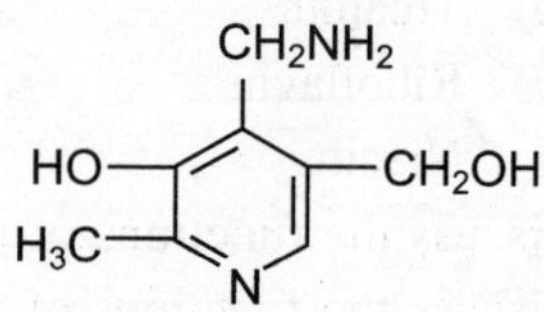

Pantothenic Acid

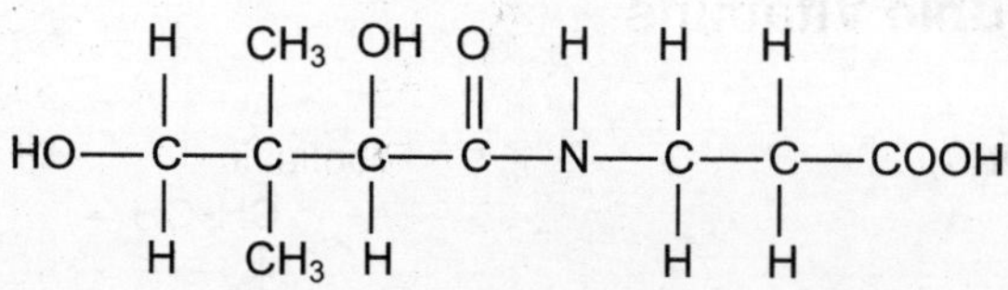

Folacin
(represented by monopteroylglutamic acid)

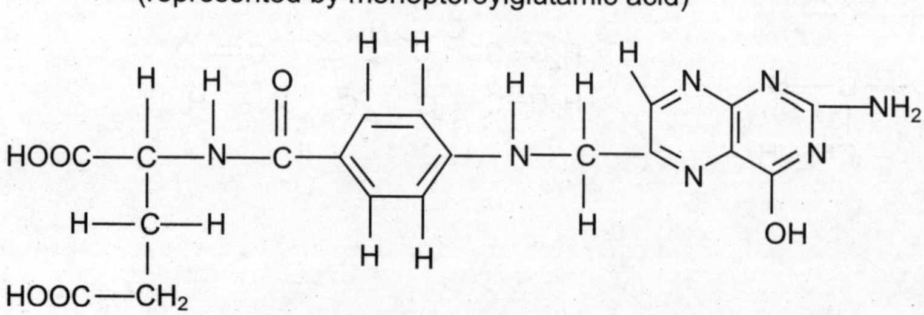

Biotin

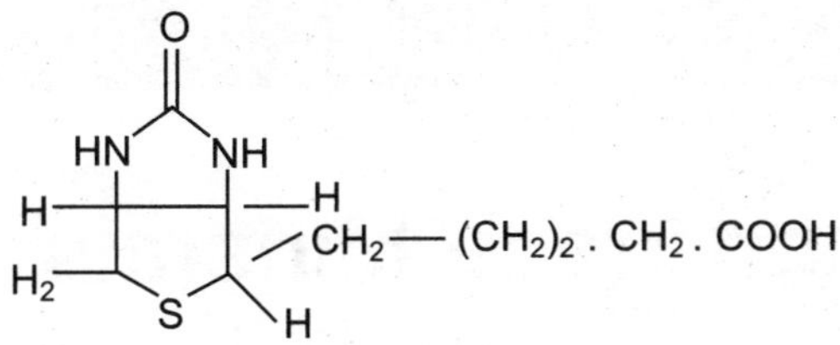

Vitamin B_{12}
(represented by cyanocobalamin)

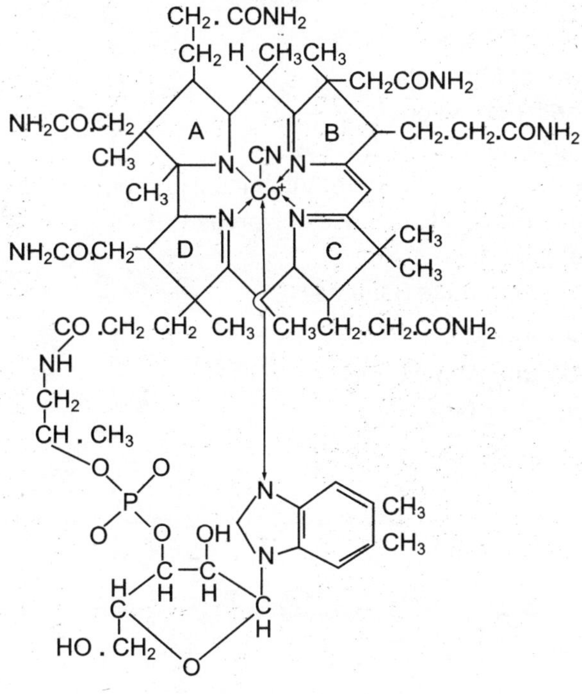

Choline

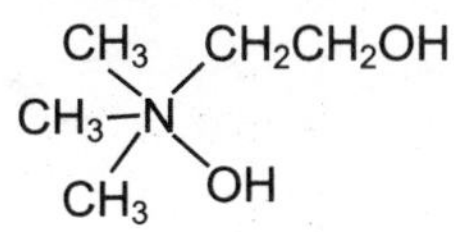

CHAPTER

10

Major and Trace Minerals

Introduction

The importance of minerals in our well-being is emphasised by the fact that iron deficiency anemia is one of the three major health problems in India.

The increase in the number of fractures in the elderly as also the incidence of high blood pressure are also pointers that focus one's attention on minerals, calcium and sodium. A liberal inake of calcium, with increased mobility and exposure to sunlight is known to improve the strength of bones and thus reduce their fragility. A reduction in sodium intake can be one of the helpful factors in reducing hypertension. Though advertisements for dietary supplements may lead you to believe that these may be the answer to the problem, it is not so. The key is to select foods to meet the body's mineral needs and to season foods moderately to avoid excess intake of salt.

Nature and Composition

As you may know from your elementary chemistry course, minerals are inorganic substances. So far we have studied nutrients, (carbohydrates, fats, proteins and vitamins), which are organic compounds.

Minerals are present in all body tissues and fluids. In bones and teeth the minerals calcium and phosphorus are deposited in protein material. Iron is found in blood as a part of the red pigment, haemoglobin. Minerals occur in foods as salts and also in combination with organic substances.

Minerals have two distinct characteristics

- Mineral elements do not provide energy.
- Mineral elements are not destroyed during food preparation.

The mineral elements found in the body form only **4 to 6 per cent** of the weight of our adult body. This means that about 2 to 3 kg of our body weight consists of minerals. Of this 90 per cent is accounted for by seven minerals (calcium, phosphorus, potassium, sulphur, sodium, chloride and magnesium). The other minerals are known as **trace elements,** as these add together to about 10 per cent of the total mineral content of the body. The mineral composition of the adult body is given in Table 10.1.

The largest concentration of minerals is found in the bones and teeth. Minerals are also found in soft tissues such as nerves and muscles and in blood and other body fluids.

General Functions of Minerals

Some minerals play an important role in the regulation of body functions. These are:

1. Maintenance of acid-base balance.
2. Control of water balance.
3. Contraction of muscles.
4. Normal response of nerves to physiological stimulation.
5. Clotting of blood.

Minerals do not act singly in their function and regulation of body processes, but work with the help of other minerals and organic compounds. A certain concentration of each element must be present for efficient functioning of the body.

Table 10.1: Mineral Composition of Adult Human Body[1]

Mineral	*Approximate amount in adult body*	
	60 kg	*50 kg*
Major Mineral Elements		
Calcium	1030 g	855 g
Phosphorus	645 g	535 g
Potassium	210 g	175 g
Sulfur	150 g	125 g
Sodium	90 g	75 g
Chlorine	90 g	75 g
Magnesium	26 g	21 g
Trace Elements		
Iron	3.4 g	2.9 g
Molybdenum	2.6 g	2.1 g
Zinc	1.7 g	1.4 g
Selenium	1.7 g	1.4 g
Fluorine	0.9 g	0.75 g
Copper	130 mg	110 mg
Manganese	130 mg	110 mg
Iodine	26 mg	21 mg
Cobalt	4 mg	3.6 mg
Chromium	4 mg	3.6 mg

1. Based on Robinson *et al., Basic Nutrition & Diet Therapy,* 7th edn., p. 151, 1993.

Some of the important tissue formations and processes in which mineral elements function in unison are discussed below. This will be followed by a discussion of each important mineral element and its specific functions.

Bones and Teeth Formation: Most of the calcium, phosphorus and magnesium and small amounts of other mineral elements are deposited in the bones and teeth. Bones and teeth are formed of tough protein material into which minerals are deposited. Most of the bone formation (ossification) in the foetus occurs in the eighth and ninth months of pregnancy. At birth, the bones are very soft, but the infant has a well formed skeleton. Throughout the growth phases (childhood, adolescence and early adulthood) the bones become long, thick and increase in hardness.

Thus bones form an important part of the body framework. Bones also serve as a reservoir of the component mineral elements. Thus the blood levels of these minerals are maintained by withdrawal of these elements from the bone. The minerals provided in the diet replace those withdrawn and thus help to maintain the bone structure. Thus even in bones, there is a continuous process of maintenance and repair of the tissue.

In the foetus, the first teeth are formed from fourth to sixth week of pregnancy. By the twentieth week, these teeth calcify. These are milk teeth and their formation is known as **primary dentition.**

Soon after birth up to about third birthday, the permanent teeth are formed, while wisdom teeth are formed between the eighth and tenth year. Before the teeth erupt, they are fully formed. Tooth enamel and dentine contain an appreciable quantities of calcium and phosphorus. These are protective layers of the teeth. As these parts do not contain blood vessels, a decayed tooth cannot repair itself. Hence the only way to ensure the health of teeth is to take care of the teeth and prevent decay.

Structural Components of Soft Tissues: Many mineral elements are found in the structural components of soft tissues. These include potassium, sulphur, phosphorus, iron and others.

As Components and Co-factors of Vitamins, Hormones and Enzymes: Various regulatory compounds contain very small amounts of mineral elements as constituents. For example, sulphur is part of many important compounds such as thiamin (a B vitamin) and coenzyme A. Vitamin B_{12} contains cobalt; the enzyme carbonic anhydrase contains zinc and the hormone thyroxine contains iodine. Calcium, as an activator, is a co-factor in the action of pancreatic lipase. Incorporation of iron into haemoglobin needs copper, while the synthesis of insulin in the pancreas needs zinc.

Muscle Contraction and Response of Nerves are regulated by the mineral elements (sodium, potassium, calcium and magnesium), present in body fluids in definite amounts. These elements regulate the movement of materials through the cell membrane. Normal response of nerves to physiological stimuli are also regulated by these mineral elements.

Control of Water Balance: Sodium and potassium are responsible for the control of water balance between the inside and outside of cells. This function is dependent on the correct concentrations of sodium and potassium. Potassium is mainly found in the fluid inside the cell, while sodium is chiefly found in the fluid outside the cell.

Maintenance of Acid-Base Balance: It is very important to maintain a constant pH in the body fluids at all times to ensure normal function of our body.

The mineral elements are responsible for the maintenance of acid-base balance. The pH of the body fluids is maintained between a narrow range of 7.35 and 7.45. This function of mineral elements in maintaining acid-base balance is discussed in detail in Chapter 11.

Dynamic Equilibrium

As in the case of other nutrients, there is a continuous turnover of minerals in body tissues; they take up minerals, synthesise new compounds and discharge waste matter. However, the healthy body maintains a very fine balance in all these processes, which is known as **dynamic equilibrium.** The levels of these minerals are regulated by hormones.

There are several ways by which this balance is maintained. One way is to release the mineral from stores in the liver and bones; the second way is to control the absorption of the nutrient according to the amount needed by the body and a third mechanism of control is to excrete the excess through the kidney. The blood levels of these minerals are regulated by hormones.

Recommended Dietary Allowances

The recommended dietary allowance (RDA) for each mineral element for the adult is given later. The allowances for growth stages of life are higher per unit body weight than the adult stage. Unlike the major nutrients (carbohydrates, fats and proteins) which have high bioavailability (about 90 per cent), mineral elements vary a lot in the percentage that is absorbed from the diet. Thus iron absorption may be as low as 5 per cent; calcium 20 per cent, while sodium is absorbed almost completely.

Absorption of mineral elements is favoured by

(*a*) **Body requirement:** If the body needs are high, as in pregnancy and growth stage of children, there is higher absorption of calcium and iron (up to 60 per cent) from the diet.

(*b*) **Stomach acidity:** Absorption of several minerals, for example, calcium and iron is improved by the presence of acid conditions. Thus absorption of calcium in the intestinal tract is enhanced by lactose, which is hydrolysed to lactic acid. The absorption of calcium, iron and zinc is improved by ascorbic acid.

(*c*) **Form in which the mineral is present in the food**: Haeme iron in animal foods is more easily absorbed in the body than iron compounds present in plant foods.

Absorption of mineral elements is reduced by

(*a*) Dietary components, which combine with mineral elements to form insoluble complexes, reduce their absorption. These components include oxalic acid, phytic acid, excess fibre and others. Minerals are also bound by some medications.

(*b*) The absorption of some minerals is adversely affected by an excessive intake of other minerals. Such a situation arises when supplements of minerals are taken. For example, intake of iron supplements hinders the absorption of zinc, while zinc supplements reduce the absorption of copper.

(*c*) Increased mobility of intestinal track due to diarrhoea, intake of laxatives, etc., reduces the time of absorption and hence the amount absorbed.

(*d*) Parasites present in the intestinal tract also interfere with the absorption of minerals. Iron deficiency anaemia in children is attributed to this factor.

Toxicity

The possibility of toxicity due to excessive intake of mineral elements from normal natural foods is **very remote.**

Excessive intake, which can be toxic, is possible only when —

(*a*) Iron pills or other nutritional supplements are taken in excess

(*b*) errors are made in substituting supplements

(*c*) Exposures to toxic levels of chemicals in an industrial plant.

(*d*) Children consume excessive number of iron pills accidentally.

Even common salt used in the kitchen can be toxic, if fed by mistake in excess to infants.

Major Minerals

Calcium

Body Composition and Functions: Bones and teeth contain about 99 per cent of calcium in the body, in combination with phosphorus, protein and other minerals. These give the skeleton structure and rigidity. In the long bones, the calcium and phosphorus is stored mainly in the ends (trabeculae), from where it can be easily taken to maintain blood calcium levels.

The remaining 1 per cent of calcium is present in the soft tissue and blood and is responsible for many regulatory functions. These functions, which it carries out along with other minerals, are:

- It is involved in normal muscle contraction, which includes heartbeat.
- Control of the transmission of nerve impulses.
- Maintenance of permeability of cell membranes to permit movement of material in and out of the cells.
- Help normal clotting of blood.
- Activate action of enzymes, e.g., pancreatic lipase as a cofactor.
- Ensure the absorption of vitamin B_{12}.

Food Sources: The best source of calcium is milk. Infants receive an excellent supply of calcium from their mother's milk. The milk of cows, buffaloes and goats is rich in calcium. The calcium in milk is accompanied by a favourable proportion of phosphorus, hence, it is very well utilised in the body. Milk products such as curd, *paneer, mava,* SMP, are good sources of calcium.

The millet *ragi* and seasame seeds (*til*) have a high concentration of calcium. Green leafy vegetables are a good source of calcium, though only a part of the calcium from these is available to the body.

Fresh as well as dried fish, especially small fresh fish, if the bones are also eaten, provide substantial quantities of calcium in the diet.

Besides these, some spices such as cumin seeds (*jeera*), coriander seeds (*dhaniya*), contain enough calcium to make a contribution, if these are used frequently in sufficient quantity, in the diet. The food sources of calcium are presented in Table 10.2.

Utilisation of Calcium

Most of the utilisation of calcium occurs from the small intestine (duodenum and jejunum) as calcium salts are more soluble in the acid medium there. As mentioned earlier, other factors which favour the utilisation of calcium are presence of vitamin D, ascorbic acid and lactose. More efficient utilisation occurs in periods of rapid growth, such as pregnancy and childhood.

The presence of substances which form insoluble salts of calcium, e.g., oxalic acid (in leafy vegetable), phytic acid (in cereal bran) and excess of fat in the diet, may hinder calcium utilisation. Excess of fibre in the digestive tract may increase faecal excretion of calcium, thus reducing utilisation.

Depending on the body's need, 10 to 40 per cent of calcium from the diet is absorbed. The level of calcium in the blood is maintained at a constant level, irrespective of the dietary intake, by the action of hormones. Parathyroid hormone stimulates the kidney to alter vitamin D to its active form vitamin D_3 hormone, when the blood level of calcium is lower than normal. Vitamin D_3 hormone raises the blood calcium level by increasing its absorption, drawing it from bones and decreasing its excretion by the kidney. Calcitonin (another hormone) inhibits release from the bone and thus ensures normalcy.

The excretion of calcium is increased on a high protein diet. If such a diet is low in calcium, it may lead to negative calcium balance.

Table 10.2: Food Sources of Calcium

Foods	*Calcium mg/100g*	*Foods*	*Calcium mg/100g*
Milk & Milk Products		*Green Leafy Vegetables*	
Cow's milk	120	Agathi	1130
Buffalo milk	210	Amaranth (*math*)	397
Cheese	790	Fenugreek (*methi*)	395
Khoya (*mava*)	956	Rape leaves	370
Skim milk powder (SMP)	1370	*Fish & Sea Foods*	
Cereals & Millets		Hilsa	180
Ragi (*nachani*)	344	Rohu	650
Amaranth seeds	510	Dry fish	500–6000
Rajgira seeds	223	*Nuts & Oilseeds*	
Pulses & Legumes		Gingelly seeds (*til*)	1450
Bengal gram whole	202	Mustard seeds (*rai*)	490
Horse gram (*matki*)	287	Cumin seeds (*jeera*)	1040
Rajmah	260	Poppy seeds	1584
Green gram (*mung*)	124	Coriander seeds (*dhania*)	630

Recommended Dietary Allowances

Calcium (Ca) requirement has been measured by long-term balance studies. Such studies among Western population, whose habitual diet contains high levels of calcium from milk, have indicated a requirement of Ca of the order of 1 g. However population groups in many developing countries live on an intake of about 500 mg without any ill effects. Long-term balance studies in such population indicate that they are in positive Ca balance even on much lower intakes. This is due to the ability of the body to adapt to different levels of intakes of Ca and maintain a positive balance. On the basis of these studies the earlier RDAs for Ca were suggested, which had given a range of intakes, as was also recommended by FAO/WHO.

In the 1989 revision, the evidence for Ca nutrition status of Indian population was examined, and it was suggested that the earlier RDA be retained. Instead of a range, a single figure for each group is suggested as shown in Table 10.3.

It may be noted that during periods of high demand such as pregnancy and lactation, more calcium intake is recommended.

The desirable intake of phosphorus was considered. Since phosphorus deficiency is unlikely in the types of diets consumed in India, adequate intake of phosphorus may not be a problem. It was suggested that a Ca: P ratio of 1 : 1 may be maintained in most age groups, except in infancy where the ratio suggested is 1 : 1.5.

Effect of Deficiency: Deficiency of calcium manifests itself, only after years of insufficient intake. When sufficient calcium is not supplied, pregnant women lose calcium from their body tissues to supply the needs of the foetus. Similarly nursing mothers lose calcium and phosphorus for the formation of milk.

Table 10.3: A RDAs of Calcium and Phosphorus (mg/day)

Group		*Calcium*	*Phosphorus*
Adult Men		400	400
Adult Women		400	400
Pregnancy and lactation		1000	1000
Infants		500	750
Children	1–9 years	400	400
	10–15 years	600	600
	16–18 years	500	500

If adequate calcium is not provided in the diet, during pregnancy and lactation, the bones of the women get porous (**osteoporosis**). A large percentage of Indian women, especially form the low income strata, suffer from osteoporosis. In later years of life, these women suffer from loss of stature, bent backs, high susceptibility to fractures of hip and wrist. These conditions, are due to loss of bone mass, which results in bending, and compression of vertebrae.

In children lack of calcium affects their growth adversely. The skeletal frame does not mineralise properly, resulting in weak bones, which are unable to support the weight of the body. Rickets, which is a manifestation of vitamin D and/or calcium deficiency, is characterised by bowed legs, enlarged joints, beaded rib joints and other deformities. The teeth are also affected in calcium deficiency and the blood does not clot normally.

Osteoporosis is a complex ailment. The factors, which contribute to weakening of the bone structure, especially of senior citizen are:

- Changes in lifestyle, leading to reduced movement,
- Lack of weight bearing exercise,
- as also poor absorption of calcium and phosphorus due to staying indoors (lack of vitamin D synthesis).

The best way to prevent osteoporosis is to maintain adequate calcium intake, physical activity to reduce loss of bone mass with age and exposure to sunlight to ensure vitamin D synthesis to aid calcium absorption.

Phosphorus

Body Composition and Functions: Bones and teeth contain 85 per cent of the phosphorus in the body. The remaining 15 per cent is found in various compounds, which contribute to body function and regulation. Thus functions of phosphorus are:

- Body building as an important component of bones and teeth.
- Fat absorption and transport with aid of coenzyme A and ATP.
- As a part of DNA (deoxyribonucleic acid) and RNA (ribonucleic acid), which are essential for genetic coding and protein synthesis.
- As a part of ATP (adenosine triphosphate) and ADP (adenosine diphosphate), which are essential for energy metabolism in the body.
- As a component of enzymes needed in carbohydrate, fat and protein metabolism.
- As a part of buffer salts, which maintain acid-base balance in the body.

Food Sources: The diet which meets the body's needs for calcium and proteins will also meet the body's needs of phosphorus. Rich sources of phosphorus include milk, eggs, flesh foods, legumes and nuts. Many processed foods and soft drinks have added phosphates.

Magnesium

Body composition and functions: Bones and teeth contain 60 per cent of the magnesium in the body.

Besides body building, magnesium has three other important regulatory functions. Along with other minerals, it regulates muscle contraction, regulation of the transmission of nerve stimuli and activates the function of many enzymes involved in metabolism.

Like calcium, magnesium is absorbed in an acid medium in the gastrointestinal tract. in fact, they compete for carrier sites in this process. It is important not to have an excess intake of these elements to avoid competition in absorption.

Food Sources: Green leafy vegetables are a rich source of magnesium, as magnesium is a constituent of chlorophyll. Plant foods are also rich in magnesium.

As no deficiency of magnesium is likely to occur in the Indian population, no specific recommendations are made for its dietary intake.

Trace Elements

Iron

Functions: Though the amount of iron in the body is only about two to three grammes, its presence is very important. Iron combines with protein for the development of haemoglobin, the red pigment of the blood. The main function of iron in haeme is to carry oxygen from the lungs to the cells and to carry back some of the carbon dioxide formed, to the lungs for exhalation.

Iron is also an essential constituent of many tissues (muscles) and of the catalysts which regulate oxidation-reduction reactions in the body.

Iron is stored in the liver, spleen and bone marrow in the form of the protein **ferritin.** Men have higher stores of ferritin than women.

Food Sources: Eggs, liver and meat contain iron in a readily available form. Among the plant foods, leafy vegetables, cereals such as whole wheat flour, rice flakes, an Italian millet, are good sources of iron. Pulses, split and whole, treenuts, *bajra,* ragi, *jowar* and parboiled rice are also good sources of iron. Table 10.4 gives the sources of iron.

Table 10.4: Sources of Iron

Food	*Iron mg/unit*[1]	*Iron mg/100g E.P.*
Leafy vegetables, dark green	2–30	5–60
Italian millet, rice flakes, whole wheat flour	25	10–20
Rice, *jowar, bajra,* ragi	1–1.5	3–6
Pulses and treenuts	1–2	5–10
Flesh foods (liver, meat), eggs	1	2–6
Other Vegetables	1	2–5
Fruits	1	1–3

1. Unit as indicated in Table 14.1.

As mentioned before, the availability of dietary iron in the body is promoted if it is in a soluble form. Acidity favours iron absorption by dissolving the iron present. The presence of ascorbic acid helps iron absorption. A high cereal diet, which has high phytate, low calcium and low ascorbic acid, tends to make much of the iron present unavailable to the body.

Utilisation of Iron: Iron needs of the body are met by –

- Use of iron released from red blood corpuscles (RBCs) over and over again.
- Absorption of iron from the diet.
- Use of the stores of ferritin.

Absorption of iron from food takes place mostly in the duodenum and the small intestine. Only 3 to 10 per cent of iron is absorbed by a well nourished adult. Higher percentage is absorbed in growth stages and by anaemic persons when need of the body is high. If the body has an immediate need for iron, it passes directly from the intestine into the blood stream. If the supply of iron is more than what the body needs, it is stored in the mucosa of the intestinal cells as ferritin. Ferritin is made up of a protein and an iron containing compound.

Diet directly supplies only about *one mg* of iron as compared to the reutilisation of iron from the breakdown products of hemoglobin which supplies 25 mg. Since most of the iron produced from the breakdown of iron compounds in the body is reutilised, iron is known as **one way element.**

Recommended Dietary Allowances

The Recommended Dietary Allowances for iron is presented in Table 10.5. It can be seen that the amount of iron needed is greater during pregnancy than any other stage of life. It helps the foetus to store iron, which last for the first few months after birth. Infants after six months of age, girls and women, who lose blood in menstruation, need more iron than boys and men of the same age. Persons, who have suffered blood loss, because of blood donation, surgery or accident, also need more iron in the dietary than their normal intake.

Mechanism for maintenance of iron balance

The body has three mechanisms for maintenance of iron balance, which prevent iron deficiency:

1. The catabolized red cells in the body are continuously reutilized.
2. The absorption of iron from the intestines is regulated according to the iron status of the body; thus there is increased iron absorption, if there is iron deficiency and a decreased absorption, if there is an iron overload.
3. The storage protein ferritin acts as a 'bank account' for iron in the body; thus the storage protein ferritin releases iron to meet excessive demands, as in the last trimester of pregnancy.

Deficiency: Iron deficiency anaemia is quite widespread in India, the prevalence varying from 45 per cent in male adults to 70 per cent in women and children. While the main etiological factor is dietary iron deficiency, folate deficiency also contributes to anaemia among young children and pregnant women.

The lack of iron results in anaemia due to insufficiency of haemoglobin, the iron containing pigment in the blood. Persons lacking iron get tired easily, feel faint due to inability of the body to carry sufficient oxygen to the cells for respiration. Iron deficiency anaemia poses a serious threat to

- the ability of children to study and participate in games,
- the ability of women to face the stress of childbearing and nursing, and
- the ability of men to work satisfactorily.

Thus, it affects the quality of life of a large part of our population. It is our duty to correct and alter this situation.

Table 10.5: RDA of Iron

Particulars	*Iron mg/day*	*Particulars*	*Iron mg/day*
Man (60 kg)	28	*Children*	
Woman (50 kg)	30	Boys 10–12 years	34
Pregnant woman	38	Boys 13–15 years	41
Lactation	30	Boys 16–18 years	50
Children			
1–3 years	12	Girls 10–12 years	19
4–6 years	18	Girls 13–15 years	28
7–9 years	26	Girls 16–18 years	30

Iron Overload

When too much iron is absorbed, large amounts are deposited in the liver, lungs, pancreas and other tissues. **Hemochromatosis** is a genetic defect, in which there is excessive absorption of iron resulting in organ damage and skin pigmentation. It may further lead to the cirrhosis of the liver.

Excessive iron storage, without tissue damage, results in **hemosiderosis**—iron storage minus tissue damage. It occurs when iron supplements are given for long periods even after it is not needed. Abnormal breakdown of red blood corpuscles (RBCs) can also be the cause of hemosiderosis.

Iodine

A small amount of iodine is required to keep our body healthy.

There are about 25 to 30 mg iodine in the body. Of this about 33 per cent iodine is present in the thyroid gland. But iodine in minute traces is found in all cells of the body. Two hormones produced by the thyroid gland, viz., triiodothyroxine (T_3) and thyroxine (T_4) contain iodine. These hormones monitor the rate of energy metabolism in the body and thus are essential for growth and development.

A deficiency of iodine is marked by a swelling of the neck with the enlargement of the thyroid gland. This condition is known as simple goitre. The ashes of dry sea plants, which contain iodine, have been successfully used as medication for prevention of goitre for centuries in India.

When mothers suffer from prolonged iodine deficiency, they give birth to babies, who are physically and mentally deformed.

The amount of iodine in plants is dependent on the presence of the mineral in the soil. In mountainous areas like the Himalayan regions, the iodine from the soil is washed away by rains and melting snow. Plants that grow in these regions are very low in iodine content. Similarly the salts, mined in these areas, known as rock salt do not contain any iodine. People in such areas used to suffer from goitre. Goitrous regions of the world are shown in Figure 10.1 But nowadays, the salt is enriched by the addition of iodine and cases of goitre are not that common wherever such enriched salt is provided.

The water of the oceans contains iodine. The sea plants and the fishes which feed on it are rich sources of iodine. Salt obtained from the sea contains iodine. Vegetables which are grown in soils containing iodine are also good sources of iodine.

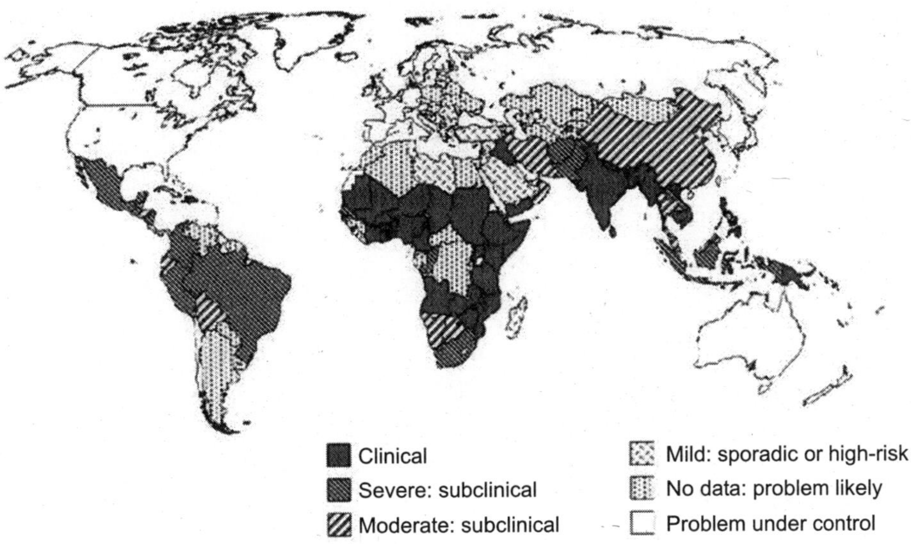

Figure 10.1: Goitrous regions of the world.

Other Trace Elements

Besides iron and iodine, a number of other trace elements are required by the human species. These are copper, zinc, selenium, cobalt, fluorine, molybdenum and manganese. Their functions are given below.

Copper is associated with iron in energy production.

Zinc is an essential part of cell enzyme systems. It combines with insulin to form a storage form of the hormone. It is important in the immune systems as part of white blood cells.

Selenium functions as an essential part of an antioxidant enzyme that protects cells and their membranes against oxidative damage and hence against cancer. In this way, it spares vitamin E. It is also credited as a protective agent against mercury poisoning in animals. Reduced blood selenium values have been reported in children suffering from protein-calorie malnutrition.

Cobalt: The only known function of cobalt is its association with RBC formation as part of vitamin B_{12}.

Fluorine is necessary for resistance to dental caries. It may have a function in prevention of the bone destruction associated with ageing.

Molybdenum functions as a catalyst component in several cell enzyme systems.

Manganese: Like other trace elements it functions as an essential part of cell enzymes.

Study Questions

1. What are the distinct characteristics of minerals?
2. List the general functions of minerals.
3. List the factors which favour absorption of calcium.
4. What are the sources of iron in the body? Why is iron called a one-way element?
5. Why is iodine important in human nutrition?
6. Write short notes on trace elements.

CHAPTER 11

Water, Fluids, Electrolytes and Acid-base Balance

Water

Body Composition: Water is the major component of our body. If you weigh 50 kg, 31 kg of that weight is water (Figure 11.1).

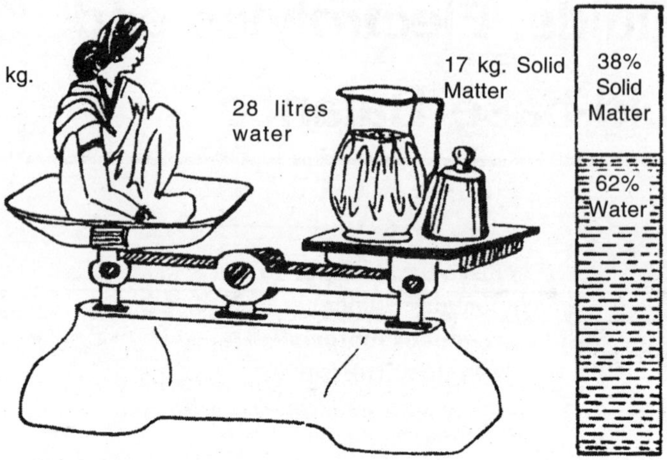

Figure 11.1: Water content of human body.

Approximately 55 to 70 per cent of the total body weight is made up of water. The percentage of water tends to decrease as a person gets older. Thus infants and children have a much higher content of water than adults. Fat individuals have less water than lean ones. Water is an essential nutrient next only in importance to oxygen. Deprivation of water even for a few days can lead to death.

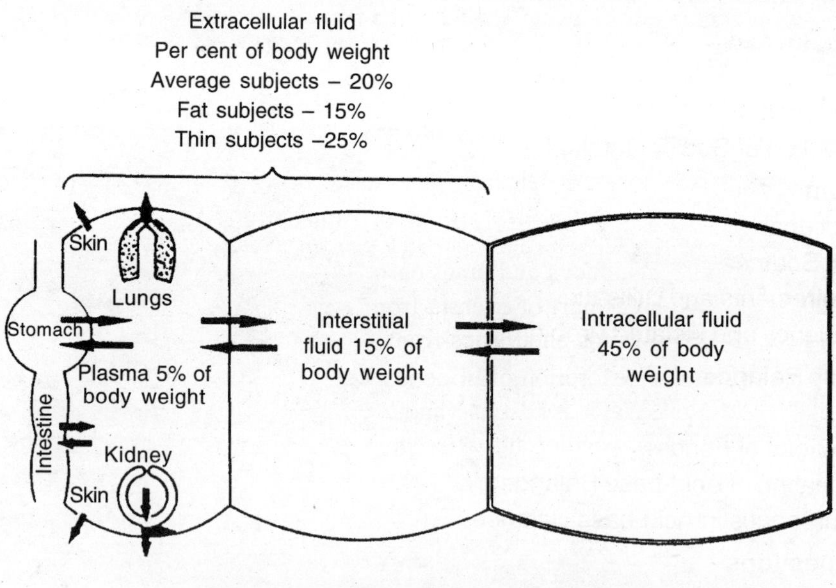

Figure 11.2: Body fluid compartments.

Water is an essential component of every cell of our body. There is a variation in the water content of various tissues. Metabolically active tissues such as brain, liver, blood and muscles contain more water than bone and fat tissue, which are less active. For example, blood plasma has 90 per cent, muscle tissue 75–80 per cent and fat tissue 20 per cent water.

Water holds innumerable body components in solution or suspension. Therefore, it is more appropriate to refer to these as fluids. The fluids, **which exist inside the cells,** are called **intracellular** fluids, which form about 55 per cent of water in the body. The rest is found as **extracellular** fluid (outside the cells). Blood, lymph circulation and interstitial fluid (fluid between cells or tissues) are part of extracellular fluid (Figure 11.2).

The fluid balance is maintained between the compartments as also between blood and interstitial fluid; kidneys are the final regulators of fluid balance.

Functions : Water serves as a building material for each cell of the body.

Water is a **universal solvent** and is able to dissolve all the products of digestion. Further as it is a **constituent** of all body fluids, it helps in the **transport of the products** of digestion to the appropriate organs. For example, **blood,** which contains 90 per cent water, **carries carbon dioxide to the lungs, nutrients to the cells** and **waste nitrogenous material** and **salt** to the kidneys. **Urine** which contains 97 per cent water has all the **waste material dissolved** in it and the body is thus able to **excrete soluble waste** products of metabolism. Water is needed for many **chemical reactions** to occur in the body. For example, the breakdown of sugar to simpler substances needs the presence of water. Water acts as a **lubricant** preventing friction between moving parts of the body. The body temperature is **regulated** through the evaporation of water from the skin and lungs.

Table 11.1: Water Balance in a Healthy Adult.

	Water intake	*Water loss*
	Water intake — 800 to 1100 ml	Urine — 800 to 1000 ml
	Water in food — 600 to 900 ml	Vapour — 600 to 1000 ml (skin & lungs)
	Metabolic water — 200 ml	Faeces — 200 ml
Total	1600 to 2200 ml	1600 to 2200 ml

Normal Losses

As depicted in Figure 11.2, kidneys and lungs carry out water from the body. Water is also lost as perspiration through the skin and as part of excreta from the bowel (Table 11.1). The volume of urine voided depends on the intake of fluids and varies from 400 to 1400 ml.

The minimum or obligatory excretion of urine is about 600 ml to keep all the solutes (salt, urea, etc.) to be excreted in solution. Water is lost as vapour through the skin (insensible perspiration) and also as visible perspiration in hot weather and after strenuous activity.

Water Balance

The body normally maintains a water balance precisely, i.e., the amount of water ingested is equal to the water excreted or lost from the body (Table (11.1). This water balance is maintained even though the fluid intake may vary widely from day-to-day. How exactly this regulatory mechanism works is not known; but certain regions of the hypothalmus are believed to regulate the intake. The water excretion is controlled by hormones.

Sources: The water we drink as such is the main source from which maximum water is obtained by the human body. In addition to this, the intake of all beverages and liquid foods that contain water, contribute water to the system. Certain metabolic reactions carried on inside the body also release water and this is another source of water.

In a water balance study it was found that of the total 2200 ml available water in the system, 1100 ml was obtained by drinking water as such, 900 ml was obtained from the diet and 200 ml obtained from the metabolic oxidation (Table 11.1).

Requirement: About 1 ml of water is needed per 1 kcal energy intake; thus about 2000 ml water is necessary when energy intake is 2000 kcal. Infants who have a large body surface area, in proportion to body weight, need 1.5 ml water/1 kcal energy intake.

The amount of water needed by an individual will depend on many factors such as the **environmental temperature, humidity, occupation and the diet.** In general, apart from water obtained in the food, an individual may need to drink about 1.5 to 2 litres of water per day. An athlete or a player, playing a strenuous game such as football or hockey, may lose several litres of water and dissolved salts during the game and would need replacement early. On the other hand, a sedentary individual would need much less water.

Problems

Dehydration: When intake of water and other fluids is less than the body needs, dehydration occurs. Dehydration is a serious medical problem, which needs **prompt attention and remedial action.** Dehydration results from excessive loss of water due to vomiting and/or diarrhoea. Infants who have a high body water content and high water requirement get dehydrated very quickly, when they suffer from diarrhoea. If the loss of water and electrolytes is not promptly made up by feeding beverages such as oral rehydration solution, coconut water, weak tea, lemon sherbet, etc., the infant may not survive.

Vomitting due to either gastrointestinal disturbances or any other cause can lead to appreciable loss of fluid from the body. Excessive perspiration due to strenuous exercise, while playing games such as hockey, football can result in losses of many litres of water. Protracted fevers can lead to appreciable loss of water due to perspiration. In all such instances where there is loss of water, it is important to **replace** the water and soluble salts lost quickly to **maintain body composition.**

Any **loss more than 10 per cent of fluid** from the body can be serious. Progressively, deprivation of water can cause poor absorption of food, delayed elimination of wastes, elevation of body temperature, failure of the circulatory system and malfunctioning of the renal system.

Oedema is accumulation of excess fluid in the tissues. It occurs when the sodium content in the extracellular fluid increases due to the inability of the kidneys to excrete sodium. Water is retained with the excess sodium, resulting in oedema. In protracted protein deficiency, the tissues are unable to ensure water balance, and the oedema, which follows, is called nutritional oedema. Other conditions, which lead to oedema, are kidney disease, cirrhosis of the liver and heart ailment.

Electrolytes

Chemical compounds, which break up into their constituent ions, when dissolved in water, are known as **electrolytes,** because each carries an electric charge. The positively charged electrolyte is known as a **cation** and the negatively charged one as an **anion.** In an electrolyte solution, the total number of cations are exactly equal to the total anions. Electrolytes are necessary to regulate the water and acid-base balance in the body.

Sodium is the principal cation and chloride the anion in blood plasma. The other cations are potassium, calcium and magnesium; other anions are bicarbonate, phosphate, sulphate, proteinate and organic acids.

In contrast, inside the cell, the main cation is potassium and the main anion is phosphate. There is a strict maintenance of concentration of electrolytes in the fluids inside and outside the cell in a healthy person. Thus sodium stays mainly outside the cell and potassium inside the cell. Any change in the level of electrolytes in the blood plasma is an early warning of disorder in the body.

Sodium

Sodium is an essential nutrient, which participates along with other minerals in many regulatory functions.

Functions: The regulatory functions of sodium include normal muscle contraction, maintenance of normal osmotic pressure, water balance and cell permeability, and transmission of nerve impulses and regulation of acid-base balance. It facilitates the absorption of sugars and amino acids, through the sodium pump.

The adult body contains about 85 g sodium; halt of it is in the extracellular fluid, about two-fifths in the bone and about a tenth in the intracellular fluid.

Food Sources: The main source of sodium in the diet is salt. It is used as a preservative in a variety of pickles. It is also used in processed foods, snack foods such as potato wafers and other savoury foods.

Other sodium compounds used in food preparation include baking soda, baking powder, monosodium glutamate (MSG) (ajinomoto).

The typical diet contains about 500 mg sodium, when **no** salt or sodium containing salts are added during preparation. Most of this sodium is present in animal foods such as milk and meats. Most of the plant foods, with a few exceptions are low in sodium.

Utilisation: About 95 per cent of sodium intake is absorbed. The sodium not utilised is excreted in the urine. Actually the sodium content of the body is regulated by the kidneys.

Requirement: Dietary deficiency of sodium does not occur in normal circumstances, as common salt is a very cheap ingredient.

Sodium, which is available from common salt (sodium chloride) in the diet, helps to maintain the fluid and acid-base balance of the body. People, who do rigorous exercises or who work in hot places such as furnaces or mines, lose salt from the body in perspiration and urine, and so need an extra intake of salt. Similarly, during the hot weather, when one perspires profusely, extra amount of salt is needed in the diet. Deficiency of salt in the diet may cause cramps of muscles, headache, tiredness or sickness.

Salt may need to be restricted in diets of persons suffering from kidney or heart malfunction.

Reduction of Sodium Intake: Hyperactivity in children has been found to be related to excessive intakes of sodium from use of processed supplementary foods.

Intake of salt in diets has increased with the increase in use of processed and readymade foods in the diet. There has been an increase in the incidence of heart ailments as also diabetes mellitus. Hence a number of health organisations recommend that most people would benefit by reducing their sodium intake. Since the taste for salt is an acquired taste, it is possible to modify it.

An intake of 3 to 5 g salt is sufficient to prepare a palatable diet. The following changes will help to reduce salt intake:

1. Do not add salt on the table to foods.
2. Reduce the amount of salt used in preparation. Try ½ to ¾ amount of the amount used earlier.
3. Use minimal amounts of oil and spices in seasoning food, so that the amount of salt needed in preparation will be reduced.
4. Prepare desserts without adding salt.
5. Use a variety of herbs and spices to flavour vegetables, meats and reduce the need for salt.
6. Use salty foods sparingly, e.g., pickles, *papad,* foods baked with soda, etc.
7. Read labels of processed foods to note presence of salt and sodium compounds and avoid those with high sodium content.

Potassium

Potassium is primarily present in the intracellular fluid (about 12.6 g/per kg), so that the body is able to conserve it.

Functions: Like sodium, potassium helps to maintain the normal osmotic pressure of the body fluids and the acid-base balance of the body. It is also involved in muscle contraction and transmission of nerve stimuli. It acts as an activator of several enzyme reactions in metabolism.

Food Sources: Potassium is widely distributed in foods. Meat, fish and poultry are good sources. Fruits such as bananas, oranges, mausambi, lemons and vegetables like potatoes, carrots, leafy vegetables and whole-grain cereals are also good sources of potassium.

Requirement and Utilisation: About 3 to 7 g per day as potassium chloride, which is the intake in ordinary diet, appears to be adequate. About 90 per cent of ingested potassium is absorbed from the intestine, the rest is excreted in urine.

Deficiency and Related Problems: Normally dietary deficiency of potassium does not occur. But persons, who take diuretics for weight reduction, may lose excessive amounts and need to consume potassium rich foods to make up the loss.

Severe vomiting, diarrhoea, diabetic acidosis may increase losses and thus precipitate a deficiency. The symptoms are the same as diarrhoea and need to be corrected promptly to avoid a fatal crisis.

Abnormal elevation of blood plasma potassium known as **hyperkalemia** occurs in severe dehydration and kidney failure, which needs immediate action. Rehydration fluids rich in sodium, potassium and glucose/sucrose help to reverse the situation and pave the way to recovery.

Acid-base Balance

pH: The concentration of hydrogen ions in a solution is referred to by the symbol pH. It is the measure of acidity or alkalinity of the solution. Neutral pH, which is the pH of water, is 7.0. The pH below 7.0 denotes acidity which increases with decrease in the pH. The alkalinity on the other hand, increases with increase in the pH.

The pH of **body fluids is maintained** in the **narrow** range between **7.35 and 7.45**, which is slightly alkaline. The maintenance of pH in this narrow range is known as acid-base balance.

Reactions of Foods: The foods which contain sizeable amounts of sulphur, chloride and phosphorus, metabolise to form anions in excess of cations. Such foods are potentially **acid** producing foods. Acid producing foods include cheese, legumes, cereal foods, coconut, eggs and flesh foods.

The foods which produce excess cations on metabolism are termed alkali producing foods. These foods contain excess cations such as calcium, sodium, potassium and magnesium. Fruits, vegetables, milk, groundnuts, etc., are alkali producing foods.

It is important to note that the sour tasting fruits (citrus and other fruits) are alkali producing foods. So the taste of the food **is not related** to its metabolic reaction.

The third group of foods which are low in mineral elements are termed **neutral foods.** These include sugar, starch, tapioca, oils, butter and other cooking fats.

Regulation of Acid-base Balance: Mineral elements act as buffer salts, which prevent change in the pH. In the body the carbonate and the sodium phosphate buffer systems are important in pH regulation. Proteins, which hydrolyse to form amino acids, containing an alkaline (NH_2) an acidic (COOH) group, are also good buffers.

Carbonic acid is the main acid produced in metabolism, which is exhaled by the lungs as carbon dioxide and water vapour. Breathing rapidly and deeply helps us to bring down the increased carbon dioxide content of the blood.

This is the basis of for the recommendations for exercises, which make us breathe rapidly and cleanse the blood.

Yoga, which teaches us to breathe deeply, ensures that oxygen reaches all the cells. Thus it helps the process of oxidation, which releases the carbon dioxide to be exhaled. The kidneys are able to excrete very acidic urine, when excess acid is produced in the body, thus preventing changes in blood pH. The kidneys act as the last regulators of acid-base balance.

Disturbances in Acid-base Balance: If the pH of body fluids drops below pH 7.3, it is called acidosis. When diabetes is not controlled, the patient who has acidosis excretes large amounts of ketones.

In severe starvation, the body fat reserves are metabolised in the absence of carbohydrate and acidosis occurs. In renal failure, acidosis occurs, as the kidneys are not able to get rid of excess acid.

If the pH increases above 7.5., it is called **alkalosis.** Any condition which leads to loss of stomach acid, results in alkalosis. Severe vomiting is one such condition. Another is excessive intake of antacids such as sodium bicarbonate. Third is loss of hydrogen ions due to renal malfunction.

Any change in pH needs immediate action to avoid disturbance in the metabolism and restore normalcy.

Study Questions

1. List the functions of water in the body.
2. Write notes on: dehydration, oedema, and electrolytes.
3. List steps to be taken to reduce salt intake.
4. What are the functions of potassium in the body?
5. What is pH?
6. What is acid-base balance?
7. How is the acid-base balance regulated in the body?
8. Write notes on: reactions of foods; acidosis and alkalosis.

CHAPTER 12

Nutrition for Fitness, Athletics and Sports

Introduction

The interest in physical fitness is very high in all the age groups of populations around the world. It may be to keep fit, healthy and thus improve the quality of life or it can be to participate in athletics and possible competition.

Our body composition, muscular ability, respiratory and cardiovascular capabilities are very closely related to nutrition and exercise. Diet and nutrition does influence performance.

Exercise for Physical Fitness

Just as eating three meals regularly is a consistent part of daily life, so should exercise be a consistent, regular part of daily life. In physical education in schools, activities that are appropriate for life-long participation need to be emphasised. This will ensure physical well-being and optimal function of the majority of students. Some of them may become athletes.

Enjoy Your Activities and Exercise

The cardinal rule of our body is conservation of energy. To keep an energy balance in adult life we need to learn to enjoy spending it. Voluntary exercise is an ideal way to use energy, as it helps us to stay in shape and look good. It helps to improve posture, build muscle strength and increases flexibility of joints. It strengthens the heart (a vital muscle) and improves circulation, which we refer to as the pink glow of health. Naturally it relieves tension and helps us to enjoy life. The reduced risk of contracting chronic diseases is an added bonus.

How to Select an Exercise Programme

The choice of an exercise programme varies from individual to individual. The word *choice* is very important for there are literally innumerable ways to attain your goal of fitness. The following are the guidelines to choose it:

1. Choose an exercise you like so that you will enjoy doing it.
2. Choose one that can be done in all seasons.
3. Choose one that can be done preferably near your residence.
4. Choose one for which you have facilities.
5. Choose one that can be done regularly.
6. Choose an exercise that involves the large muscles in the body.

Physical Fitness Movement

The awareness about and interest in physical fitness is increasing in our people. It appears it is no longer a fad but a welcome trend. The longer one follows some type of regular exercise, the more committed one becomes. Walking and soft workouts have enabled more persons to participate, who are not athletically inclined. Many of these persons are middle-aged adults who control health problems with moderate exercise. They thus feel more in control of their lives.

Beginning an Exercise Programme

It is important to begin an exercise programme with a proper plan. Strong motivation is necessary to pursue an exercise programme on a long-term basis. Some of the basic guidelines for beginning are:

1. Record weight, height, chest, waist and hip girth.
2. Initiate the programme gradually. As little as 3 to 5 minutes may suffice, for those who have been sedentary, especially older persons. Increase the period to 20 to 30 minutes over 3 to 4 weeks.
3. 3 to 5 minutes warm-up period, which consists of smooth, stretching exercises, should precede intense exercise. At the end of intense exercise, decrease the intensity slowly to allow the body to cool down.
4. Aerobic exercises are most helpful to increase physical fitness.
5. Persons, who have chronic ailment or are overweight, should consult their doctor and check blood pressure, cardiovascular function, muscle and joint function before starting. The doctor may help to select the exercise programme and goals to be set.

Requirements for Moderate Exercise

Fluids and Oxygen

Fluids: More water is needed with increase in exercise. The need to replace fluid losses during exercise is well recorded. All cellular activities take place in an aqueous medium. Water carries nutrients and waste products via blood stream to and from the cells. Thus **sufficient blood volume is a must** to ensure loss of heat produced through skin and sweat. Water is lost from the body through sweat and respiration. Water for sweat is taken from blood, resulting in reduced blood volume, which may endanger heart function. Significant fluid losses may reduce sweating and blood flow, disturbing body temperature regulation. A water loss of 4 to 5 per cent reduces work capacity by 20 to 30 per cent; a 10 per cent loss may result in circulatory collapse.

The fluid losses in exercise depend on the duration and intensity of exercise as also the ambient temperature and humidity. Normal sweat production, without exercise, is 500 to 700 ml per day. It may increase to 8 to 12 litres per day with prolonged exercise in humid conditions.

Electrolytes: Though sweat contains electrolytes, chloride, magnesium and potassium, performance is not disturbed by electrolyte losses. In hot months, during training, a dilute salt solution (1/2 teaspoon salt per liter) may be used as a rehydration drink to correct excessive sweat losses (American College of Sports Medicine, 1984).

During exercise, as heat is released with energy production, the body temperature rises. One sweats in an effort to control body temperature. The loss of water due to sweat must be made up to avoid **dehydration.** The amount of water needed in hot summer months is much more than in cool weather.

Oxygen: Breathing ensures a constant supply of oxygen to the body. The need for oxygen increases with exercise, as more oxygen is needed to release extra body energy. The ability of the body to provide the oxygen needed is known as **aerobic capacity**. The aerobic capacity is dependent on the fitness of tissues involved in oxygen intake and transport — **lungs, heart and blood vessels** and the body composition.

Body Fitness is measured in terms of aerobic capacity. Aerobic capacity is the ability of the body to provide the increased demands for oxygen and use it during exercise. As it varies with the body size, it is measured as the amount of oxygen consumed per kilogram body weight. Thus it is an indirect measure of the health of the respiratory system.

Body Composition: As mentioned in the energy balance chapter, the muscle mass (lean body mass or the active metabolic tissues) in the body uses larger part of the oxygen. The aerobic capacity is dependent on the percentage of lean body mass and body fat. Body composition is determined by these two components of body weight.

Nutritional Needs for Exercise

Nutrient Reserves

Any exercise activity increases energy expenditure. Proper diet is an essential prerequisite for good performance be it for athletic competition or for just keeping fit. It is important to have **nutrient reserves** to meet the demands during periods of exercise. If the reserves are used up, the body cannot meet its needs and fatigue and exhaustion may occur. As we know, carbohydrates and fats are the basic suppliers of these energy reserves, as very little is drawn from protein.

Carbohydrate is the major nutrient to provide energy for exercise. Our body has two sources of carbohydrate reserves—the glucose in the circulating blood and the glycogen, stored in muscles and liver. For an active person, the diet needs to provide 55 to 60 per cent of total dietary calories in the form of **complex** carbohydrates as they break down more slowly and help maintain blood sugar levels more evenly. Secondly, starches are more readily converted to glycogen to maintain this reserve store.

Fat: There is no basis for increasing the level of fat in the diet. The total fat should not exceed 20 to 25 per cent of the total dietary calories. Vegetable oils, which are rich sources of essential fatty acids, should form a part of the total fat intake.

Protein: It is important to meet one's recommended dietary allowance (RDA) for protein. This adds up to about 10 to 15 per cent of the total calories from protein. No additional protein is needed, as it is not meant to serve as an energy source.

Vitamins and Minerals: They are essential only in the process of energy release as co-factors. In general, the efficient use of vitamins and minerals by the body is increased due to exercise. Hence exercise *per se* does not increase the need for vitamins and minerals.

The athletes, who need more energy, take larger amounts of good food, which increases their intake of vitamins and minerals. The only groups that need to focus special attention in this respect are adolescent and female athletes, who may need iron supplements, if their blood iron levels are very low.

Exercise and Energy

Kilocalories: Physical activity needs energy, *i.e.*, kilocalories. The energy needed for various exercises is given in Table 12.1.

The amount of energy used in exercise varies with —

(*a*) the intensity of the exercise
(*b*) the duration of the exercise
(*c*) the sex, age, weight of the individual

(*d*) the state of the individual and

(e) the level of training.

In addition, it is affected by the rest taken during the exercise and the environmental conditions, such as temperature, humidity, the surfaces involved, the obstacles or physical difficulties, etc. (such as hilly terrain during cross country running).

Effects on the System. The need for calories is increased. Exercise helps to regulate appetite. Exercise is the only way to regulate the person's body system and to regulate the body fat content. Lack of exercise tends to raise the body's fat set-point, resulting in more fat stores. It is lowered when a person exercises regularly.

Table 12.1: Approximate Energy Expenditure in Some Aerobic Activities[1]

Activity	*Kilocalories per hour*	
	Male (60 *kg*)	*Female* (50 *kg*)
Sitting, inactive	66	55
Walking, moderate	167	139
Walking, brisk (5.6 km/hr)	281	235
Bicycling (8.8 km/hr)	198	165
Bicycling (16.0 km/hr)	449	374
Dancing (moderate)	220	183
Golf	277	231
Swimming, moderate	290	242
Swimming, vigorous	537	447
Tennis, singles	396	330
Runnings (8.8 km/hr)	519	433

1. Modified from Robinson, *et al., Basic Nutrition and Diet Therapy*, 7th edn., 1993, p. 128.

Nutrient Ratios: As mentioned earlier, active persons, even athletes or any other sports persons need the same amount of protein and fat as an inactive person of the same body size.

Complex carbohydrates are the fuel of choice before the exercise period and during the recovery period, which follows. The recommended ratios of energy nutrients to support physical activity are:

Carbohydrates	:	60 to 70% of total kilocalories
Fats	:	20 to 25% of total kilocalories
Proteins	:	10 to 15% of total kilocalories

Athletic Performance

Nutritional well-being is important for all physical activities. Just as we save money, when we intend to take a trip, so must our body stock reserve fuel before participating in athletic and sports activities. Many school children, high school and college students take part in competitive games, even endurance races. Therefore, they need to know the dietary input that helps to improve their performance. Table 12.1 gives approximate energy expenditure in some aerobic activities.

Energy: Athletes may need 3000 to 5000 kcal for most sports. Children and teenagers need adequate energy to ensure normal growth and additional energy to meet needs during training and contests. Athletes gain unnecessary weight when they are not training or participating due to not reducing energy intake to sedentary levels. This is true of dancers, soldiers, mountain climbers and others, whose extra energy need for their professional activity is periodical.

Preparation for Athletics/Sports

Carbohydrate: There is need to increase muscle glycogen stores prior to the competition. This is known as **carbohydrate loading.** The carbohydrate intake (mainly starch from grains) is increased slowly in the week before the event, beginning with 350g and increasing it to 450 to 500g in four days. The day before the event the intake is reduced to normal, and complete rest is recommended for the day. Carbohydrate loading is used only by persons engaged in endurance activities such as marathons, long distance running, cycling, walking, swimming and cross-country skiing. Those involved in short intense activities may find carbohydrate loading a hindrance to their performance, as it leads to a feeling of heaviness, due to water retention. Children and teenagers should not attempt carbohydrate loading. Even athletes should restrict it to three or four times in a year.

Precontest/Pregame Meal: Eat a light meal of about 300 kcal, two to four hours before the game/contest. It should be mainly cereal preparation, which is high in complex carbohydrate, low in protein, with little fat or fibre in it. This permits the body to digest and absorb and store it as glycogen. Foods, which one can choose from, include *pohe* with toned milk or curds, *chapati* and *dal; idli-sambar, upma,* bread, *bhakri-zunka,* etc.

Nutrition During Performance

The fluid and nutrient needs during a contest/game depends on the intensity and duration, as also ambient temperature and humidity.

The athlete cannot depend on thirst to meet fluid needs. The athlete should drink 400 to 500 ml cool water two hours before the competition, another 400 to 500 ml 15 minutes before the event. He/she should drink 100 to 150 ml every 20 minutes, depending on the event and climate. He/she should continue to drink fluids after the event until the preevent weight is restored. Plain cold water is normally the fluid of choice to ensure rehydration, except for endurance competitions or training rounds.

Ergogenic Aids

Winning is the aim of all competitors in sports. Naturally they would like to use any substance that can aid their activity. These substances are known as **ergogenic** (work producing) aids. Most of these are worthless, except the steroids. The consumption of steroids is dangerous. These steroids are synthetic sex hormones. They have two functions:

(*a*) Tissue growth (anabolic) and
(*b*) Masculinisation (androgenic).

These are used to increase muscle size, strength and performance. Athletes often take these in mega doses of 10 to 20 times that of normal body production. It is **illegal** to use steroids and those who use these are disqualified from participating in Olympic games.

The use of steroids is undesirable as it affects the health of the athlete adversely. The undesirable physiological effects include **stunting normal skeletal development, liver injury, damaging the heart, sterility and many more.** The steroid user undergoes undesirable changes in his/her personality such as being **too aggressive, mood swings from depression to violent rage,** etc. Becoming **drug dependent** can be a **serious handicap** to normal life and health. In view of these long-term harmful effects, sports persons should shun the use of hormones as aids to boost their performance. The adults who guide them — their parents, teachers, trainers and others — must ensure that the youngsters are encouraged to develop long-term goals for a healthy competition and life-long health rather than succumb to short-terms fame, followed by loss of health, unhappy disposition and loss of normal, dignified human existence. The aim of sports is to improve one's physical, social and ethical standards. This basic principle must guide all athletes and sportsmen.

Study Questions

1. How should you select an exercise programme?
2. Write short notes on:
   (*i*) Basic guidelines to begin an exercise programme.
   (*ii*) Body's needs during exercise.
   (*iii*) Nutritional needs for exercise.
   (*iv*) Preparation for participation in athletics.
   (*v*) Ergogenic aids and their effects on the body.

CHAPTER

13

Disorders of Nutrition

Introduction

Malnutrition is a health problem found in all developing countries like India. Undernutrition or lack of adequate diet is a form of malnutrition which is most widespread. The causes of undernutrition are many and often interrelated.

Poverty resulting in low purchasing power is one of the main causes of undernutrition because poor families cannot buy adequate food for themselves.

In some communities, especially in rural areas, nutritious food such as milk may not be available throughout the year. Thus, sometimes even though families can afford to buy nutritious food, non-availability may lead to malnutrition.

Ignorance of the relation of foods to health is another reason for the prevalence of malnutrition. For example, sometimes protein rich foods such as milk, eggs and fish are not fed to the child on the assumption that they are harmful to the child, even though the, family may be producers of milk or catching fish themselves.

Increasing urbanisation is another cause of malnutrition. A number of families flock from villages to cities, hoping to find better means of livelihood. Often, living conditions for such families are even worse than what they had in the villages. Overcrowding, insanitary environmental conditions, poor hygiene, contaminated water supplies are some of the problems encountered. In addition, not having enough food; decreases resistance to infections, and exposes the family members to frequent attacks of diarrhoea and other diseases. This intensifies the problem because what little food is consumed is not absorbed but lost.

In poor communities, because both parents have to work to maintain the family, the children, especially the younger ones, do not have anybody to take care of them and feed them at regular intervals. Often, an elder child, who may only be a few years older than the infant, is left to take care of the young ones. Without supervision by adults, the children are not fed properly and may develop symptoms of one or more deficiency diseases.

There is thus a vicious circle which encompasses poverty, ignorance, poor housing, disease and infection and unless this is broken by improving the economic condition of the low socio-economic groups, malnourishment of a huge sector of the population of the world cannot be eradicated. Figure 13.1 illustrates the close relationship between health, economics and social progress. It shows how poverty engenders disease which in turn engenders more poverty.

Foods contain a number of nutrients. When sufficient quantities of the right type of foods are not eaten, many essential nutrients are not available in adequate quantities to the body. This leads to the development of several deficiency diseases. Some of the common deficiency diseases found are Protein-Energy Malnutrition (PEM), vitamin A deficiency, anaemia due to lack or poor absorption of iron, and vitamin B complex deficiency.

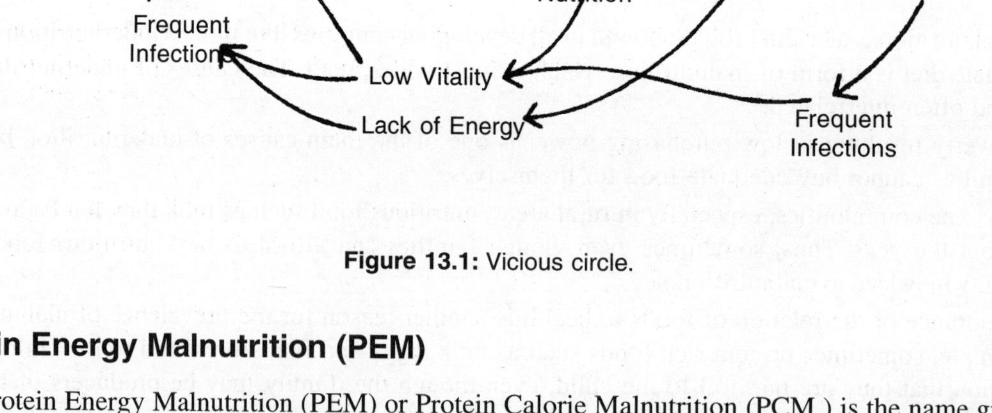

Figure 13.1: Vicious circle.

Protein Energy Malnutrition (PEM)

Protein Energy Malnutrition (PEM) or Protein Calorie Malnutrition (PCM) is the name given to various degrees of nutritional disorders caused by inadequate quantities of protein and energy in the diet. This is one of the most widespread deficiency disease in India and covers abroad spectrum ranging from marginal deficiency with loss of weight and poor growth to a severe deficiency in which the body may have developed oedema or may have wasted away. Such deficiency occurs mainly in children below five years of age, when they are weaned from mother's milk and the diet substituted does not supply sufficient protein and energy or protein only. When such lack has been prevalent for a long time in the community, the parents' may fail to note the low weight and stunted growth of the children.

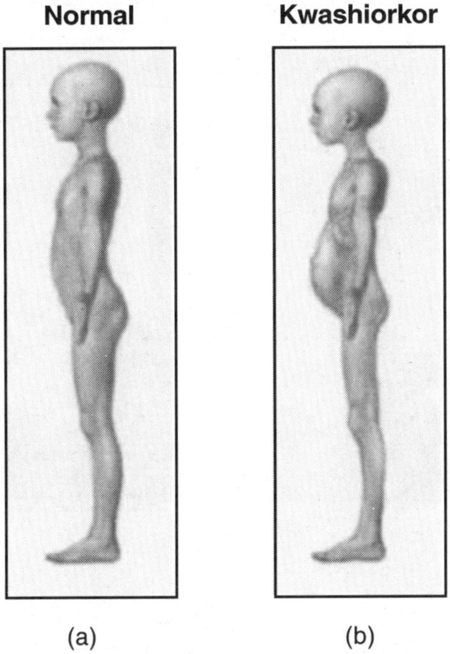

Figure 13.2: Kwashiorkor (a) normal, (b) Kwashiorkor.

One of the names of the disease associated with protein energy malnutrition is 'Kwashiorkor', a term used by Cicely Williams in 1934 to describe this condition while working in West Africa. Kwashiorkor means "the sickness a child develops when another baby is born", in the language spoken in Ghana. Kwashiorkor occurs when there is not enough protein in the diet but calories or energy in the form of carbohydrates is available in sufficient quantity.

However, when both protein and energy are insufficient, over prolonged periods, a condition known as 'marasmus' occurs in children.

In nutritional marasmus, there is also growth failure so that there is stunted growth. In addition, because of their being not enough protein and calories in the diet, the protein from the body tissues is used up for energy so that the child is all skin and bone. The child has an alert and hungry expression but may not necessarily look miserable.

Kwashiorkor is characterised by growth failure, swelling of legs and feet (oedema), wasted muscles, a miserable expression and changes in the colour of the skin and hair. The hair changes to a light colour and becomes so soft that it can be easily pulled out. The skin develops rashes and also becomes lighter in colour (Figures 13.2 a, b, c, & d).

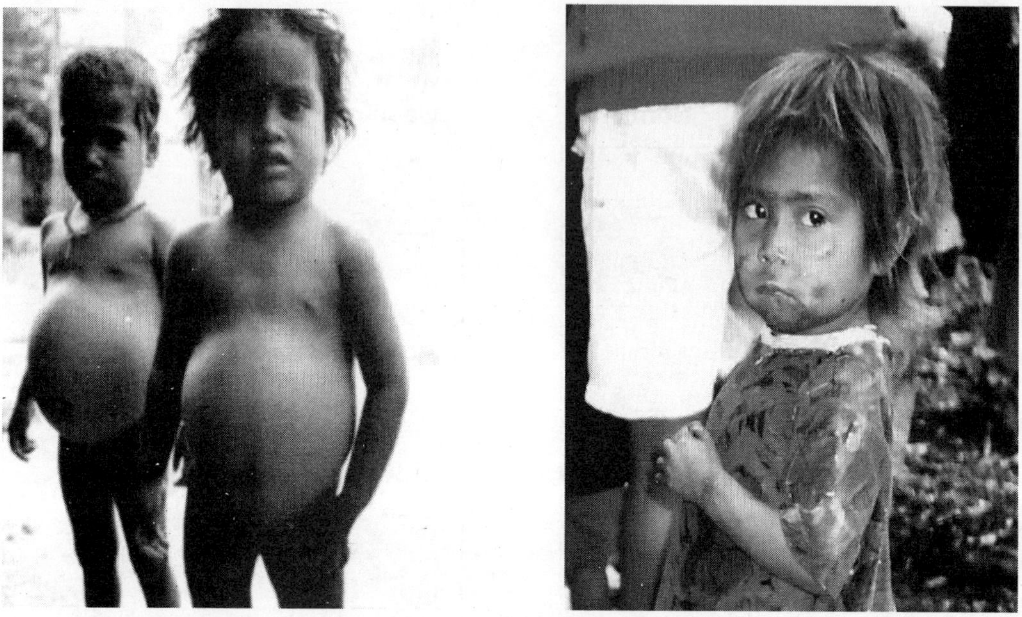

Figure 13.2: (Contd...) (c) Kwashiorkor, (d) recovery.

Both Kwashiorkor and Marasmus can be complicated with other infections due to intestinal parasites and bacteria.

The reasons for the prevalence of protein calorie malnutrition are not difficult to find. Poverty as has already been discussed is the prime factor. The families do not have enough income to purchase the necessary nutritious foods. Ignorance of the relation of foods to health and nutritional well-being is another possible cause of protein calorie malnutrition. Apart from this improper distribution of foods due to controls, lack of proper transport and other such reasons make it difficult for consumers who can afford to buy, to get the necessary foods.

In rural communities, especially, the children are nursed by mothers over long periods and supplementary foods essential to prevent PEM are not provided at the proper age. Sometimes even when supplementary foods are fed to the infant, they are insufficient and may not contain enough protein and calories. Bottle feeding has become a part of life in many communities. However, many mothers do not have any knowledge of the precautions one has to take in using this method of feeding infants. Bottles and nipples are not washed properly after every feed; sometimes the milk is allowed to stay in the bottle over long periods allowing growth of pathogenic organisms. These unhygienic feeding habits are predisposing factors which lead to diarrhoea and other intestinal disorders. In many households, the wage earner is served the food available in precedence over the needs of infants who may actually be in greater need of more protein and calories.

Prevention of PEM through Dietary Management

Eradication of poverty, increase in purchasing power of the population and nutrition education remain the most effective means of the prevention of PEM. Once there is enough economic freedom, a number of ways such as those given below can be used to combat the menace of PEM.

(*a*) Prolong breast feeding as much as possible but at the right stage start feeding supplementary foods.

(*b*) Make use of locally available vegetable and animal protein foods for feeding the child.

(*c*) Educate the mother and other members of the family about the correct diet for children.

Vitamin A Deficiency

Besides Protein Energy Malnutrition (PEM) another principal nutritional problem is vitamin A deficiency. A direct result of vitamin A deficiency is impairment of vision ultimately leading to blindness. It is estimated that 9 million are blind and 45 million are visually handicapped in India. Maintenance of the blind costs the nation Rs. 81 crore and loss of production is estimated around Rs. 1080 crore (Directorate of Health Services, Government of India). The number of people who have become blind due to nutritional deficiency of vitamin A runs into several lakhs. This deficiency is seen particularly in the rice eating southern and eastern belts of India.

Vitamin A deficiency is found more in children than in adults. Among children, the male child seems to be more affected than the female child. Pregnant women are also, however, susceptible to this deficiency. Recent survey of children estimates that 3 to 8 per cent of all pre-school children and 10 to 15 per cent of all school children suffer from vitamin A deficiency. The average percentage of all children suffering from this deficiency works out to ten. As long as children are breast fed which is usually from six months to one year, there is no sign of vitamin A deficiency. However, in the lower socio-economic groups, once the breast milk is withdrawn, the diet does not seem to supply enough of this vitamin.

Vitamin A is necessary for growth, and lack of it could result in stunted growth and abnormalities of bones and teeth. Deficiency of the vitamin also leads to dryness of the conjunctiva of the eye and cloudiness of the cornea. At this stage night blindness may be observed. Severe deficiency of vitamin A results in the cornea becoming dry and losing its transparency thus having a hazy appearance. During the next stage the cornea become soft and may fall off resulting in total blindness (Figures 13.3a and b).

The principal causes of vitamin A deficiency is lack of adequate supply in the diet. Though vitamin A is present only in animal foods its precursor beta-carotene is present in green leaves, ripe mangoes and other fruits. In fact, experiments have shown that an intake for 15 days of green leaves by pre-school children whose diets were deficient in vitamin A improved their Serum vitamin A level. Poor absorption of vitamin A and carotene due to lack of fat in the diet, gastro-intestinal disorders, liver disease and other metabolic abnormalities can also result in vitamin A deficiency.

Attempts have been made to distribute vitamin A and D in capsule form and skim milk powder fortified with vitamin A through health centres to children especially in rural areas to prevent vitamin A deficiency. These have not been very successful because it is not possible to find the same pre-school child every two or three days to feed these supplements.

As vitamin A is stored in the liver for prolonged periods, attempts have been made to administer orally massive doses such as 60,000 mcg of vitamin A to school children half yearly. Experiments carried out during the past seven years have shown that 84 per cent of the children were protected from vitamin A deficiency when such massive doses were given. Oil preparations containing the vitamin were effective and had very little toxic effects. In view of these findings, the Family Planning Department of the Government of India has launched a programme in several regions of this country where there is deficiency of vitamin A to administer massive dosage of vitamin A to pre-school children at annual intervals.

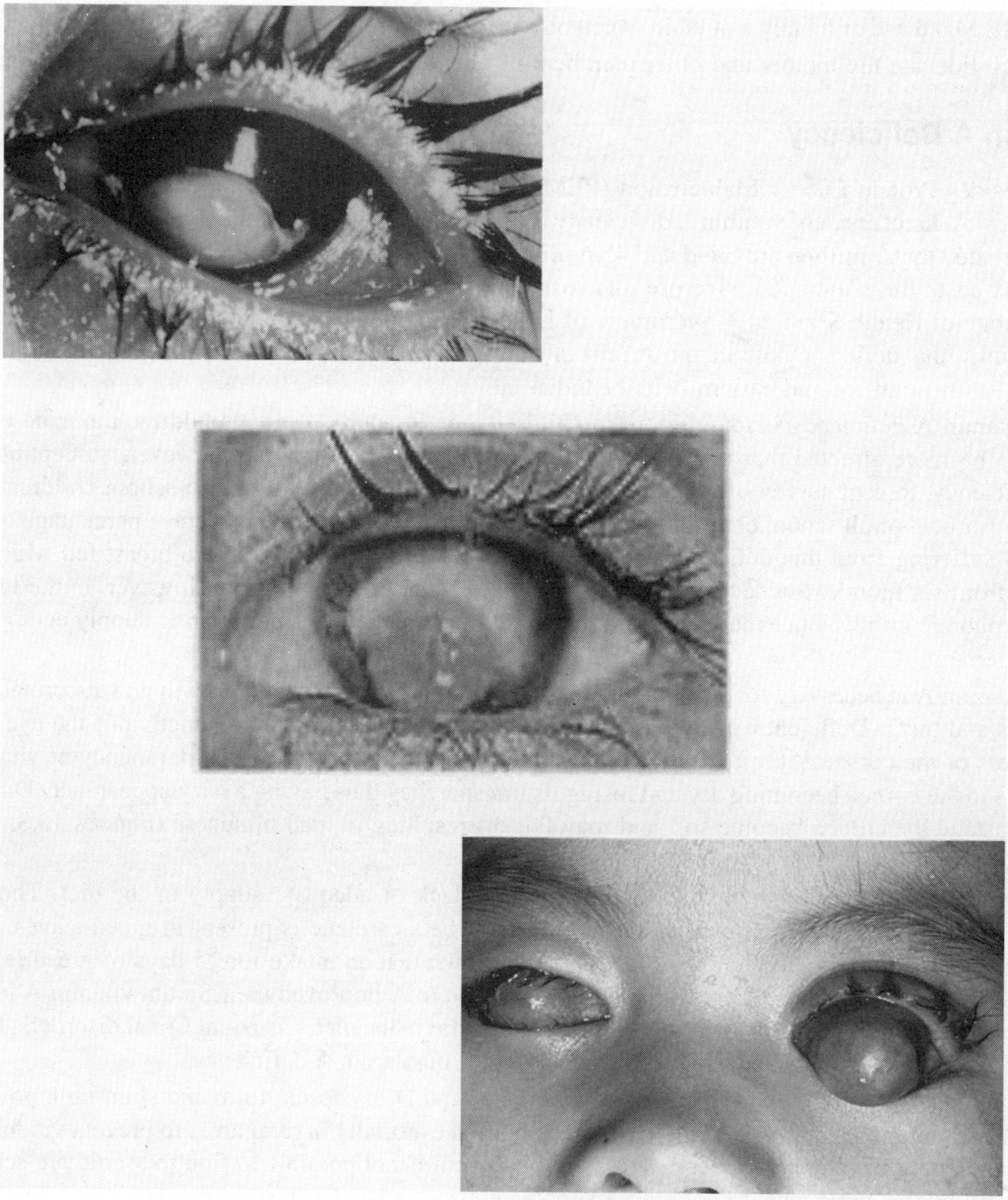

Figure 13.3: Vitamin A deficiency.

Iron Deficiency Anaemia

Iron deficiency anaemia is a major nutritional problem in our country. The age groups affected are women at reproductive age, pregnant women and pre-school children especially from low income groups (Figures 13.4 (a) & 13.4 (b)]. Its prevalence ranges from 60 to 70 per cent in women and children, and 30 to 40 per cent in adult males and older children in most parts of the country.

Deficiency of iron causes anaemia, a condition in which there is a decrease in the haemoglobin content of the red blood cells (erythrocytes), and there is an alteration in their size and shape. Hence haemoglobin content of blood has been used to study the incidence of anaemia. Determination of haemoglobin level in the blood of large numbers of people in different age groups in many parts of the world, has helped to establish standards with which the results of field studies can be compared.

Haemoglobin studies of large numbers of school children in India, have shown that more than 50 per cent of them have haemoglobin levels less than 10.8 g per 100 ml. Similarly the haemoglobin levels of more than 50 per cent pregnant women, attending rural health centres, was found to be less than 10 g per 100 ml.

The major cause of anaemia in our country is iron deficiency due to inadequate intake of dietary iron and/or its poor absorption, from the cereal based diets consumed by people. Iron intake in the diets of low socio-economic groups has been found to be around 20 mg per day in adults and 6 mg per day for pre-school children. These amounts of iron intake are considered to be marginal due to the high phytate content of the diets, which render part of the iron unavailable to the body. However, it has been observed that if sufficient amounts of vitamin C and calcium are provided, iron can be absorbed even in the presence of phytates.

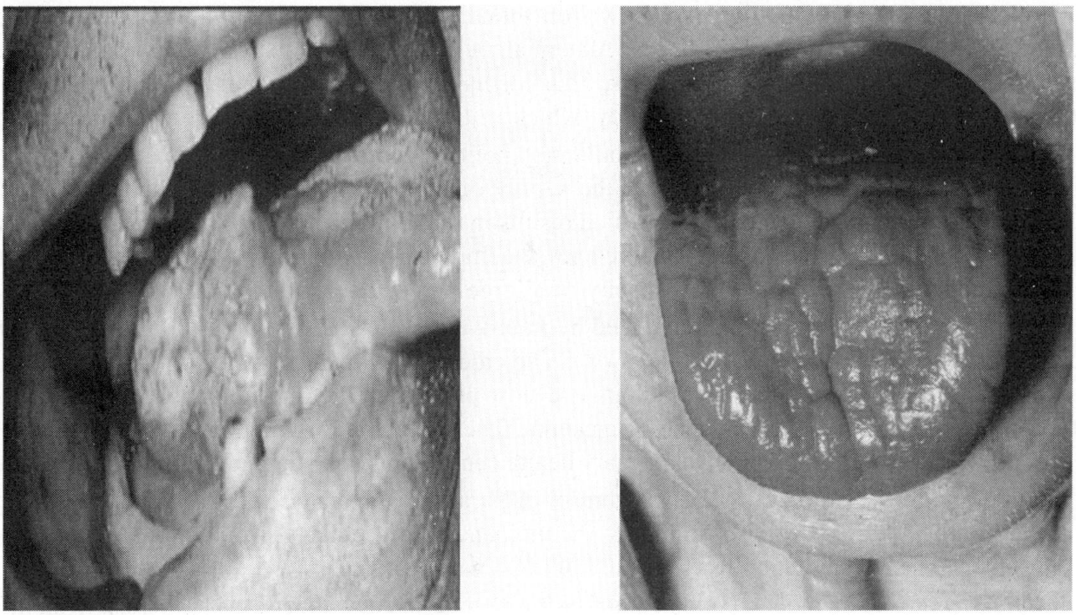

Figure 13.4: (a) Anaemia

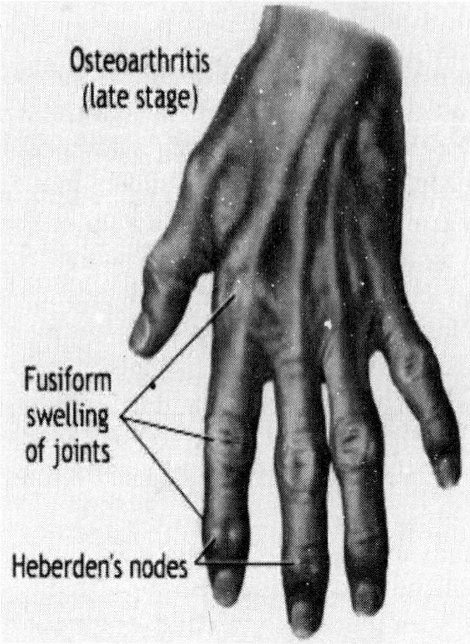

Figure 13.4: (b) Anaemia

Loss of iron through sweat is possible and in a tropical country like India, it has special relevance. Loss of blood through hook-worm infestation is another cause of iron deficiency. The infestation appears to be more in wet areas than dry areas. In such areas anaemia is found to be present in all age groups and sex groups, including men. Low iron intake coupled with hook-worm infestation thus poses a serious community health problem. Anaemia could also be due to loss of excessive blood in menstruation and during child birth in women. Haemorrhages, due to accidental injury or other causes, could also deplete haemoglobin from the body, which if it is not replaced, could lead to anaemia.

Anaemia develops slowly and is usually not noticed in early stages. In anaemia, since the haemoglobin level in the blood is reduced, the supply of oxygen to the cells is reduced. Therefore, physical activity is considerably lowered, which results in reduction in working capacity of the person. If we consider the high prevalence of iron deficiency anaemia, we may realise the magnitude of economic loss in the India, due to reduced work capacity of a large percentage of the population.

The incidence of anaemia can be reduced by improvements of dietary habits. These are inclusion of leafy vegetables, which provide iron; vitamin C and calcium, and pulses, which provide protein, iron and B vitamins. Since change in dietary habits is a slow process, some interim public health measures have been taken to reduce the incidence of anaemia. These include distribution of tablets containing iron and folic acid to pregnant women at primary health centres and iron supplements to school children.

In addition to these programmes, the control of parasites associated with blood loss (like hook-worm) need to be given top priority to reduce the incidence of anaemia. It would also be necessary to improve environmental sanitation to eradicate infection with parasites.

Another practical method to combat and prevent iron deficiency anaemia is to increase iron intake in the diet through fortification of a universally consumed dietary article with iron. In the Indian context, salt has been indentified as a suitable vehicle for fortification, as it is consumed by all in a fairly uniform amount. The iron fortified salt has been found acceptable in trial experiments. It has been tested among anaemic children and rural and urban communities. It was observed that the prevalence of anaemia was reduced significantly, when iron fortified salt was consumed over a period of 12 to 18 months. The fortified salt is now being introduced in two districts of one state through public distribution system. The results obtained in this trial will guide the ultimate introduction of iron fortified salt in the country.

Thus a mufti-faceted approach is being used to control and prevent the incidence of iron deficiency anaemia.

Vitamin B-complex Deficiency

The overall prevalence rate of vitamin B-complex deficiency is estimated to be about 20 per cent in India (Figure. 13.5).

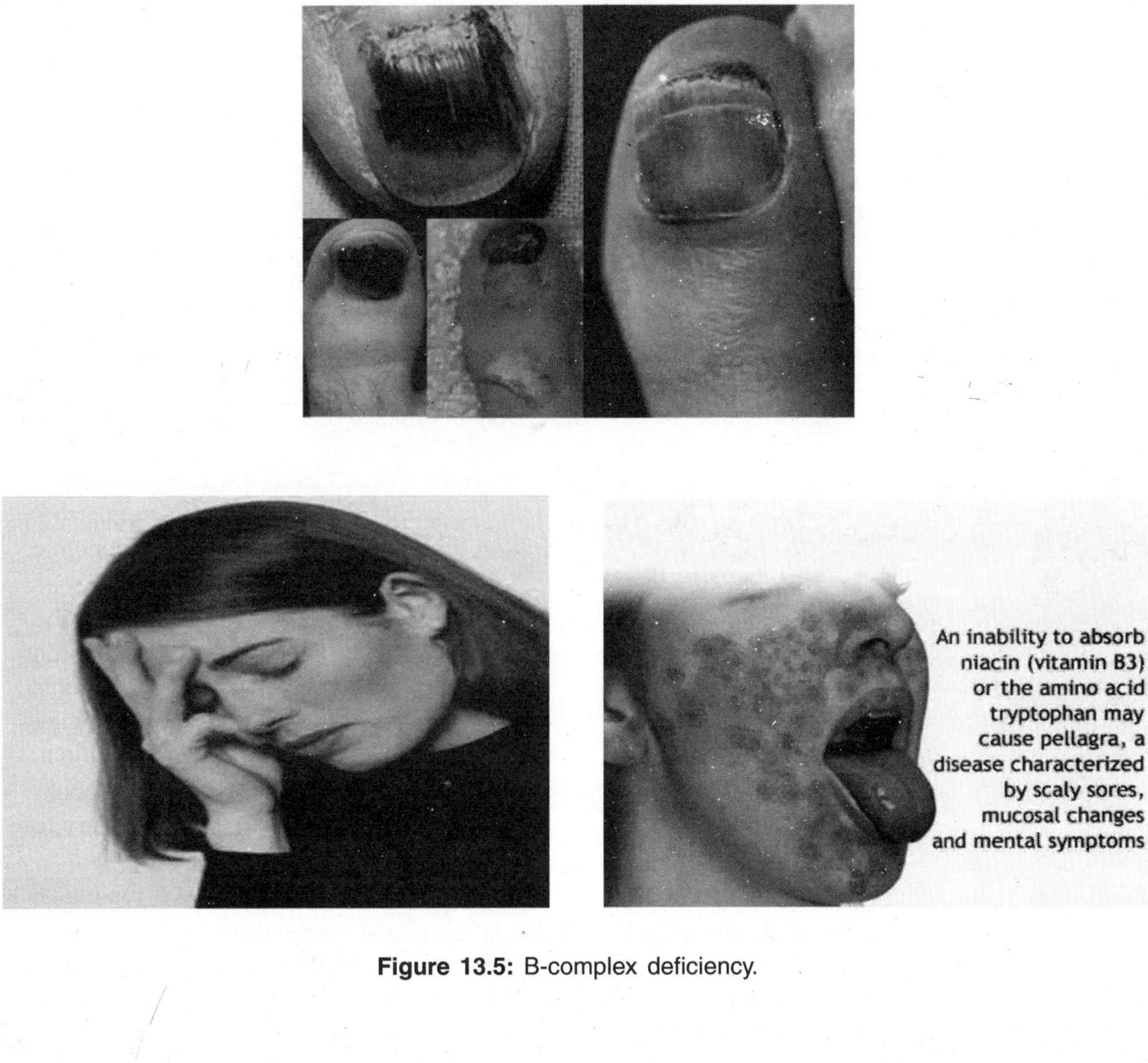

Figure 13.5: B-complex deficiency.

Some of the common symptoms of vitamin B-complex deficiency are sore mouth, sore tongue and erosion at the angles of the mouth. These symptoms are widespread in the community, more so among the ill fed children of the low socio-economic groups.

Low intake of these vitamins in the diet is the primary cause of deficiency. This is compounded by gastro-intestinal infections, such as diarrhoea and dysentery, in which even the little vitamins ingested, may be flushed out before absorption. During pregnancy and lactation, the need for the B vitamins is increased, if there is no extra intake of the vitamins in the diet, deficiency symptoms may occur. It is observed that chronic alcoholics suffer from thiamin deficiency, as the need for thiamin increases with ingestion of alcohol.

Food processing methods affect the vitamin content of the products. For example, thiamin and niacin are partially lost in refining and polishing of cereals, such as rice and wheat. Parboiling helps to conserve these vitamins and in regions of the country like Kerala, where parboiled rice is consumed, incidence of thiamin deficiency, is rare. However, marginal deficiency could still exist in homes in rice-eating areas, if practices such as excessive washing of rice before preparation and discarding the water in which rice is cooked are still prevalent.

Beri-beri, a disease caused by thiamin deficiency, used to be endemic in the coastal parts of Andhra, especially where the rice polished in mills was used. But recent surveys show that there is not much evidence of the disease. The enactment of laws making under-milling compulsory and improvement in the technology of milling may be one of the reasons for reduction of this deficiency. Another reason possibly is the change in dietary habits of the people, such as inclusion of foods such as wheat and wheat products, which contain thiamin, in the diet.

Beri-beri, which is caused by deficiency of thiamin, can affect children as well as adults. The most serious victim is the baby of a mother, who does not secrete enough milk and has little thiamin in her milk. In such thiamin deficient infants, one of the symptoms is the *visible cry* in which the child appears to be crying, *without* making any noise. The disease occurs between the first and fifth month and it strikes suddenly and could result in death, if no adult is looking after the child, when the mother is away at work. Little siblings, who may be in-charge, may not realise that the infant is crying and is in need of nourishment.

In adults, thiamin deficiency could result either in dry beri-beri or wet beri-beri. Dry beri-beri is characterised by arms and legs wasting away, losing their sensation. Wet beri-beri is accompanied by swelling of the limbs and impaired function of the heart; it could ultimately result in death due to cardiac failure.

Riboflavin deficiency is frequently observed in children and some adults among the low income groups in India. The symptoms of this deficiency are cracks in the skin and corners of the mouth, known as *cheilosis*. These cracks have a raw appearance and are slow to heal. The eyes turn red blood shot due to the cornea becoming crowded with capillaries. There is a tendency to avoid bright light. This is known as *photophobia.*

The deficiency of niacin occurs, when the staple cereals are highly refined and intake of *dals* and legumes is meagre. Niacin deficiency is called *pellagra* (rough skin) and it affects the skin, the gastro-intestinal tract and the nervous system. There are rashes on the skin (*dermatitis*), which at times can affect the whole body (Figure 13.6). *Diarrhoea* is another symptom, which is frequently observed. The effect on the nervous system results in lack of alertness, anxiety and irritability. This could slowly develop into a situation in which the person affected may become mentally confused and could even lead to insanity. These severe effects on the nervous system are termed *dementia.* If the deficiency is not corrected in time, it could result in death.

Sporadic incidence of *pellagra,* a disease occurring due to severe deficiency of niacin, is reported from regions, where *jowar* (sorghum vulgare) is the staple. *Jowar* is not low in niacin and tryptophan, the amino acid from which it can be synthesised in the body. The studies carried out at the National Institute of Nutrition, Hyderabad, seem to indicate that amino acid imbalance (high leucine/low iso-leucine) may be the cause of *pellagra* prevalent in the regions, where *jowar* is the staple food. This is more so during lean periods when *jowar* may be the only source of nourishment and other foods to supplement the staple are not available. New strains of *jowar* with lower concentrations of leucine have been developed to prevent the sporadic occurrence of *pellagra.*

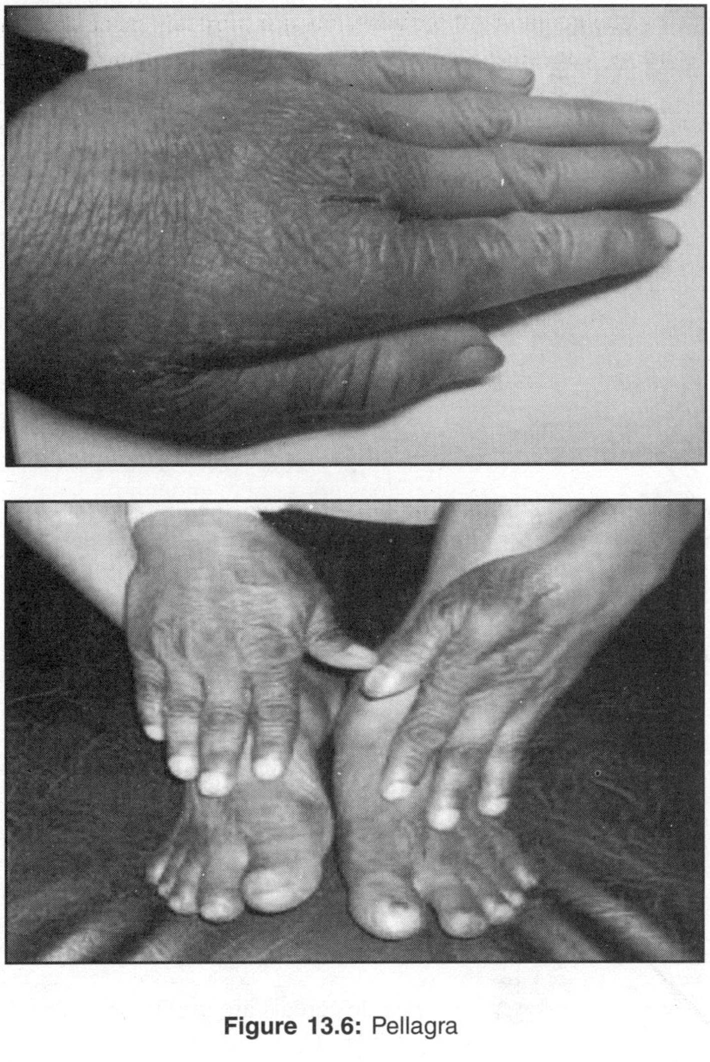

Figure 13.6: Pellagra

Thus thiamin deficiency could be corrected by taking care to see that the rice is either undermilled or parboiled. Inclusion of other foods rich in thiamin such as wheat and wheat products, could help remove thiamin deficiency. Use of milk and milk products and other foods, which are rich sources of riboflavin, could prevent riboflavin deficiency. Groundnuts are a rich source of niacin and very much liked by most people. Use of a combination of cereals, pulses and inclusion of groundnuts, would help prevent B-complex deficiency.

Iodine Deficiency Disorders (IDD)

Iodine deficiency in man leads to a number of disorders, which include goitre, cretinism, mental retardation, deaf-mutism, neuropsychic retardation and myxoedema in elderly. From the socio-economic point of view, endemic neuropsychic retardation may be the most important of the iodine deficiency disorders. One is often struck by the number of superficially normal-looking persons in the endemic regions, who on closer observation are found to be mentally subnormal or have mild defects in their motor function or have both these lacks simultaneously. It has been observed that large numbers of cases of mild or moderate retardation in intellectual, motivational or neuromotor maturation occur in conjunction with endemic goitre. In order to focus attention on this multifaceted nature of iodine deficiency, these disorders are now referred to as *iodine deficiency disorders* and not goitre.

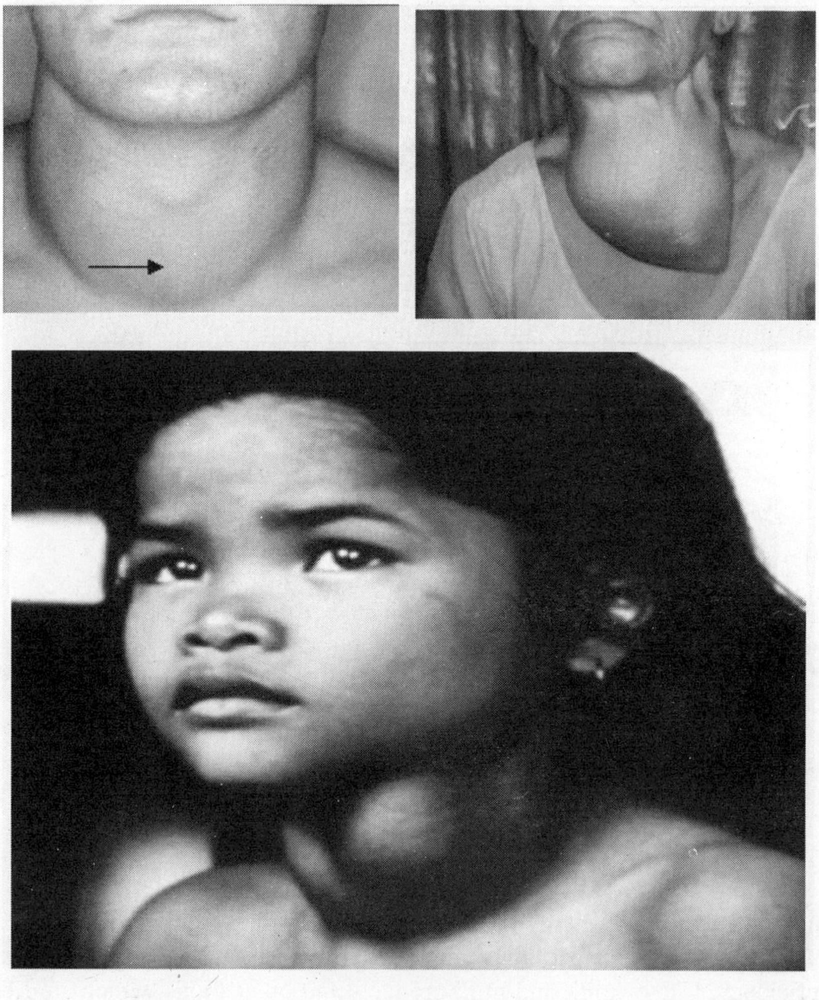

Fig 13.7: Goitre

According to official estimates, 145 million people in India live in the goitre-endemic regions, and 40 million are actually suffering from goitre. Apart from the sub-Himalayan states, which were always known to be goitre-prone, recent surveys have shown the presence of endemic pockets in Andhra Pradesh, Madhya Pradesh, Maharashtra, Bihar, Gujarat end Kerala as well. In all endemic goitre pockets have been observed in 17 states to varying extent.

In the endemic areas of goitre, a number of disorders are observed in children. There is retardation of physical growth, as also lack of mental development. A number of deaf-mutes have also been observed in these area. The ultimate sequel is occurrence of *cretinism* in children born to women, who were so severely depleted that they could not provide iodine for proper development of the foetus. *Cretins* are dwarfs. Cretins have low basal metabolism, and suffer from muscular weakness, dry skin, mental retardation and their skeletal development is arrested. If desiccated thyroid is given to such infant, early enough, there is noticeable improvement in physical development, mental retardation may be less severe, but any damage, which may have taken place in the central nervous system, cannot be reversed.

Goitre results in enlargement of the thyroid gland, as is seen in Figure 13.7. Girls and women are more susceptible to goitre than boys and men.

The simplest way of eradicating iodine deficiency is by addition of iodine to the diet. Salt is a very convenient vehicle for addition of iodine. This procedure is inexpensive and within the technological capability of our country. It has been used since the 1950s. The efficacy of use of iodised salt to reduce the prevalence of IDD has been demonstrated under Indian conditions. However, there have been some difficulties in the distribution of iodised salt and the progress in eradication of this deficiency has been slow.

In view of the high incidence of the deficiency and its deleterious effects on the health of future generation, there has been a new momentum in the implementation of iodine prophylactic programmes in the developing world. In India, the government decided to extend the salt iodation programme to cover the entire country by 1993 in a phased manner.

In view of the high incidence of anaemia in the country, now attempts are being made to fortify salt with both *iron* and *iodine*. The technological aspect of this process have been successfully completed. The doubly fortified salt is going to be field tested in Uttar Pradesh and Andhra Pradesh. When these studies are successfully completed; we can hope to eradicate *two debilitating deficiency* diseases—IDD and anaemia, by use of fortified salt. It will be our duty to educate the public about the importance of using the fortified salt.

Study Questions

1. Discuss the reasons of malnutrition among Indians.
2. What is PEM? Can it be prevented in the home?
3. Write short notes on:
   (*a*) Vitamin A deficiency
   (*b*) Iron deficiency anaemia
   (*c*) Causes of anaemia
   (*d*) Vitamin B-complex deficiency
   (*e*) Iodine deficiency disorders
   (*f*) Cretinism
   (*g*) Fortification of foods.

Practical Work

(*a*) Plan and prepare nutritionally adequate meals for under-nourished toddlers and pre-school children by use of multi-mixes (at least five simple preparations) steamed, soft-cooked and boiled foods.

(*b*) Plan supplementary foods for pre-schoolers, school children and pregnant mothers at low cost.

PART - III

Meal Planning and Management

CHAPTER 14

Food Guides for Selecting an Adequate Diet

Introduction

The RDA are designed to serve as a guide for planning nutrient intakes of population groups. While the RDAs are of considerable value to the professional nutritionist, the RDA have little meaning or utility to the average consumer. Therefore, some effective ways have been devised to interpret recommended daily intakes of nutrients and food composition in a meaningful and useful way to assist the consumer in making nutritionally wise food choices. These are known as food guides.

A diet, which provides all the essential nutrients in sufficient quantities to meet your needs, is an adequate or balanced diet. You need a plan to select an adequate diet so simple and attractive that everyone including you, a young student as also the elderly family members can understand and follow it. The experts have devised such a plan. This practical plan, known as a food guide, helps to ensure good nutrition through proper food selection.

The focus of food guides has been on meeting nutrient needs by selecting various types of food to support optimal growth and development and resistance to disease.

During the past several decades, nutritional deficiency diseases in India have decreased and infectious diseases have been brought under control, health has improved, and life expectancy at birth has increased. But at the same time, chronic and degenerative diseases such as heart disease, cancer, hypertension and diabetes have become leading causes of death and disability in India.

It is felt that the food group approach, exemplified by the basic five food groups represents a model of moderation, a simple and easily applied guide which enables individuals to make nutritionally wise food selections, consistent with their needs.

Development of a Food Guide

Several factors have to be considered in developing a food guide for a large country like India. Some of the relevant factors are:

- Foods plentifully available and normally used in the dietary.
- Normal meal pattern.
- Recommended dietary intakes of nutrients for Indians.
- Need to emphasise some foods because of prevailing nutritional deficiencies in the country.

As you know, food availability and meal patterns vary from one country to another. Therefore, a food guide for one country, such as the Basic Four used in the USA, is not suitable for use in India, where meal pattern, food availability and cost are different. This is one of the reasons for developing a food guide for India.

In developing a food guide, the foods are classified on the basis of their use and the major nutrients which they provide. Such a classification can serve as a guide for the selection and use of foods. For example, cereals, *dals,* and leafy and other vegetables are such classes. Most preparations use oils and fats as a seasoning, and jaggery or sugar as a sweetener. These foods, which enhance food acceptability, can be one of the food groups. This is how the food guide is developed.

The five food groups suggested by ICMR and their nutritional contribution is presented in Table 14.1.

Table 14.1: Nutrient Contribution of the Five Groups

Food Group	*Foods Included*	*Main Nutrients*
1.	Cereals and their products – Rice, wheat, jowar, bajra, ragi, maize, other millets and their products	Energy, protein, iron, thiamin, niacin, fibre
2.	Protein foods – *Dals*, legumes, milk, eggs, fish, poultry, meat and their products	Proteins, energy, calcium, iron, B-complex vitamins, invisible fat, fibre
3.	Protective vegetables and fruits – (*a*) All green leafy vegetables, orange-yellow fruits and vegetables	Carotenoids, vitamin C, iron, calcium, folic acid, fibre
	(*b*) Vit. C-rich fruits and vegetables	Vitamin C, carotene, fibre
4.	Other vegetables and fruits – All gourds, beans, peas, potatoes, onions, etc., all other fruits — banana, apple, melons, grapes, etc.	Supplementary sources of minerals, vitamins and fibre
5.	Oils, fats, sugars and their products – Oils, ghee, butter, vanaspati, sugar, jaggery, jams, syrups	Energy, fat, essential fatty acids Energy

Adapted from ICMR Special Report Series 1991.

Food Guide for Selecting an Adequate Diet

All the foods we use in our daily meals are divided into five groups in the food guide for India. This is presented in Table 14.1. The food groups are chosen because of the specific nutrients contributed by each to the total diet. The food group approach involves grouping foods together on the basis of similarity in composition and nutritive value. Each food group provides certain nutrients. About 40 different nutrients are known to be essential for normal nutrition. If one gets the proper amount of eight key nutrients (that is protein, vitamin A and C, thiamin, riboflavin, niacin, the minerals calcium and iron) through intake of given number of servings of natural foods from each of the food groups, it is expected that the intake of all other nutrients, will be sufficient to meet body needs.

As you may observe, the first column in the table indicates the food group, the third column specifies the amount in one serving, and the last column indicates the minimum number of servings to be taken to meet your nutritional needs. If sufficient amounts of foods from each of the five groups are included in the day's diet, the nutrient requirements of the body will be met. Such a diet is a balanced diet, as it meets the person's nutritional needs. This guide offers the advantages of simplicity in food choices. It is also reasonable assurance of a nutritionally adequate diet.

Let us study each food group in details, so that we can use the food guide as a practical tool. The food guide is presented pictorially in Figure 14.1.

Table 14.2: Food Guide for India (1) (2) (3)

Food Group	*Foods Included*	*Size of Serving*	*Suggested No. of Servings*
1.	**Cereals and Breads** The staples, rice, wheat, *bajra, jowar,* maize, ragi and their preparations	25 g	9–16
2.	**Protein Foods**		
	Dals, legumes, nuts and oilseeds	25 g	
	Milk and milk products	150 g	3–5
	Eggs	1 No.	
	Fish, poultry, meat	30 g	
3.	(*a*) **Protective Vegetables and Fruits** All green leafy vegetables, orange, yellow vegetables and fruits	50–75 g	1–2
	(*b*) **Vit. C Rich Vegetables and Fruits:** Amla[4], guava, drumstick, orange, papaya, mausambi, etc.	50–75 g	1–2
4.	**Other Vegetables and Fruits** All the remaining vegetables such as fruit vegetables, gourds, immature beans and peas, potatoes, onions, etc. Fruits such as bananas, melons, sapota, grapes, apples, etc.	50–75 g	3 or more
5.	**Oils, Fats, Sugars**		
	Oils, ghee, butter, *vanaspati*	5 g	5 or more
	Sugar, jaggery, murabbas, syrups	5 g	5 or more

1. Adapted from ICMR Special Report Series 1991.
2. Mudambi, Sumati R., *Food for Fitness, Nutrition Education* 2, SNDT Univ. Publication, 1971.
3. Mudambi, Sumati R. & M.V. Rajagopal, *Fundamentals of Foods & Nutrition,* Wiley Eastern, Limited, New Delhi 1990, pp. 24–25.
4. Only 10 g will suffice.

Group 1: Cereals and Breads

The first food group includes preparations of cereals and millets, which are the staple foods in India. These foods provide more than half our body's daily need for energy and proteins. In addition, if the whole grain or its flour is used in the preparation, these foods can be a valuable source of thiamin (one of the B vitamins) and iron.

The foods in the group include rice, wheat, *jowar, bajra, makka* (maize or corn), ragi or *nachani,* and cereal products such as *rawa* (*suji* or semolina), rice flakes (*pohe, aval*), *senvaya* (vermicelli), etc. (Figure 14.2).

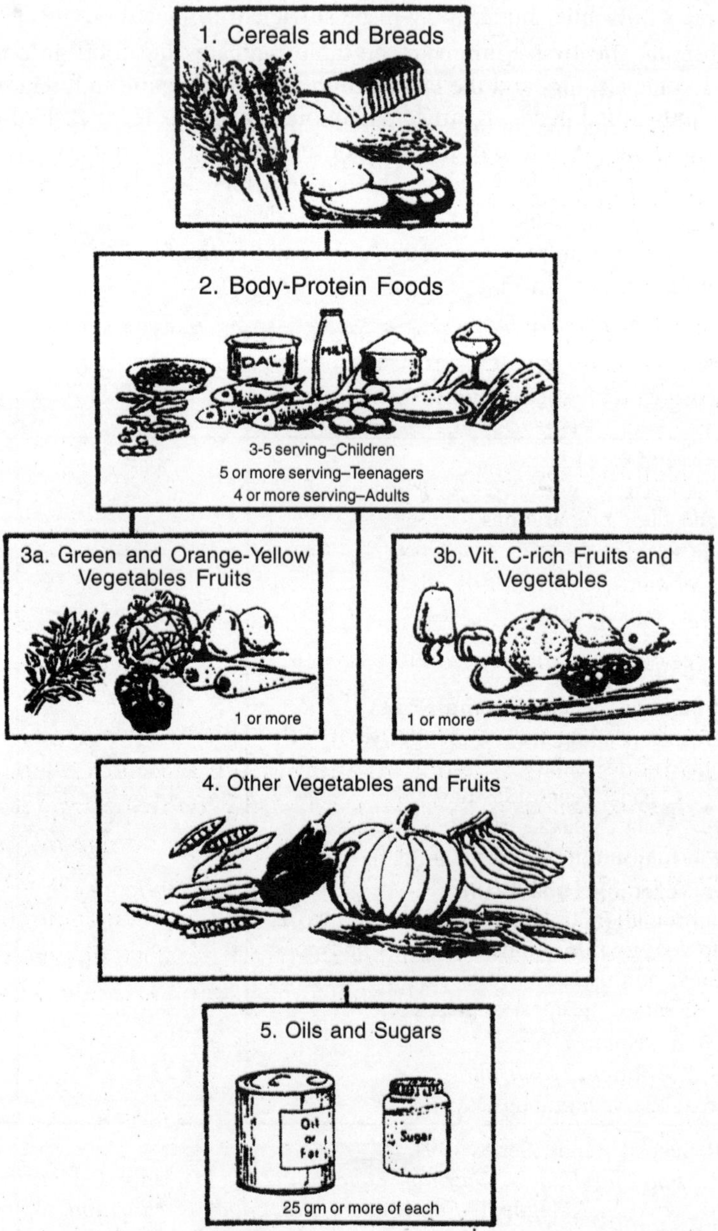

Figure 14.1: A daily food guide.

Serving Size: One serving of these foods is any preparation made from 25g of any cereal or millet. This is equal to half a katori of cooked rice, one medium chapati, two phulkas, two or three puries, half a medium roti or bhakari, two slices of bread, two tablespoons of rice flakes (dry, not soaked), or two tablespoons of ready-to-eat cereal.

Suggested number of servings: A sedentary person may need about ten servings. Those who need more servings of foods in this group are:

- Teenagers.
- Expectant mothers (latter half of pregnancy) and nursing mothers.
- Persons involved in heavy physical work such as lifting and carrying heavy loads, agricultural work, pulling *rikshaw,* etc.
- Players who practice for hours games such as badminton, tennis, squash, *hututu* etc.
- Persons whose hobbies involve intense physical exertion for some hours each day.

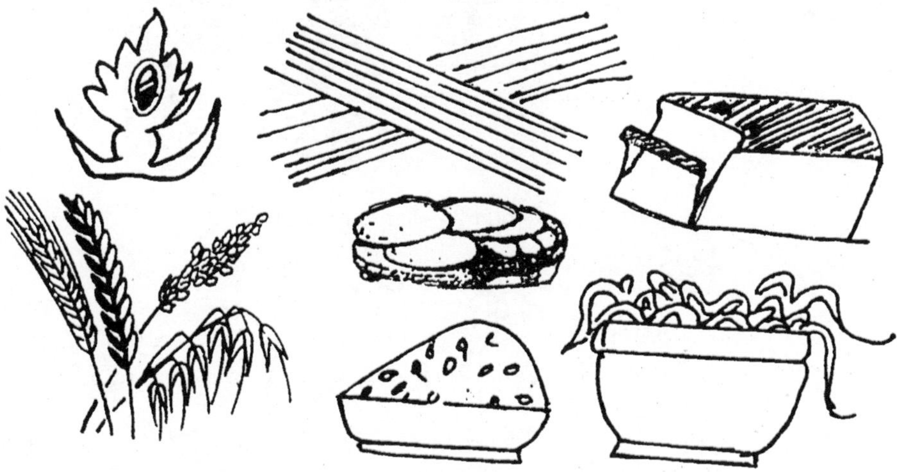

Figure 14.2: Group 1 — Cereals & their products.

Expectant mothers, in the latter half of pregnancy, need two servings more than their normal intake, while nursing mothers may need four servings more than their normal intake.

Group 2: Protein Foods

This group includes the major sources of proteins in our dietary, such as *dals,* whole pulses, milk, eggs, fish, poultry and meat (Figures 14.3 & 14.4). A third or more of our protein requirement is met by these foods. These foods are not only good sources of proteins, but also of minerals and vitamins. *Dals,* eggs, and meat are good sources of iron. In addition, milk is a very good source of calcium and riboflavin. Milk, eggs and liver are rich in vitamin A. These foods also supply part of our requirement of the B vitamins. The foods in this group are varied in their composition. Therefore, the **serving size** of these foods varies as given below:

Dals and whole legumes or pulses	25 g
Milk and milk preparations	1 medium cup or 150 ml
Egg (medium size 50–52g)	1 No.
Fish, meat and poultry	25 to 30 g

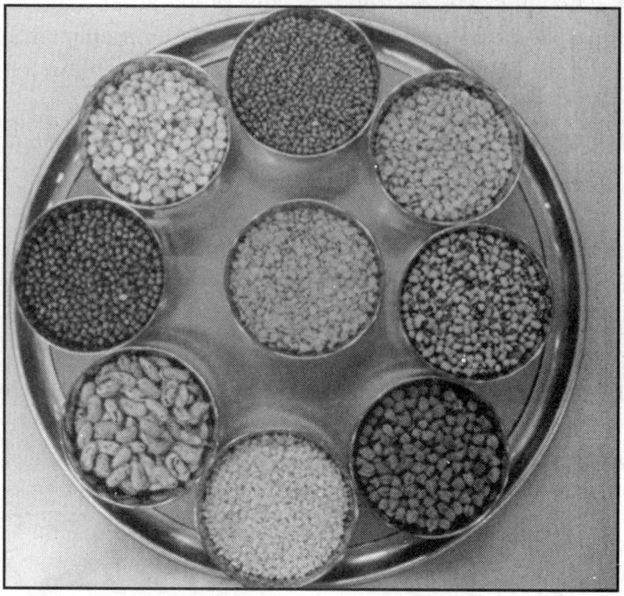

Figure 14.3: Group 2—Plant protein foods.

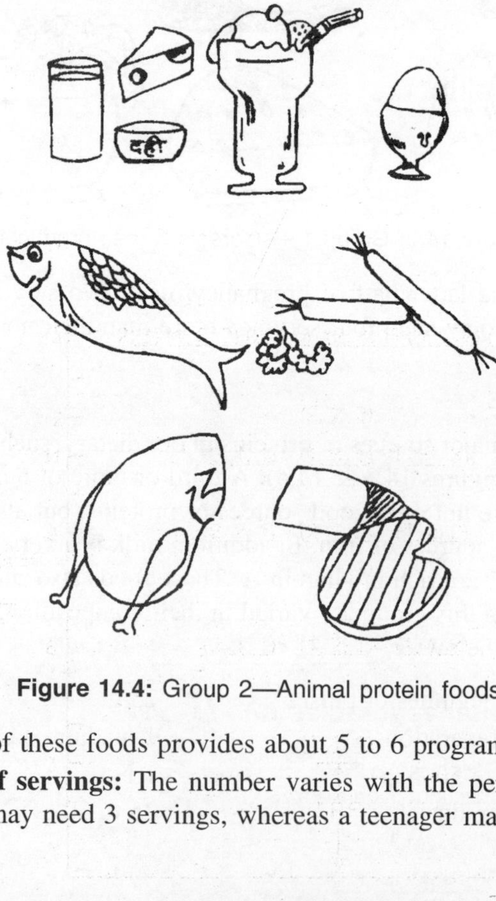

Figure 14.4: Group 2—Animal protein foods.

One serving of each of these foods provides about 5 to 6 programmes of protein.

Suggested number of servings: The number varies with the person's age and body size. For example, an adult woman may need 3 servings, whereas a teenager may need 5 servings.

Group 3: Protective Vegetables and Fruits

The protective vegetables and fruits are rich sources of beta-carotene or provitamin A and ascorbic acid or vitamin C. To emphasise these sources, the group is divided into group 3(a) and group 3(b).

Group 3(a) — Vitamin A Rich Green and Yellow Vegetables and Fruits

This group is a rich source of pro-vitamin A, and includes all dark green leafy vegetables such as *math* (amaranth), *palak* (spinach), *methi* (fenugreek), radish leaves, colocasia leaves, etc. It also includes light green leafy vegetables such as cabbage, onion tops, and lettuce, and yellow-orange vegetables and fruits such as carrots, pumpkin, mangoes, papaya, oranges, cantaloupe (*turbuz*), apricots, etc. (Figure 14.5).

All of these vegetables and fruits share one common component, which brings them together in one group. This component is the yellow plant pigment beta-carotene, which is a precursor of vitamin A. One serving of this group provides 75–120 per cent of our day's need of vitamin A. In addition, the dark green leafy vegetables provide about 50 per cent need for vitamin C.

Serving size: One serving is 50 g fruit, or half a *katori* of cut vegetables or fruit.

Suggested number of servings: It is suggested that one or more servings a day be included from this group. In practice, you can include dark green leafy vegetables three times a week, yellow — orange vegetables two times a week, and light green vegetables two times a week.

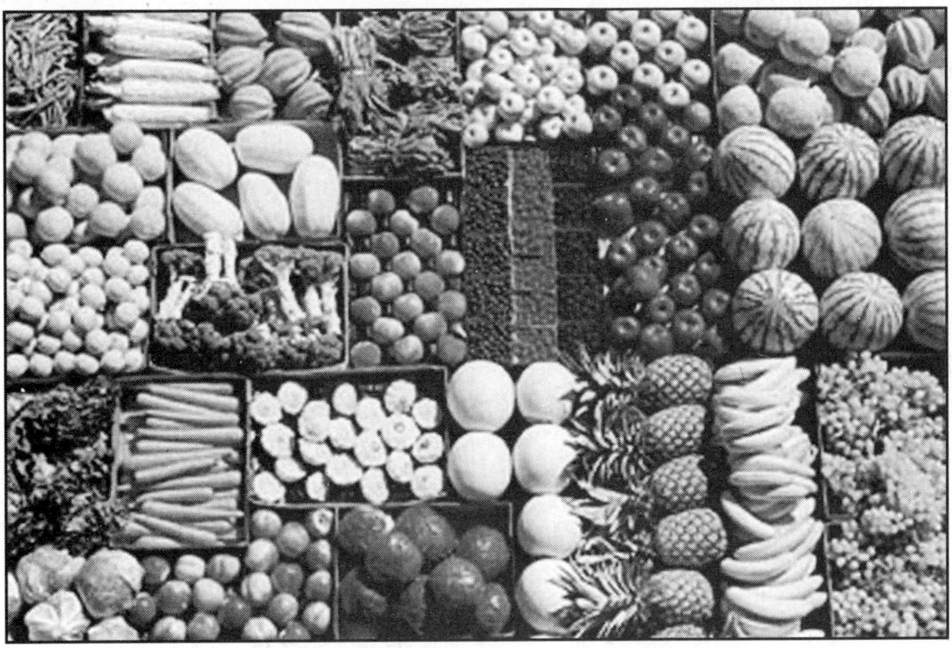

Figure 14.5: Group 3(a) & (b) Protective vegetables & fruits.

Group 3(b) — Vitamin C Rich Vegetables and Fruits

In this group we have rich sources of ascorbic acid, which is also known as vitamin C. A tropical country such as India has a number of rich sources of vitamin C, which are not found in temperate regions, and hence are not mentioned in the Western food guides. For example, the richest source of vitamin C in the tropics is *amla* (Indian gooseberry), which contains ten times as much vitamin C as any citrus fruit. Guavas, cashew apples, *bor,* cabbage, and drumsticks (both leaves and pods) are excellent sources of vitamin C, and contain 3 to 6 times the amount provided by citrus fruits.

Besides these, we have a variety of citrus fruits such as oranges, *mausambis,* pummelo, grapefruits, etc., and other fruits such as papaya, mangoes, pineapples and tomatoes, which are also good sources of vitamin C (Figure 14.5).

Serving size: Generally, one serving is a 50 g portion or half a *katori* of cut vegetable or fruit. There are some exceptions to this serving size, when we choose a very concentrated source. For example, you need only one *amla,* or 25 g of guava or cashew apple to comprise a serving.

Suggested number of servings: One or more servings a day is suggested. One serving provides half or more of our day's need for vitamin C. Please remember that some vegetables and fruits are good sources of both beta-carotene and vitamin C. Some examples of these are cabbage, drumstick leaves, amaranth, oranges, mangoes and papaya. If you choose one of these, you will take care of the servings from both group 3(a) and group 3(b).

Group 4: Other Vegetables and Fruits

All the vegetables and fruits not mentioned as part of Group 3(a and b) are included in this group. The members of this group are:

Fruit and flower vegetables — cucumber, cauliflower, *brinjal,* capsicum, ladies finger, etc.

Gourds — ash gourd, bottle-, snake-, bitter-, ridge-, sponge gourd and others. Immature **beans and peas** — french beans, cluster beans, *chawli,* red gram (tender), *walpapdi*, etc.

Roots and tubers — beetroot, radish, potatoes, yams, onion, etc.

Other Fruits — bananas, melons, grapes, apples, jackfruit, plums, berries, *chikus* (sapota), *pears,* plantain, *litchis, seetaphal, ramphal,* pomegranate, etc. Some of these are depicted in Figure 14.6

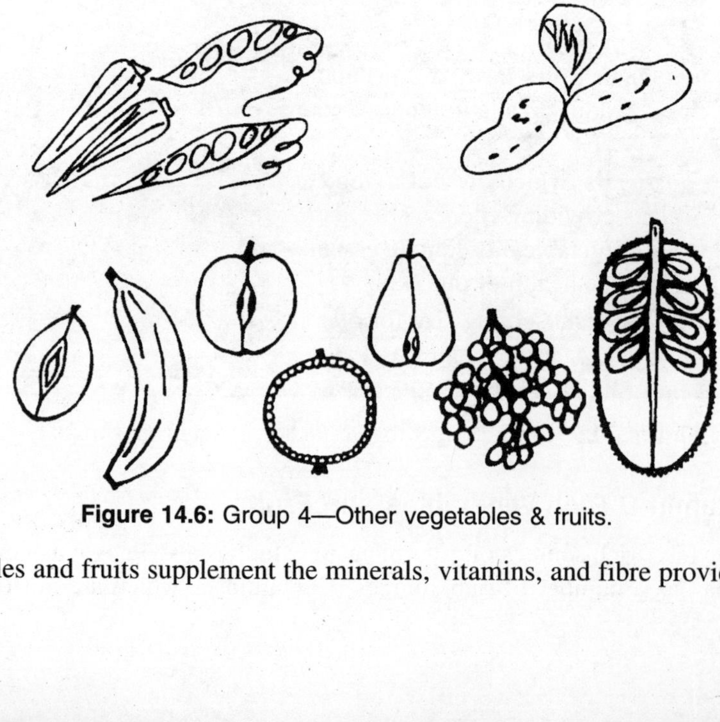

Figure 14.6: Group 4—Other vegetables & fruits.

These vegetables and fruits supplement the minerals, vitamins, and fibre provided by Group 3 in our dietary.

Serving size: One serving is a 50 g or half a *katori* of cut vegetable or fruit.

Suggested number of servings: It is suggested that you should include at least three or more servings from this group each day.

Group 5: Oils, Fats and Sugars

There are two major classes of foods included in this group: **oils and fats** including oils, ghee, butter and *vanaspati,* used as a spread, seasoning or shortening and **sugars.** Sugar, jaggery and preparations such as jams, syrups, etc., are included as sugar serving (Figure 14.7).

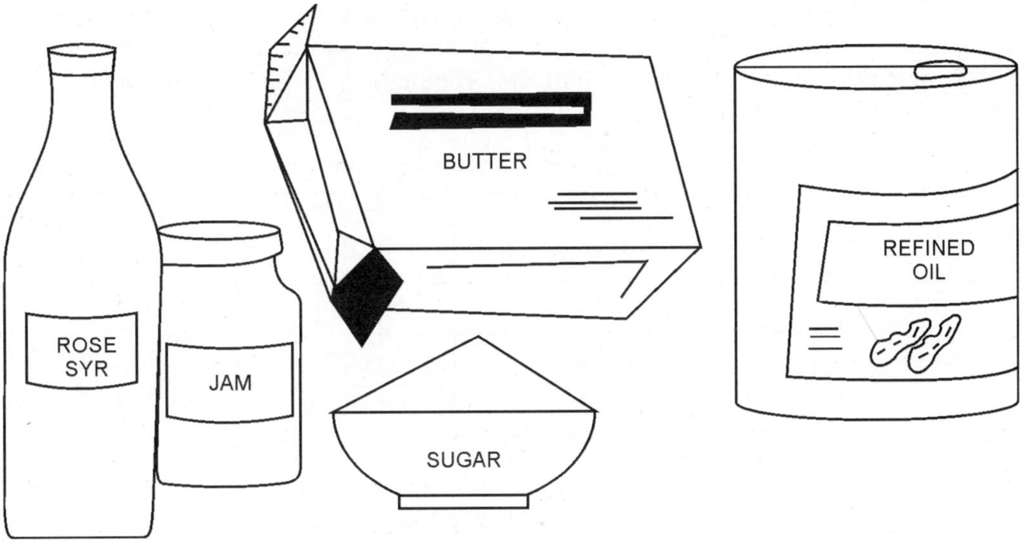

Figure 14.7: Group 5: Sugars, oils and fats

These foods enhance the taste and acceptability of any preparation. All these foods provide energy. Sugars are a readily available energy source, while oils and fats are a concentrated energy source.

In contrast to sugars, which are not a good source of any essential nutrients, oils and fats have other functions besides providing energy. Oils and fats are necessary to transport and utilise fat-soluble vitamins in the body. Vegetable oils contain essential fatty acids, which are necessary for growth in the young and to maintain the health of our skin.

Serving size: A typical serving size for oils, fats and sugars is 5 g, or about a teaspoon, since we use a teaspoon to add sugar to beverages and also to serve oil or ghee.

Suggested number of servings: Since it is not an essential component in nutritional planning, there is no recommended amount for sugar.

Generally, four to five servings a day of fats and oils is suggested. We must include about 10 g or two servings of vegetable oil to meet our need for essential fatty acids. The remaining servings needed can be taken as ghee, butter, or *vanaspati.*

The total amount of oils and fats in the diet will vary with our total energy needs and our energy intake from the other food groups. We must remember that high fat diets are harmful to our health.

Therefore, the ICMR Advisory Committee (RDI, 1991) suggested that the intake of dietary fat be 20 per cent or less of the total calorie intake for adults and 25 per cent for young children.

In summary, how much do we need of these foods? The answer is simple: only as much as is required to meet our nutrient and energy needs and to make the food palatable.

Nutrient Density

Several investigators are individually studying ways to develop an easy-to-use index of nutritive quality of individual foods. One of these is **nutrient density.** Foods which provide nutrients at a greater proportion to need than energy are considered to be nutrient-dense with respect to those nutrients. It is the ratio of the percentage of the recommended allowance of the nutrient to the percentage of the energy requirement in a serving of the food. For example, a serving of cow's milk (150 ml) provides 100 kcal, 180 mg calcium and 0.29 mg of riboflavin. The nutrient density is calculated as given in Table 14.2.

Table 14.2: Nutrient Density Calculation

	Energy Kcal	*Calcium mg*	*Riboflavin mg*
RDA (Man)	2400	400	1.40
Milk — 1 serving	100	180	0.30
Percentage of RDA from milk	5	45	21
Nutrient Density		9.0	4.2

Thus milk is an excellent source of calcium, as it provides 45 per cent of the RDA in one serving and of riboflavin (21 per cent of RDA); while it accounts for only 5 per cent of RDA for energy. Thus the nutrient density of calcium in milk is 9.0 and riboflavin 4.2.

Practical Aspects of Food Selection

While you select foods from each food group, pay attention to the practical aspects of so that you get the most nutrients for each rupee spent for food.

In Group 1, the cereals and breads group, the amount of iron and thiamin in the food preparations varies with how **refined** the grain or flour is. The *chapatis* made from whole wheat flour contain six times as much thiamin as bread made from the same amount of refined wheat flour. Parboiled rice and rice flakes contains more iron and thiamin than milled polished rice. This knowledge can help your selection of foods from this group.

In the protein foods group, there is a wide choice of foods. Group 2 includes all types of *dals* such as *tur, chana, mung, urad, masur* and whole pulses or legumes such as *chawli, rajma, wal, matki, chana,* etc. As you may know, oilseeds such as groundnuts and *til* (sesame) also belong to the legume family and are included in this group. You can choose those *dals* and pulses, which are available at the most reasonable cost. Though all *dals* and legumes are good sources of B-vitamins, *mung* contains more thiamin than others. Groundnuts are a very rich source of niacin.

Milk is another important part of Group 2. Milk is used in a number of preparations, such as tea, coffee, butter-milk, curds, *basundi,* etc. To know the total servings taken, we need to estimate the amount of milk used in these preparations. We may use 15 to 25 g per cup of tea, and 30 g in coffee. A cup of butter-milk may contain 40 to 50 g of milk, while a cup of *basundi* may be made from 2.5 to 3 cups of milk. So you must note the amounts used in order to estimate your total milk intake.

Similarly, when you use eggs in a custard or pudding, you will have to note the recipe and portion eaten to estimate the protein intake. When you buy meat, poultry and fish, note the fatty tissue and bone, and estimate the lean part per kilogramme. If you use these in a curry, record the total volume and the amount served per person to estimate the protein intake.

In Group 3 and Group 4, the cost per serving depends to a great deal on the particular vegetables and fruits selected. The edible portion of vegetables and fruits varies immensely. Estimating the edible portion is important, since this affects the cost per serving.

In Group 3(a), leafy vegetables are sold as a bunch. The entire bunch is not edible; as tough stems and damaged leaves are removed. The amount removed varies with the quality and the variety of the leafy vegetable. A good quality spinach has 90 per cent edible portion while fenugreek *(methi)* may have only 50 per cent.

The edible portion of vegetables and fruits from Group 3(a) and Group 4 also varies greatly. *Amla,* tomato, capsicum, french beans, cluster beans, beetroot, radish, etc., have a 90 to 98 per cent edible portion, while peas, oranges, papaya, mango, and banana have only a 50 to 75 per cent edible portion.

Individuals on a weight reduction regimen should use foods of low nutrient density sparingly, as they provide mainly energy and very little of essential nutrients.

Finally, regular physical activity is extremely important in normal digestion and other body functions in maintaining desirable body weight and in regulating appetite.

Food cost: One of the questions that worries us is: will nutritious food be more costly than our present dietary? The answer to this question is an emphatic **NO.** We can afford nutritious food.

Vegetables and fruits are the foods, which have the greatest variation in price. Those, which are in season, cost the least. The price of a particular variety is lowest at the peak of its season. What is less well known is that **at the peak of the season, each vegetable and fruit has the highest nutrient content, flavour and taste.**

There has been extensive research in this aspect and it has been proved that the **nutrient content and yield** of any plant food, whether it is spinach, beans, oranges or mangoes, **is highest at the peak of the season**. When you buy seasonal foods, you buy the best in terms of quality and nutrients at a reasonable price.

Another point to note is that inexpensive varieties are often more nutritious. Inexpensive fruits such as *amla* and guava are excellent sources of vitamin C, while costly fruits such as apples and grapes are poor source of this vitamin.

Many vegetables and fruits can be grown at home in each season. The home products can be a valuable source of nutrition and improved quality of the diet.

Moderation is a good rule as far as the foods in Group 5 are concerned. As sugar is only a sweetening agent, we would be well advised to consume it in reasonable amounts. If we take too much of it, we will not have place for foods that supply varied nutrients. And although oils and fats play an important role in the dietary, high fat diets are recognised to be harmful to our health.

Use of the Food Guide in Meal Planning and Evaluation

The food guide is a practical tool to use in meal planning and evaluation. Please note the following important points when using the food guide in meal planning:

1. Select foods from each of the five broad food groups.
2. Choose at least the minimum number of servings from each of the food groups.
3. Make choices *within* each group. Please remember that foods in each group are *similar but not identical in food values.*
4. Try to include *at least one food* from Group 2 in each meal.
5. Use seasonal vegetables and fruits to ensure good nutrition at low cost.

The nutritive value of menus planned, using the food guide, for an adult woman and an adult man are given in Tables 14.3 and 14.4. On scrutiny of these tables, it is evident that the nutrient content of the menu is equal to or greater than the recommended dietary allowances (RDA) for an adult woman and man.

Table 14.3: Nutrient Content of Menu for an Adult Woman

Food Group	*Foods and Servings*		*Amount g*	*Energy Kcal*	*Protein g*	*Vit. A value mcg*	*Iron mg*
1.	Rice	(4)	100	340	7		3.0
	Chapati	(5)	125	425	15		14.4
	Bread	(2)	40	98	3		0.2
2.	*Dal*	(2)	50	170	11		2.9
	Milk	(1)	150	100	5	240	0.3
	Egg	(1)	50	86	7	300	1.0
3.	(*a*) Amaranth	(1)	50	22	2	2760	13.0
	(*b*) Guava	(1)	50	24	–		1.0
4.	Brinjal	(1)	50	15	1		0.4
	French beans	(1	50	12	1	65	0.9
	Potato	(1)	75	73	1		0.5
5.	Jaggery		15	57	–	–	1.7
	Sugar		25	100	–	–	–
	Oil		20	180	–	–	–
	Vanaspati		15	135	–	112	–
	Ghee/Butter		10	90	–	73	
	Total intake			1927	53	3,550	39.3
	RDI			1900	45	3,000	32.0
	Excess or deficit			+27	+8	+550	+7.3

You can meet the dietary needs of different members of your family by using the food guide. For example, teenagers can take more servings from Group 1, 2 and 5 to meet the high energy requirements of body building and growth.

Besides using the food guide to plan meals, you can use it to evaluate your present dietary and to modify it, if necessary. It can also be used to check the diet plans of institutions for nutritional adequacy.

The dietary score card is presented in Table 14.5. Five points are awarded for a serving in Groups 1, 2, 4 and 5, with ten points given for a serving in Group 3. The maximum scores for each food group are also given.

This dietary score card can be used to evaluate any menu or diet plan by the following steps:

Table 14.4: Nutrient Content of Menu for An Adult Man

Food Group	*Foods and Servings*		*Amount g*	*Energy Kcal*	*Protein g*	*Vit. A mcg*	*Iron mg*
1.	Rice	(4)	100	340	7		3.0
	Chapatis	(6)	150	510	18		17.2
	Bread	(2)	4 slices	196	6		0.4
2.	*Dal*	(2)	50	170	11		2.9
	Milk	(2)	300	200	10	480	0.6
	Eggs	(2)	100	170	13	600	2.1
3.	(a) *Palak*	(1)	50	13	1	2,790	5.5
	(b) Orange	(1)	50	24	–	0–550	0.1
4.	Brinjal	(1)	50	12	1		0.4
	Cauliflower	(1)	50	15	1		0.7
	Potato	(1)	75	75	1		0.5
5.	Jaggery		20 g	76	–		2.2
	Sugar		20 g	205	–	–	–
	Oil		25 g	225	–	–	–
	Vanaspati Ghee/Butter		20 g	180	–	150	–
	Total intake			2,406	69	4,570	35.6
	RDI			2,400	55	3,000	24.0
	Excess or Deficit			+6	+14	+1,570	+11.6

Table 14.5: Dietary Score Card

	Food Group	*Points Per Serving*	*Maximum Score*
1.	Breads and Cereals	5	45
2.	Protein Foods	5	15
3.	Protective Vegetables and Fruits	10	10
4.	Other Vegetables and Fruits	5	20
5.	Fats, Oils and Sugars	5	10
		Total	100

1. Check if all five groups are included in the meals.
2. Add up the score for each group.
3. If the total score for any group is higher than the maximum permissible score, count only the maximum score for that group.
4. Add the total score and evaluate as follows:

    100 Excellent

    90 Good

    Less than 90 Need to include the missing groups.

You can add more foods from all groups to the minimum servings suggested, in order to make the meals satisfying. One word of caution. Be moderate in the amount of food you take from each group, even if you like a particular food very much. Otherwise, you may not be able to include sufficient amounts of foods from all the food groups.

Also, snacks are an important part of meal planning. The term snack is applied to a wide variety of foods, which are eaten between meals. A number of snacks are offered and eaten at tea, social meetings/get–togethers. The choice of these foods can be important in meeting one's nutritional needs.

Plans for Food Budget

In practice, one must make daily menus for a week and base the food purchase. This step is essential whether the plan is for a single person, a family or an institution. The food purchase is guided by nutrient needs and also the food budget. Planning helps to make the best use of the available money to meet the needs of the family members.

The food choices within a group can be guided by one's food budget. The steps, which help to get the best returns for the food money include:

- Buying the staple foods, *dals* and pulses in bulk, when the prices are competitive, just after the harvest.
- Buying milk and milk products from government dairy outlets.
- Buying fruits and vegetables from main markets at competitive rates.
- Buying seasonal vegetables and fruits.
- Buy sugar, jaggery in bulk from wholesale dealers.
- Buy oil from wholesale depots in bulk.
- Make butter and ghee at home.
- Buy spices in bulk and prepare the spice mix at home.

There are several government programmes, which subsidise foods for the various socio-economic stratas. These include rationed foodgrains, foods given to children in grade schools to ensure attendance, school lunch programmes and supplementary feeding of expectant and nursing mothers. These programmes help to meet the nutritional needs. Some of these reduce the food budget of the family.

Nutrition Education

Nutrition education is a very important input to help people to select an adequate diet. Children learn food selection for diet from their parents. It is good to remember that there is a lot of good in the practices of present-day regional groups that have enjoyed good health and longevity.

In nutrition education, people must be encouraged to retain the existing beneficial food habits and add other foods which may help to meet their nutritional needs. Successful nutrition education reinforces the existing cultural pattern and brings about only qualitative improvement by using available foods.

At present nutrition is taught in limited number of faculties. It should form a part of primary school curricula. The need to prepare authentic, accurate teaching material for use in teaching at all levels can never be overemphasised. It is the responsibility of each person, who learns this subject, to contribute to this effort.

Fallacies about Foods and Nutrition

A fallacy is a false or wrong idea. Wrong ideas about effect of food on health may be spread deliberately by those, who wish to promote their products. Food fallacies exist because of ignorance of basic scientific information about the subject. Food quacks exploit this ignorance to sell their products.

In each region, people have a number of beliefs. These are passed on unquestioned from one generation to the next. It may be wise to consider those in the light of scientific knowledge. Some may have a sound basis, others not.

Some Misconceptions about Carbohydrate in the Diet

Potatoes **are fattening.** No particular food is fattening or otherwise. All energy intake in excess of the body's need is stored as fat. Potatoes provide about a kilocalorie per gram, about the same as cooked rice. It is the oil, used in seasoning or frying that contributes to the extra calories of the potato recipes.

Honey is said to contribute significant amounts of minerals and vitamins. This is not supported by facts.

Similarly, it is said that jaggery contributes more nutrients to the diet than white sugar. Actually it does not, for the amount consumed in the diet is very small.

Sucrose (sugar) is injurious to health, because it is pure refined food. This not true. It is the cheapest sweetener available and hence used in infant milk formulas and in medical preparations. When used in moderation, it is an important source of quick energy. Used in ORS, it is life saving. It is present in many foods in nature such as apples, peas, honey, oranges, etc.

Maida is nutritionally poorer than *atta* (whole wheat flour). This is true.

When grains are milled and refined, the outer coat of the grain is removed. Thus the high quality protein, minerals, B vitamins, all the vitamin E found in the embryo are lost. But the whole wheat flour used to make *chapaties,* millet flours (*bajra, jowar, ragi,* etc.) used to make *roti,* contain all the nutrients in the grain. It is important to know these facts.

General Fallacies

It is said that cooking or processing vegetables results in loss of nutritive value. It is not a correct statement. Cooking and processing improves the texture and flavour of vegetables. The loss of vitamin C in home cooked vegetables is only **minimal** (10 to 15 per cent), if the cooking water is retained.

It is said that water is: "fattening". Water has no energy value. Even if it is held in the tissues, it cannot be converted into fat.

"Natural Foods", "Health Foods" and "Organic Foods"

Most of the food items we buy are natural foods, as these are grown in our garden, or on a tree or produced on a farm. Almost all foods are organic as they contain compounds having carbon, hydrogen and oxygen. Most of the foods we eat provide the nutrients needed, so these can be called health foods. But when these terms are used to describe some foods, the intended meaning is different.

Thus when food is called "natural food", it contains no added chemical, such as preservative, emulsifier or antioxidant.

Food grown on soils fertilised with manure, compost or vermiculture, without addition of any chemical as fertiliser, pesticide or herbicide are called "organic foods". These are generally more expensive than those produced otherwise. But scientific study to evaluate the difference in major nutrient content has shown none. A few minor variations occur indicating that the use of chemical fertilisers can help introduce trace elements as needed but organic fertilisers cannot. Thus there is no advantage due to the use of organic fertilisers.

A food labelled as "Health food" implies that it must have some health-giving attributes, which other foods do not have. This is not the case. Hence the use of the term "Health Foods" is inaccurate.

Study Questions

1. What are the factors which you should consider for developing a food guide?
2. List the five groups into which foods can be divided.
3. Define a balanced diet.
4. List the foods you include in your daily meals. Check and see if you use the amounts of food indicated in the daily food guide. If you don't list the foods that are missing or present in smaller amounts.
5. List the steps to be taken to conserve the food budget.
6. Why is nutrition education important?
7. Write short notes on:
    - Food fallacies.
    - Misconceptions about carbohydrate foods.
    - Organic foods.

CHAPTER

15

Meal Planning for the Family

"I never knew a man who did not like a kitchen fire,
Nor a woman, if she be away awhile, but would tire
Of inns and servants and would long to be
Back in her own kitchen, buttering toast and making tea."

(Grace Nell Crowell 'Kitchen' from White Fire, the South West Press, by permission of Mrs. Crowell and The Turner Company, Dallas, Texas)

MEAL PLANNING involves deciding what to eat each day at each meal. It takes thought, effort and use of knowledge acquired in the earlier chapters. As the family's well-being and health are dependent on how well they are fed, it is a challenge to every meal manager to meet it. It proves to be a satisfying and rewarding experience, when done well.

Each day we eat three meals and perhaps an additional snack. The various members of the family partake of these meals. We need to plan the meals to ensure that the needs of each family member are met. The plan can be flexible to take advantage of lower prices of seasonal foods, and to meet the needs and choices of your family. But it has to be a plan. Meal planning can be done by the family as a joint project. The family members can discuss the meal plans, the food budget and the actual preparation and help in making the plans work. Such co-operation will lead to greater acceptance and enjoyment of the meals. In Figure 15.1, the four steps involved in meat planning are pictorially depicted.

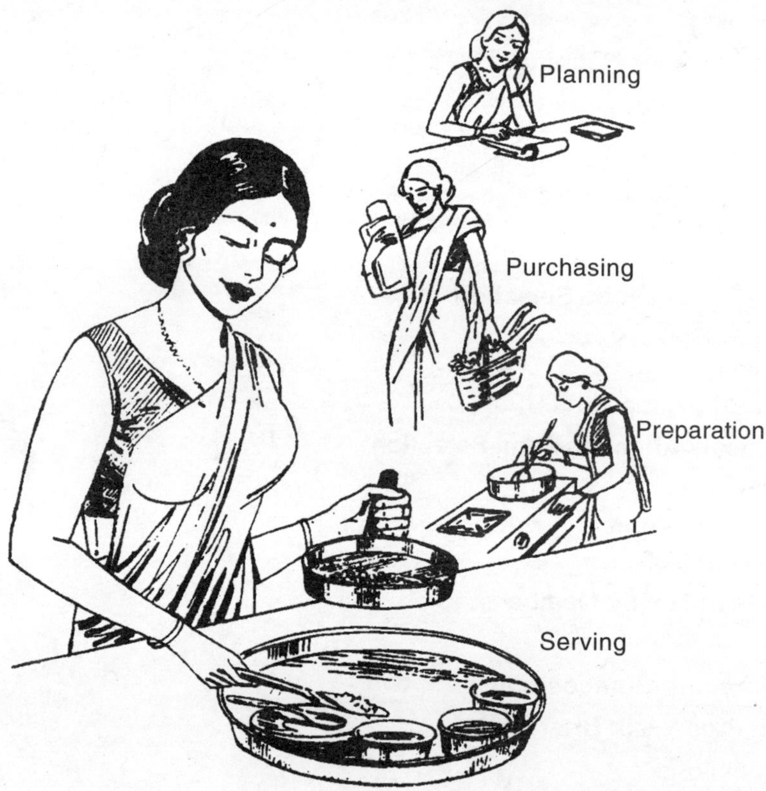

Figure 15.1: The family's meals — planning, purchasing, preparing and serving.

Meal Planning

You must take into account the family members, their ages and occupation in planning family meals. The food guide presented in Figure 15.2 will help in selecting foods. This will help you to decide the amounts of foods needed from each group. As you learnt earlier, there is a large variety in the kinds of foods within each food group, so it is possible to choose foods, which the family members like from each group. It is important to use seasonal vegetables and fruits, as these are not only of high quality, but are available at reasonable price.

The selection will also be guided by the schedules of the family members. All that you eat and drink at home or outside, the cup of tea/coffee taken daily, the snacks served at meetings, the *chana-dana,* which children eat in short recess, all form part of the daily food intake of the members. Planning for these or at least an awareness of these, makes it easier for you to pick the foods that add up to meet the needs of various family members.

Meal planning is intimately connected with food purchase. In purchasing food, consider the space available for storage and the conditions of storage. For example, if the space is limited, you may have to purchase food often. If you have a refrigerator, you can buy vegetables and fruits once a week. Thus now often you purchase foods is dependent on the space and conditions of storage.

Objectives in Meal Planning

In planning meals your aim is:

1. to satisfy the nutritional needs of the family members, according to their age and occupation.
2. keep expenditure within your family's food budget.
3. to decide amounts of foods to be purchased from each food group.
4. to consider family size and composition.
5. To consider food storage space, conditions of storage, and decide how often you need to purchase various foods.

In order to translate the meal plan into meals that meet the family's needs, the following additional steps have to be taken —

6. Prepare a food purchase list, taking the food preferences of members into account.
7. Use methods of preparation, which retain nutrients, without sacrificing palatability.
8. Serve meals, which are appetising and attractive and fit in the schedule of the members.
9. Manage the time, energy and available materials efficiently, with the help of the family members.

If you make a weekly plan for all meals, you can save time, energy and money. It will also help you to avoid monotonous meals.

Nutritional Adequacy

The first prerequisite of a good meal plan is that it should meet the nutritional needs of the whole family. This objective can be achieved by selecting foods according to the daily food guide (Figure 15.2). Thus each meal must include:

Cereals and their products	To provide energy and proteins.
Dals, milk, egg, fish or meat	To supply proteins, B-vitamins and some minerals.
Protective vegetables and fruits	To provide vitamins A & C, minerals and fibre.
other vegetables and fruits	To supplement nutrients provided in Group 3
Sugars, oils and fats	To provide energy, satiety and improve palatability.

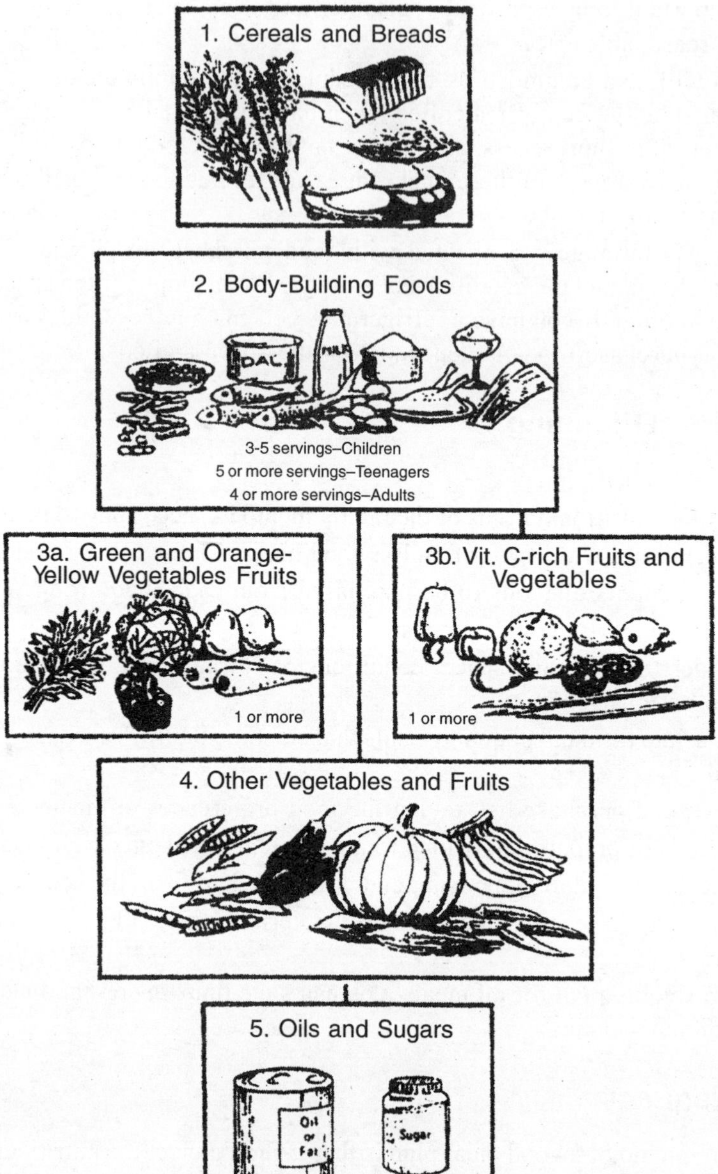

Figure 15.2: A daily food guide.

If you include the suggested number of units from each group, you can be reasonably assured of meeting needs for protein, vitamins and minerals. The variety chosen within a group will be determined by the taste preferences of the family members.

Specific requirements for various periods of the life-cycle are made in the recommended dietary intakes. These can easily be fulfilled by using more units from the food groups, which provide these nutrients. For example, a teenager may need six units from group two to meet his protein needs for growth and maintenance, but an adult may need only three. An older person may be served the carrot salad in grated form, while other members may be served carrot sticks; salads may be made without oil seasoning for an overweight member, while others can have their salad seasoned. These are some of the practical ways to suit the family meals to the nutritional needs of individual family members.

Food is a basic necessity of life. It is important that sufficient part of the monetary resources are set aside to meet the food needs of the family. If the allowance for food is low, there is a greater need to plan meals carefully and to get the right foods to ensure nutritional adequacy for each member of the family.

Food Costs

You must remember that the price of food is not related to its nutritional contribution to the diet; it is ruled by the law of demand and supply. The economics of food consumption is a broad subject, but it is important to plan meals and buy food wisely so that maximum benefit is derived from the money spent. First of all you must decide the total amount of money you can spend for food purchase. Then you can select foods, which can be bought with the available money. Let us consider the economic sources of various nutrients.

Energy Foods: In Table 15.1 you can find the comparative cost of 100 calorie portion of various foods. As you may observe, grains as well as starchy roofs are economical sources of food energy. Grains supply proteins in addition to energy.

Fats, oils, sugar and jaggery, which are used to make food palatable, are also sources of energy, but these are expensive. Butter, ghee and *vanaspati* are good sources of Vitamin A.

Protein Foods: Table 15.2, the cost of supplying five grammes of protein from various foods is indicated. As you can see *dals,* whole beans and peas are the cheapest protein foods. Dehydrated fish may be another inexpensive source. If you live near a river or the sea, fresh fish may be available at competitive cost. Less expensive cuts of meat also can be used as protein. In the rural areas, eggs and poultry is produced at home by some, thus ensuring economy.

Table 15.1: Comparative Cost of Energy-supplying Foods

Food	*Cost/kg or liter*[1] *(rupees)*	*Quantity supplying 100 Kcal*	*Cost of 100 Kcal (paise)*
Wheat	22.00	30g	0.66
Rice	30.00	30g	0.90
Jowar, Ragi, *Makka*	38.00	30g	1.14
Sugar	29.00	25 g	0.75
Oil, Refined	80.00/lt	11g	0.92
Vanaspati	60.00	11g	0.75
Butter	275.00	13g	3.59
Ghee	286.00	11g	3.08
Milk, toned	28.00/lt	150g	4.20
Eggs	36/dozen	1.4 eggs	4.20

1. Based on retail prices in Pune, May, 2011.

Table 15.2: Comparative Cost of Protein Foods

Food	*Cost/kg or liter*[1]	*Quantity supplying 5 g protein*	*Cost of 5–6 g protein (paise)*
Dal, any one	36.00–74.00	25 g	0.90–1.85
Pulse	45.00–55.00	30 g	1.35–1.65
Wheat	22	50 g	1.10
Rice	30.00	75 g	2.25
Milk, toned	28.00/lt	150 g	4.20
Eggs	36/dozen	1 egg	3.00
Meat/Fish	100.00/kg	30 g	3.00

1. Based on retail prices in Pune, May, 2011.

As you know, the choice of foods used will depend on your food acceptance pattern. Milk is an important source of protein, though an expensive one. Some milk is needed at every stage of life.

Vegetables and Fruits: Vegetables and fruits are important sources of minerals and vitamins. Green leafy vegetables are a rich source of provitamin A, vitamin C, and the minerals calcium and iron. The fruits *amla,* guavas, citrus fruits, pineapple and tomatoes are a good source of vitamin C. Some vegetables and fruits are seasonal, while others are available throughout the year at a competitive cost. Various greens are available throughout the year at very little cost. Vegetables and fruits at the peak of the season are not only inexpensive, but are of high quality in terms of acceptability and nutrient content. Tables 15.3 and 15.4 give the cost of supplying a fourth of day's need for provitamin A and vitamin C from various vegetables and fruits.

Table 15.3: Comparative Cost of Vitamin A Foods

Food Source	*Cost/100 g*[1] *EP (paise)*	*To provide 1/4 RDI*[2]	
		wt. in gm	*Cost in Rupees*
Vegetables and Fruits—green and yellow			
Green leafy vegetables	3.50	8–15 g	0.28–0.52
Cabbage	3.00	62 g	1.86
Carrots	3.20	40 g	1.28
Orange	3.00	66 g	1.98
Mango	3.00	27 g	0.81
Fats			
Vanaspati	6.80	25 g	1.70
Butter	27.60	20 g	5.52
Ghee	28.00	18 g	5.00
Animal foods			
Milk	2.8/lt	375 g	10.50
Eggs	6.00	1 egg	3.00
Liver	10.00	15 g	1.50

1. Prices of Foods in Pune, May, 2011.
2. EP—Edible portion.
3. RDI—Recommended Dietary Intakes.

In the rural areas it is possible to grow the vegetables and fruits needed in one's kitchen garden. In some parts of India it is customary to plant fruit trees around the house as soon as one plans to build a house; thus ensuring a supply of fruit for the family.

The food budget of rural agricultural families is different from that of the city dwellers. the staple foods are normally available from the farms. With a little planning, they can produce the *dals,* vegetables and fruits also for home consumption, so that the quality of their diets may improve.

In estimating food cost, it is good to note that a number of non-food items are purchased at the food store, for example, toilet soap, hair oil, cleaning agents and equipment. These may appear on the bill, and must be subtracted from the total to get a correct idea about money spent for food. But the money spent for snacks at work or in the school must be added to the food costs of the family.

Factors Affecting Food Selection

Food Acceptance: Each one of us has certain foods we like; certain foods we do not like. But food tastes can be cultivated. As we move from one place to another, we can enlarge our acquaintance of foods, by trying the foods of that place. It helps us to enjoy our new environment. Learning new ways of **using** availables foods is another way of bringing variety in meal planning.

Tradition: Most of our food selection is influenced by tradition, be it national, regional or family traditions. A lot of traditional selection is based on experience, but sometimes some poor practices become part of a tradition and must be dispensed with.

Table 15.4: Comparative Cost of Vitamin C Foods[1]

Food Source	*Cost/100 g EP[2] (Rupees)*	*To provide 1/4 RDI[3]*	
		wt. in g	*Cost in Rupees*
Amla	4.80	2 g	0.10
Guava	2.50	6 g	0.15
Coriander leaves[4]	5.00	22 g	1.10
Cabbage[4]	3.00	22 g	0.66
Capsicum[4]	2.00–4.00	22 g	0.44–0.88
Knol-khol/bittergourd[4]	4.00	30 g	1.20
Drumsticks[4]	100	22 g	22
Cauliflower[4]	4.00–6.00	45 g	1.80–2.70
Banana	3.00–4.00	60 g	1.80–2.40
Mausambi	3.00	25 g	0.75
Tomato	1.00–4.00	50 g	0.50–2.00

1. Based on prices in Pune, May, 2011.
2. EP-Edible Portion
3. RDI-Recommended Dietary Intakes.,
4. Amount of cooked vegetable is indicated.

It is a good practice to evaluate traditional food selection in the light of knowledge of nutrition. Thus we can retain good foods habits and change those that result in poor selection.

Food Misinformation: Food is an important topic of conversation, articles in newspapers, magazines and even books. You see and hear about it in advertisements too. Some of this information may be useful, but a *large part* may not be. False ideas about food are common, as also wrong information. But many of these originate in ignorance. But as you learn about food composition you will be able to use this knowledge to guide food selection. It is your duty to spread the knowledge gained to others so that they discard false ideas about food, which interfere with their food acceptance and health.

Other Factors Affecting Meal Planning—Skill in Food. Preparation: Skill in food preparation is an essential part of an acceptable, enticing meal. Skill in food preparation is acquired by practice. Ingenious combinations improve acceptability of foods, add to variety and thus make food enjoyable. For example, some dark green leafy vegetables have strong flavour, which can be diluted by addition of other, milder foods, or modified by addition of other ingredients. *Methi* leaves are bitter, if ground *dal* or *besan* is added to it the bitter flavour is diluted and the mild flavour of the product is enjoyable; similarly addition of grated coconut or jaggery also makes the flavour of the finished vegetable acceptable. It is this skill that makes the flavour of the finished vegetable acceptable. It is this skill that makes a hot soup at home more appetising than a meal at a first class restaurant. One can develop skill by observing people who perform well and by practice. It is important to try and perfect the skills acquired, until it becomes a habit.

Variety: The enjoyment of food can be enhanced by learning ways to prepare dishes from other regions of India and foreign countries. If a new dish prepared once a week, the monotony in meals is avoided.

Availability of Foods

It is important to study the seasonal variation in availability of foods. In each season one can find some foods from each group. Using seasonal foods reduces cost. Some vegetables and fruits can be grown in the kitchen garden. Some foods like beans, rice, wheat can be purchased soon after the time of harvest, when the price is reasonable, and stored for the whole year.

Home Production: If some of the vegetables and fruits are grown at home, these need to be used in meal planning. Some of the fresh condiments such as coriander leaves, curry leaves, green chillies, mint and different leafy vegetables can easily be grown at home.

In rural areas where most of the staples are produced at home, meal planning helps to decide realistically the amount of food the family should retain for home use, so that the needs of the family are met. It also helps to decide what vegetables and fruits can be grown economically to improve the family's meal pattern, without adding to the food cost. When fruits and vegetables are produced in excess of the family needs, the surplus can be sold.

Schedules of Family Members: When planning a meal pattern, one needs to think of the schedules (time-table) of the family members,—meal times and the number of meals eaten at home and those that are eaten away from home. If packed lunches are made for the man of the house and children at school, the menus need to be modified to ensure that the items can be packed and the menu is appetising even when cold.

Time available for meal preparation and the help available, in food preparation, be it from children or hired help, may affect the choice of foods bought and the menu.

Family Size and Composition

The *family size* affects the foods that can be served. It is known that the money spent for food per person decreases as the family size increases, when the family income remains constant. Such is the case when there are several closely spaced children in the family. As the money available to the family does not change with the size of family, a larger part of it has to be spent to meet the food needs. Staples such as wheat, rice, *jowar* are bought in larger amounts, but the amount of milk, vegetables, fruits bought may decrease. Thus the quality of the diet is lowered. In extreme cases, it may not be possible to meet the food needs of the family members resulting in partial starvation. As this happens to a large number of families, which migrate to cities in hope of improved living conditions, it is important to emphasise the relation of family size to family's food intake and health and promote small family norms, in the interest of better health and survival. Table 15.5 indicates the availability of milk as related to the per capita income.

Family composition affects the kinds and amounts of food needed and the pattern of meals served. For example, when children are below five years of age, more milk is needed, the number of meals are more, as the child cannot take large amounts at a time. As the child grows the meal pattern changes to accommodate the school hours and the need to pack lunch or snack may arise.

Adolescents in the family need more food than adults, as they need large quantities of food to support growth and their activities. The food needs of the adult members will depend on how active they are. Older members of the family need lesser amounts of food, but may need change in consistency, due to faulty teeth or lack of teeth.

As festivals call for special menus, it is important to note these in making the food list.

Table 15.5: Income and Milk Purchased per Head

Per capita monthly income (in rupees)	*Milk purchased (ml. per head per day)*
< 100	245
101–160	316
161–240	377
241–400	441
> 401	618

Planning Process in Brief

It is necessary to plan on a monthly basis. There are five main steps in meal planning:

1. Make a list of foods from each food group, that are available in the market.
2. Check the prices and decide which of the foods from each group fit in the food budget on the basis of the number of family members.
3. Estimate the day's needs for all the family-members on the basis of the Daily Food Guide and calculate the month's food needs from it.
4. Make a list of foods to be purchased monthly, fortnightly, weekly and daily.
5. Plan menus to meet the daily needs of the family.

It is possible that some changes have to be made towards the end of the week to use up foods, which may not keep. Sometimes an additional guest may result in change of menu.

If the homemaker must prepare food, the plan should be made with economy of time and energy in view. Making a food list ahead of time helps in conserving shopping time. Some dishes may be made ahead of time, e.g., making *halwa* or *laddu* the day before the party. The plan must be related to facilities available for food preparation. Some amount of standardisation occurs in the meal plans of each family, which helps in efficient management of meals.

Study Questions

1. List the objectives in planning meals. How can you ensure nutritional adequacy in meals?
2. Discuss how to meet the nutritional needs at minimum food costs.
3. What are the non-nutritional factors, which affect meal planning? Discuss.

CHAPTER 16

Meal Planning for Various Age Groups

MEAL PLANNING for the family has been discussed earlier. It was mentioned that the needs of individual family members must be considered in estimating the food needs of the family. As the family consists of various age groups in various physiological states, let us consider the needs of each stage of life, starting with adulthood.

Adulthood

Adulthood represents the steady state in life, when a person would have completed his/her growth in terms of body size. The nutritional needs are for maintenance of body functions. The energy needs in adulthood are mainly to sustain body functions and activity. The protein requirement is to make good the wear and tear and the losses, which occur as a result of normal life processes. Thus adult stage is taken as a norm and requirements in other stages are discussed in relation to it.

Adulthood also represents the productive stage of life. Therefore, it is important that the nutritional needs of an adult be met adequately, so as to keep up vitality and a positive attitude in life, which are essential for optimum productivity.

Changing Food Habits: Each of us have foods, which are our favourites. These are served on special occasions such as birthday, parties or other celebrations. Though one should take the likes and dislikes of family members into account in meal planning, we should not allow our preferences to rule our diets. Allowing people to develop a restricted food pattern may lead to a poorly balanced diet and could be a social disadvantage. Trying to like new foods enlarges one's food enjoyment, social experience as well as diet.

Food Selection: The selection of foods is made according to the daily food guide. The amounts of foods included from the various groups will depend on the body size and activity of the individual. Thus a labourer, who is very active may need more cereals and oils and fat to meet his/her energy needs as compared to a sedentary person, who is involved in desk work. The foods selected need to be used in the day's meals, which fit into the daily schedule of the person.

Breakfast an Important Meal: The first meal in the day is important as about 12 hours elapse between dinner and breakfast. About one fourth to one third of the day's food should be taken for breakfast. Rural agricultural families normally have a hearty breakfast. But in the cities the pattern varies from region to region. Some regions have a certain definite pattern of breakfast and some preparations are clearly associated with breakfast, e.g., *idli-chatni, upma* are considered as breakfast foods in Tamil Nadu and Kerala, roasted *ragi* flour and milk, in Mysore, *dahi-pohe, doodh-pohe* in western Maharashtra, *paranthe* and *lassi* in Punjab, etc.

In many urban families, it is customary to eat the fluid and soft dishes (such as rice, *dal, dahi,* salads, etc.) in the meal at about 8.30 to 9 a.m. and pack and carry other items of the meal (such as *chapati,* bread and butter, sandwiches, vegetables, *chole, usal,* pickle, etc.) in a lunch pack to work. Thus in the cities, whatever food is eaten before leaving home for work constitutes a breakfast. It usually consists of a cereal preparation, *dal*/fish/meat preparation, and butter milk/milk, vegetables, etc.

Many persons, especially housewives and girls omit breakfast to reduce their food intake. But it is known that a person, who eats a good breakfast, performs better at work and is likely to eat less during the day. A person who skips breakfast has a tendency to take snacks or eat more at lunch and dinner, thus increasing the total food intake. Protein content of snacks is usually low and the satiety value is also low. Further comparative studies have shown that those who have good breakfasts have a greater work output and are more alert.

As many people in the cities and villages have to carry packed lunch, or select one from a limited menu in snack counters, it is very important to plan breakfast to supply foods, which are sufficient both in quality and quantity.

Lunch Often a Poor Meal: About one-third of day's food intake should be contributed by lunch or the noon meal. Lunch should be counted as a part of food plan for the day, and not just a snack to stave off hunger till dinner time.

A good lunch should provide protein and protective foods, not just starchy foods. A common eating pattern of many office workers is to have any available snack such as *samosa, batata-vada, pakodas,* etc., or bread and butter and tea at the office canteen or at a cafe nearby. This is sometimes improved when milk or a milk product like *lassi*, cold milk drink is taken instead of tea. Too often the lunch pack from home may consist of *chapati,* bread and butter or *puri*-jam, *chapati*-pickle or *chutney,* or potato *bhaji,* which are accompanied by a cup of tea/coffee. While these foods may be more filling than the snack bought at work, they meet energy needs, without supplying much protein and protective foods. It is important to include a serving of protein foods at lunch. Selection of vegetables or fruit may help meet part of the need for protective foods.

Lunch, whether served at home or packed and carried to work, or purchased at the place of work, should be planned or chosen with care. A missed meal is not easily made up. Consistent neglect of this important meal may affect the individual's performance at work, behaviour with colleagues and attitude to life adversely.

The lunch should be planned in relation to the other needs, so that it supplies a fair share of the day's nutrients through the foods selected. A suggested daily food plan for the three meals is given in Table 16.1. The lunch can be sent with a dabawala or carried personally.

Dinner: This is the main meal of the day, which may be served at noon or night, depending on the family's schedule or custom. It is good to plan a menu for dinner which helps to balance the total intake in terms of energy, protein as well as other nutrients for the day. One may prepare an additional vegetable and salad, one may also add a dessert or sweet, to add to the variety. The active members may eat more heartily of the cereal dishes, while the person who has to watch his weight may eat more of salads and vegetables. As this is a leisurely meal, which is eaten by the family together, it contributes much to the feeling of belonging, enjoyment of the company and relaxation.

Snacks: It has become an accepted practice in most offices and factories for workers to have a tea break. Most of the canteens and cafes, which serve tea and coffee, also serve snacks, most of which are shallow or deep fat fried preparations. Thus the tea break provides an opportunity to eat as well as drink. The choice of the snack may decide if it will provide only energy or energy plus other nutrients. Dishes such as *batata-vada,* vegetable patties, *pakodas* may contribute little but calories, and may dull the appetite, while *dahi-vada, idli-sambhar, misal,* sweetened milk, *lassi,* icecream, *chana-dana,* fruits, may provide some nutrients in addition to energy.

It is not possible and desirable to make rigid rules about between meals eating. It may be wise to choose such snacks as add to the nutrient intake, especially when these are intended to meet wholly or partly the need for a meal. Some suggestions for these snacks are milk or milk beverages, cereal-*dal* or *dal*-milk or cereal-milk mixed dishes, salads and fruits.

Table 16.1: Food Plan for a Day.

The daily food plan	*Sample menu*
Milk (2 servings) *Dal* (2 servings) Vegetables (3 servings) Fruit (1 serving) Cereals (10 servings) Sugar Oil, fat	**Breakfast** *Shira/upma,* milk, banana, tea **Lunch** Rice, *chapati, dal,* vegetable beans, carrot and cabbage mixed salad, *dahi/lassi*
Breakfast Cereal and milk, fruit **Lunch** Cereals, *dal,* two vegetables, dahi **Dinner** Cereals, *dal,* leafy vegetables, *dahi.*	**Tea** Tea, bread and butter **Dinner** Rice, *roti, dal,* leafy vegetables, dahi

Nutrition During Pregnancy and Lactation

Pregnancy and lactation are two stages of life when an adult women's needs are increased. She has the responsibility of supporting the growth of the foetus internally during the nine months of pregnancy and later externally by nursing the infant. Since the growth needs at the commencement of life are crucial, good nutrition is a must for the expectant as well as nursing mother. A number of tissues are formed to protect and sustain the foetus. During pregnancy the mother has to meet her own needs and the needs of the growing foetus. There is additional need for the growth of other related tissues and to build-up fat stores to cushion the foetus, prior to birth, and to supply part of the energy needed for milk formation during lactation. Thus the need for all nutrients involved in tissue synthesis is increased during pregnancy (Figure 16.1).

Adolescent mothers, who have not completed their own growth, may need additional foods to meet their own growth requirements. If these are not met, their health may be affected, which may indirectly affect the welfare of the foetus. If the mother's diet has been adequate before pregnancy, she may be in a better position to meet the demands of pregnancy.

No mother would like to injure the health of her baby through poor food habits. However, nutritional studies have shown that many women attend to the needs of other family members at the expense of their own needs. The situation does not change during pregnancy. Thus pregnant women are often the most poorly fed members of the family. In her effort to take care of others, she does not take time to sit down and eat. When she is very tired she is unable to eat. If the food supply is limited, she is the worst affected, as she feeds all other members and eats what is left. It is important that the family should plan the arrival of the baby so that the pregnant mother does not suffer from lack of food both in terms of amount and kind. The expectant father must try to ensure that the expectant mother gets the right amounts and kinds of foods, so that the health of the foetus does not suffer.

Energy Needs

The Advisory Committee of the Indian Council for Medical Research recommends an increase of 300 calories per day in the latter half of pregnancy. As growth of the foetus is very rapid in the second half of pregnancy, it is important that the increased need for energy is met.

Enough energy food should be supplied to ensure that the dietary protein is used for building new tissues, and not to meet need for energy. During first part of pregnancy the demand for extra energy is small and is taken care of by the reduced activity.

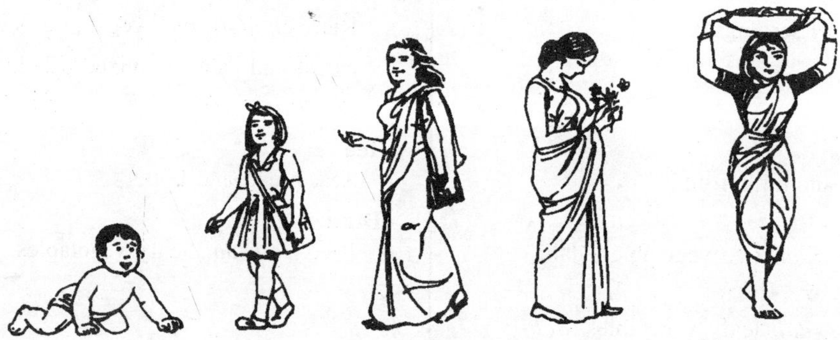

Age – 7-8 months	9 years	25 years Sedentary	Pregnant	Moderate Activity
Calories – 865	2050	1900	2200	2200
Protein – 14g	36 g	45 g	59 g	45 g
Body Weight – 8 kg	25 kg	45 kg	55 kg	45 kg

Figure 16.1: Energy and protein needs vary with age, occupation and physiological stage.

If the mother is within a few kilogrammes of the ideal weight for her body build, a gradual weight gain of up to 9-10 kg appears to be desirable. Under weight mothers may be encouraged to gain more weight, while those gaining too much weight may be advised to restrict their weight gain during pregnancy. Exact factual data about the most desirable weight gain and the significance of different rates of gain is not available.

The additional energy is used for building of new tissues, which is evident from the higher basal metabolic rate accompanying it, and also for the movement and activities of the larger body in the later part of pregnancy.

Protein Needs

Additional protein is necessary for growth of the foetus, new maternal tissues and to prepare the mother for lactation. The ICMR recommends addition of 14 g of protein daily during the second half of pregnancy.

The protein should be of good quality, e.g., milk, eggs, fish, meat, etc. Good quality may be achieved by combining sources of protein in the diet. Some of it could be supplied by milk and milk products.

Mineral Needs

The need for minerals, which form a part of body structure is increased with pregnancy. Calcium and phosphorus are needed for formation of bones and teeth. The teeth formation starts early in prenatal life, so it is important that the mother gets sufficient calcium from the beginning of pregnancy.

Iron is needed for the synthesis of additional volume of blood and other tissues formed during development of the foetus. The store of iron is built in prenatal period, because milk, the infant's main food during first three to four months after birth, is deficient in iron. It is now a common practice for the doctor to give expectant mothers a prescription for an iron salt. Though this is true, foods rich in iron should be emphasised in the diet. The mother will need to continue to eat a diet high in iron after delivery also, to make up for some of the losses at the time of childbirth. A number of foods traditionally prepared for feeding a nursing mother in the early part of lactation are rich in iron.

Iodine: There is an additional need for iodine at this stage in life. If mother's iodine intake is low, the infant may suffer from cretenism, a disease which is characterised by retarded physical and mental development. The iodine deficiency disease in adults is simple goitre.

In areas where the soil and water are deficient in iodine, the use of iodised salt is recommended.

Craving for Certain Foods: This may be due to psychological need for attention. It may be satisfied, if these do not conflict with the meeting of nutritional needs.

Nausea and vomiting may be common in early part of the pregnancy. A high carbohydrate diet, consisting of bland preparations, given as small frequent feedings, is likely to be beneficial. It is advisable to avoid strong flavours, e.g., strong coffee or tea, spicy and oily foods.

Constipation: Constipation is one of the complaints in pregnancy, because the enlarged uterus may press against the intestines and prevent normal movement. There is a tendency to decrease or minimise physical activity. This is not advisable, as exercise not only helps elimination but also keeps the body fit. Generally, some of the aids to regular elimination, which help in all stages of life, may be practised everyday to maintain good health in pregnancy. These are:

1. Drink more water. A glass or two taken before breakfast are often helpful. Some people find warm water more helpful than cold.
2. Eat the right foods. Include plenty of vegetables and fruits, especially green leafy vegetables, fresh fruits, raw salads, whole-grain preparations.
3. Eat at regular hours. Eat slowly.
4. Take some exercise daily to help movement, improve breathing and help the body to relax. A number of exercises can be performed regularly. Walking is a good and easy exercise.
5. Develop regular toilet habit. Early in the morning or, after the first cup of tea is a good time for a bowel movement.

Meeting the Dietary Needs of the Nursing Mother

It is recommended that the diet of a nursing mother should supply 700 calories in addition to her normal needs. This helps her to meet the demands of extra energy for lactation. Additional protein and other nutrients are also needed. The additional amounts recommended are indicated in the list. The increase in requirements is related to the amount of milk produced (Table 16.2).

Intake of high quality protein helps in improved secretion of milk. The intake of minerals, calcium, phosphorus, iron, iodine and vitamins, A, D, B-complex and C should be increased during lactation.

Table 16.2: Additional Amounts of Nutrients Recommended During Lactation

Nutrient	*Additional amount recommended*
Energy	700 kcal
Protein	20 g
Calcium	600 mg
Iron	nil
Vitamin A	400 mcg retinol or 1600 mcg beta-carotene
Thiamin	0.3 mg
Riboflavin	0.4 mg
Niacin	5.0 mg
Vitamin C	40 mg

Table 16.3: Additional Foods for Nursing Mother

Foods	*Amount*	*Calories*	*Protein*
Plan 1			
Wheat, *jowar, bajra* or ragi	90 g	305	8–11g
Dal, pulse, milk, fish or egg	1 S	100	5–6g
Garden cress seeds (*haliv*)	20 g	90	5
Leafy or orange yellow vegetable/fruit	50 g	25	2
Oil, any fat, butter or ghee	20 g	180	—
	Total intake	700	20–24
Plan 2			
Cereals	75 to 100 g	260–340	5–10
Dal/Pulse	20–25 g	85–100	5–6
Milk	1C	120	6
Garden cress seeds	10g	45	2
Amaranth or any dark green leafy veg.	75 g	35	3
Oil, fat	10–20 g	90–180	—
	Total intake	635–715	21–27

Modification of Normal Diet. A modification of the normal basic diet is worked out for a nursing mother. It may be observed that additional amounts of protein and energy foods are included in this diet. In most regions, it is customary to feed the nursing mother additional amount of fat (ghee) which supplies energy and vitamin A or some special preparations (Lahia, laddus of *methi, mung,* garden cress seeds), which contain sources of protein, iron, calcium and vitamins B. It is advisable to analyse the nutritional contribution of such products, so that one can emphasise those, which help to meet the additional need for nutrients (Table 16.3).

Factors Involved in Milk Secretion

Besides optimal diet others factors affect milk production. The mother's desire to feet the baby is a very important factor. A mother, who subconsciously thinks of nursing as an imposition on her personal freedom, or something which may affect her figure adversely, may not be able to nurse her baby. Her subconscious reaction may affect secretion of milk adversely. It may not be inopportune to mention that these fears are baseless. Normal lactation helps the mother to regain her natural figure effortlessly. A mother, who does not nurse her baby, may need to exercise more vigilance to avoid losing her figure, than a mother, who is able to nurse her baby.

A calm, quiet life favours maximal secretion of milk. Fear, worry, grief, anxiety, excitement, anger, tend to retard milk secretion. While moderate exercise helps milk secretion, excessive exercise depresses it. A comfortable seat, a calm atmosphere, freedom from pre-occupations and quiet are essential during nursing a baby. It is important for the nursing mother to have a happy family, which gives her emotional support during this stage of life, which is physically and psychologically very demanding and imposes restrictions on her personal freedom. This was well appreciated by our forefathers. The custom of sending an expectant mother to her parents and her stay with them for three to six months after delivery, used to ensure pleasant atmosphere for the mother and child.

Nutrition During Infancy

Proper feeding of infants is necessary to ensure normal growth and development. Infancy is the period of most rapid growth when one considers the period from birth to adulthood. The foundations of future health is laid during the first year of life. Breast milk is the first normal food for the baby. It provides the nutrients needed in a proportion suited to the infants rapid growth needs. This is a period in which the capacity of the stomach of the infant and ability to digest various foods components changes rapidly (Figure 16.2). Therefore, breast feeding is thought to be very important during this period. Each child grows according to his/her potential and individual progress is noted to record growth and development.

Nutrient Requirements

The need for energy is highest per unit of body-weight in the first year of life, as compared to the subsequent years of growth up to adulthood. The high energy needs in due to high basal metabolic rate, the energy requirement for growth and activity. The energy need decreases from second year to adulthood. The energy need for activity is very much variable, with an active infant using 40 per cent of the total energy and quiet babies using only 15 per cent of the total energy for activity.

The Indian Council of Medical Research recommends that calorie allowance for 1–6 months be 118 cal per kg and 7–12 months 108 cal per kg. When these energy needs are compared with those of an average young adult, which are from 40–50 calories per kg body-weight, the high energy needs of an infant become apparent. The relatively high need for energy of an infant is understandable, when we note that an average infant doubless his birth weight in the first five months of life and trebles it by the end of the first year.

Satisfactory weight gain is one of the simple indications of successful feeding of the baby.

As the body growth is rapid, it is accompanied by building of large amounts of body tissues. It is necessary to provide protein of high quality to sustain this rapid building process. As the body growth includes the building of strong bones and teeth, the infant's need for the minerals, calcium and phosphorus is high. Breast milk or Cow's milk supply these minerals in sufficient amounts, if an adequate quantity is taken daily. As the infant grows older, other sources such as green leafy vegetables and ragi are added to the diet to meet calcium needs.

During the last trimester of pregnancy, the well-nourished foetus builds up iron stores, so that at birth the infant has sufficient iron, stored to meet his/her needs for the first four to five months of life. Milk, which is the first food of the infant, is considered a complete food, but it is low in iron. A food supplement, which supplies iron, needs to be added, to the infant's diet, by the age of five to six months, when it is needed.

When the mother is well fed, the breast milk furnishes sufficient amount of vitamins, the only exception being vitamin D and perhaps vitamin C. The same is true for substitute milk used in infant feeding, except the fact that it contains insufficient amounts of vitamin C. Therefore, sweet lime, orange juice or some other juice high in vitamin C is usually added as one of the first supplements to the infant's diet. The other supplement is a vitamin D concentrate, which is added in the form of fish liver oil.

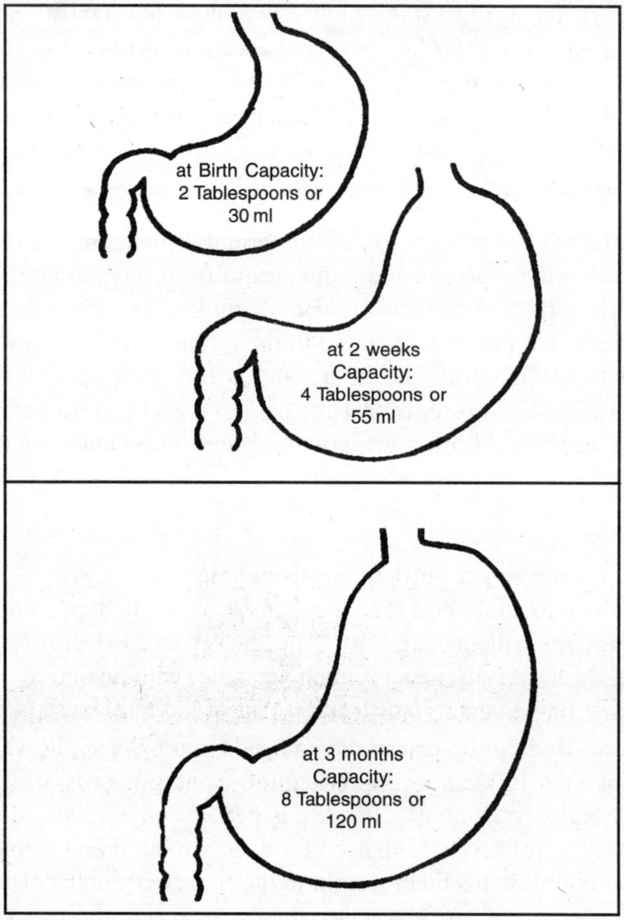

Figure 16.2: Baby's stomach–actual size at different ages.

Water

An infant is sometimes referred to as a bubble of water, due to its high proportion of body water. A baby has a high surface area per unit of body-weight, breathes faster, and therefore loses a lot of water, especially when he is dressed in warm clothing in warm, humid weather. He needs more water than adults to excrete body wastes. Therefore, an infant needs about 160 ml of water per kg per day. Though most of the needs is met by milk, it is necessary to give boiled, cooled water between feedings.

Breast Feeding

Human milk is more readily assimilated than cow's milk, for it is produced to suit the baby's digestive system. Breast milk is free from contamination, and is available at the right temperature without effort.

Breast feeding prolongs the period of natural immunity to virus diseases. These include mumps, measles, polio, some kinds of pneumonia and some infantile diarrhoeas. Babies fed on breast milk are also less likely to develop constipation and certain common infant allergies. Breast feeding does make possible an exceptionally close and harmonious relationship that is enjoyable and satisfying to both infant and mother. It should also be mentioned that in the case of a major disaster, which disrupts the supply services (water, milk, electricity, etc.), a baby's survival may depend on breast feeding. Another consideration in this atomic age is the presence of radioactive fallout as strontium–90. The consensus of scientific thought is that the amount of contamination in breast milk is likely to be smaller than in formula milk.

Human milk is specifically made to meet the needs of human infants. The best commercial formulas therefore are modified from cow's/buffalo's milk to approximate the known composition of human breast milk.

Unfortunately, even today, the increasing trend towards bottle feeding results in increased infant sickness and mortality, due to (i) ignorance of the basic rules of sanitation, (ii) insanitary preparation and poor handling of bottles and milk formula, and (iii) use of milk substitutes of poor nutrient content.

Though the mortality rate for artificially fed infants has been greatly reduced, it is still high for this group, especially in the lower economic groups. This may be due to lack of water for cleaning, high ambient temperature, lack of facilities for making the formula and lack of refrigeration. Mothers in this group do not have proper instructions in formula preparation and storage of prepared formula. An adequate diet, exercise, rest, and freedom from anxiety are important during prenatal period as well as during lactation.

Colostrum

The secretion from the breast in the first few days after delivery, is called colostrum. It has a high protein and vitamin A content and confers an immunity to certain infections during the first few months. It aids the development of the digestive enzymes. Therefore, it is important that the new born is breastfed from the first day and should be fed colostrum within an hour after birth.

When Breast Feeding is not Advisable

Breast feeding must be discontinued when:

1. Mother suffers from chronic illnesses such as tuberculosis, epilepsy, insanity, chronic fevers, severe anaemia, nephritis or cardiac disease.
2. The infant is weak or unable to nurse due to cleft palate or harelip.
3. Temporary stoppage of breast feeding is advisable when the mother acquires an acute infection, which the baby has not yet got. In such a condition the mother must empty out the breasts at regular intervals manually or with a pump, to prevent the milk supply from drying up.

There are no other reasons to stop breast feeding. It must be continued even if child has loose stools, is vomiting or has any minor or major illness.

When the child is unable to suck because of illness, breast milk can be expressed and fed.

Bottle Feeding

When a child needs to be bottle fed, most widely used substitute for human milk is cow's or modified buffalo's milk. The substitutes differ from human milk in composition. Table 16.4 gives comparison of human milk with milk of other species.

It may be noted that the protein content of these is about three times that of human milk. The type of protein present is also different. The fat content is similar in the milk of these species. Human milk contains about twice as much lactose as cow's or buffalo's milk. The energy supplied per 100 ml is about the same. Cow's milk contains more than three times as much mineral ash as human milk. This creates a high solute load for the kidneys to excrete. This problem is corrected by diluting the milk. Sugar is added to counteract the effect of dilution on energy supply.

The modifications made in cow's or buffalo's milk to prepare commercial formulas are:

1. Protein content is usually lowered; if possible, protein is treated to produce soft curd.
2. Carbohydrate such as glucose or sucrose is added.
3. Butter fat is reduced, if need be.
4. Calcium level is reduced by dilution.
5. Vitamins A, D and ascorbic acid are usually added.
6. Iron may be added.

Table 16.4: Composition of Milk from Various Species (per 100 ml)[1]

Nutrients	*Human milk*	*Cow's milk*	*Goat's milk*	*Buffalo's milk*	*Ass's milk*
Energy (kcal)	65	67	72	117	48
Protein (g)	1.1	3.2	3.3	4.3	2.1
Fat (g)	3.4	4.1	4.5	8.8	1.5
Carbohydrate (g)	7.4	4.4	4.6	5.0	6.5
Minerals (g)	0.1	0.8	0.8	0.8	—
Calcium (mg)	28	120	170	210	80
Phosphorus (mg)	11	90	120	130	—
Iron (mg)	—	0.2	0.3	0.2	—
Vitamin A (mcg)	42	52	54	48	—
Thiamin (mcg)	20	50	50	40	60
Riboflavin (mcg)	20	190	40	100	30
Niacin (mcg)	—	100	300	100	100
Vitamin C (mg)	3	2	1	1	10

1. Nutritive Value of Indian Foods, 1971.

Supplementary Foods for Infants and Toddlers

Introduction of First Solid Foods: The age at which the first solid is introduced and the types of food given is dependent on who decides this–the parents, grandparents or other relatives. It also depends on whether the family has access to a pediatrician, a family doctor, a health visitor, or a primary centre nurse. The advice will vary from one region of India to another.

In most regions there is a feast to celebrate this occasion. The first solid foods are normally introduced at five to six months of age. The foods given are cereals, cereal-milk or cereal/*dal* preparations such as *suji halwa,* rice-milk, *upma,* rice-*dal, khichdi, pongal,* bread, rice flakes/*poha,* etc. Fruits such as ripe banana, mango, papaya, which are soft and pulpy are also given. Well cooked, non-fibrous vegetables such as ashgourd, potato, pumpkin are fed along with rice.

It is important to make this transition to solid foods an enjoyable one. The amount of food offered and swallowed in the beginning is a teaspoon or so. It is normal for the infant to bring the food out, for the ability to swallow is developed very slowly. The infant enjoys this transition, if the mother is relaxed at the time of feeding and the food is not forced. The infant can accept the food better, if it is not distracted by other activities while feeding.

The number and kinds of foods given are slowly increased as the child approaches the first birthday. By the end of the second year, the toddler is able to partake of the normal family meals.

The Kinds of Foods Given

The first food fed is normally cooked cereals, which are prepared for the family or prepared baby cereals may be purchased. The cereal must be thoroughly cooked, if coarse, it should be strained. The cereal at first is mixed with milk, curd, buttermilk or *dal* soup. The amount given is gradually increased to four or five teaspoons by the seventh or eighth month.

Dal: Soft cooked *dal* (*varan*), *dal* soup can be mixed with rice and fed. Mixed preparation such as *khichdi* or *pongal* (rice and *mung dal*), *idli* (rice and *urad dal*), *dhokla* (*chana dal* and *dahi*), and any similar preparations can be fed by seven to eight months of age.

Fruits, Mashed, Strained: Fruits such as banana, mangoes, papaya, etc., are started at about five months of age. Cooked or baked apples may also be fed after removal of skin and other fibrous parts. Mild flavoured fruits in small amounts are a good choice to begin with.

Vegetables: Cooked and mashed or strained vegetables in small amounts can be added a little to the cereal by six to eight months. By the end of first year, the consistency of vegetables fed to the baby should be changed over gradually to chopped or coarsely mashed cooked vegetables. The baby needs to learn to like different flavours and textures. The addition of vegetables and fruits helps to achieve this objective.

Egg: Egg yolk can be given to the infant between the age of four to six months of age. The yolk contains protein, iron and vitamins which are valuable additions to the baby's diet. Hard cooked egg yolk seems to agree well with the babies. A very small amount is given in the beginning. The white of the egg is given only by the end of first year, as some babies are allergic to it.

Fish and Meat: Cooked ground and strained fish and meat may be given about the same time as egg yolk at five to six months of age. The fish or meat serving may be alternated with egg yolk and *dal.*

Feeding Schedules: Modern trend is to have flexible feeding schedules and not rigid. These are based on signs of hunger in the individual infant rather than on fixed hours of feeding. After the first few weeks, a healthy infant will develop a self-regulated feeding schedule of her/his own. The number of feeds will reduce to about six by the time the infant is six months of age.

A very small amount of each new food should be added to the infant's diet. New foods should be introduced gradually, one at a time to permit the infant to get used to it. The foods should be of soft, smooth consistency. It is normal for an infant to bring out the food in the beginning until the ability to swallow is established. The child should be encouraged to try new flavours and textures.

The amount of feed should be increased as the number decreases. By the beginning of the second year, the baby will have three to four meals. The foods included for a good daily diet for a one year old child are given in Table 16.5.

Table 16.5: Diet for One Year Old Child.

Milk	2 to 3 cups	Fruit for Vitamin C	1 serving
Dal	2 tablespoons	Other Fruit	1/4 cup
Egg	1	Rice*	1/4 cup (cooked)
or Meat or Fish	2 tablespoons	*Chapati*/bread	1/2 to 1 *chapati* or sliced bread
Cooked green or yellow vegetable	2 tablespoons	Butter/ghee *vanaspati*	1 teaspoon
Other vegetables including potatoes	2 tablespoons	Fish liver oil	Enough to supply 5 mcg (200 I.U.) vitamin D

**Rawa,* ragi, *jowar, pohe* or any other cereal could wholly or partially replace rice.

Helping Children to Develop Good Food Habits

Most of the problems of food acceptance begin in the toddler stage. The problem starts with the mother, who thinks that the child should be well fed, and tries to feed the child more food than it needs. The child will show a marked decrease in appetite in the second year, because the child grows at a slower rate in the second year as compared to the first year. So it is important to give small portions of food and let him/her enjoy food. Allow the child some freedom to decide when he/she is satisfied. Allow some flexibility in choices and help the child form good food habits gradually. Learning is a slow process and is helped by the adults having patience and a sportive attitude, never by bribe, admonition or punishment.

Toddlers

Children can share family meals, by the time, they are two years old. A few alternatives may be needed, when the family makes highly spiced food. It is advisable to keep foods, which are too fatty or too sweet out of the child's menu. Such foods may fill his limited space, without providing the nutrients needed. The child may be encouraged to eat sweets towards the end of the meal, so that he/she may not eat these to the exclusion of other foods.

It is good to give appetising beverages such as fruit juices and milk to the children. It is good to serve part of his milk needs in the form of soups, *kheer,* custard or icecream. Fruits are ideal snacks. Crisp crackers or toast are liked and the child can eat these without help, which helps him to feel independent.

Indications of Good Health

Some indications are visible, and can be measured and recorded, others are qualitative, and not easily recorded.

The most common measurable criterion is regular gain in weight. At birth an average healthy baby weights about three to three and half kg. A little loss of weight is observed in the first few days, but it is regained within two weeks. From this point, the child gains weight regularly. It doubles its birth weight between four to six months of age and triples it by the end of 10–12 months. Therefore, slow weight gain or stationary weight is the first indication of something amiss in the infant care.

Other signs of good health are rosy cheeks, bright eyes, firm layer of subcutaneous fat, normal eruption of teeth, good sleep and regular elimination. A healthy baby is a happy baby.

Meal Planning for School Children and Adolescents

Once the child starts going to school, the attention of the parents is diverted to his/her school work and food becomes a secondary matter. As a result the nutritional needs of the child of school age are often overlooked. If the child was well-nourished as he entered school, the effect of neglect during school years does not show up for some time.

The nutritional needs do not change very much during school years except for a gradual increase in food intake to meet the needs of the growing body. But going to school does mean that the meals and activities have to be planned to fit in the school schedule. It is necessary to eat one meal away from home, wich may be a box lunch or snacks bought at school.

Food Needs of the School Child — 6–12 Years Old

At this stage it is important to ensure that each meal carries sufficient amounts of protein, minerals and vitamins. The food needs are increased in keeping with the child's growth rate and activity. The kinds of food needed are the same as those for younger children but the amounts needed are increased. The children of this age can take most of the foods served in the family meals, except highly spiced or fried foods, strong tea and coffee. The child can take all fruits at this age, including those which have seeds as guavas and grapes which were not suitable at a younger age. He can eat many foods, which need biting and chewing such as popped cereals, roasted groundnuts and bengal gram, roasted corn on the cob, *amla,* bor, etc.

Spacing and Time of Meals

Children usually need four or five meals. The child should be encouraged to get up about half an hour before breakfast. About twenty minutes may be needed for the meal. When the child goes to school, its a good idea to allow about half an hour between breakfast and school time for the child to get ready. Lunch time should be midway between breakfast and dinner. Some children need a mid-morning as well as, a mid-afternoon snack.

Breakfast the Neglected Meal

With the need to adjust to the school time, the first meal is either scanty or omitted entirely. This is a hazard from the nutritional point of view. For a missed meal is hard to make up. There are many reasons why a child does not have a good breakfast. The breakfast may not be ready in time and therefore the child may not be able to eat it and reach the school in time. The child may not get up in time and therefore the breakfast may be hurried. If the child does not go to bed in time, it is difficult for him to get up early enough to find time to get ready for school and eat a good breakfast. The child's ability to attend classes and learn his lessons at school may be affected, if he is hungry during school hours, due to a poor breakfast.

Breakfast can be a very enjoyable and varied meal. Some of the traditional breakfasts from some regions are given in Table 16.6.

Table 16.6: Regional Breakfast

Region	*Breakfast foods*
Punjab	*Parantha* and *lassi*
Maharashtra	*Shira* and milk, *Dahi-pohe, Doodh-pohe*
Madras	*Idli chutney, Dosa Chuteney* & Coffee, milk beverage
Mysore	Ragi preparation and butter milk
Modern pattern in all regions	Bread and butter, egg, fruit, milk.

A good breakfast should include some cereal or cereal *dal* preparation, some milk and fruit. However, if the fruit is preferred at some other time in the day, it may be omitted from the breakfast.

Lunch

This meal may have to be eaten away from home, which is a major change for the child at this stage. It requires considerable planning and management to ensure that a child is well fed even when she/he eats away from home. The foods, which must find a place in the packed lunch include—(a) cereal preparation such as *chapati, upma,* bread, etc., (b) pulse or milk product, which may be *usal, dal, til chutni,* curd, *lassi*, milk or roasted groundnuts, (c) vegetable preparation or fruit. You can make one dish, which contains foods from all the three groups, in which oil, butter, ghee, sugar and/or jaggery are hidden or visible ingredients. Some preparations, which are children's favourites, are:

- *Masalabhaat* (made with rice, *mung dal* and vegetable–cabbages, carrots, peas).
- *Thalipeeth* (made from a mixture of cereals and pulses flour and vegetables.
- *Dahi-bhaat,* tomato or cucumber slices and lemon pickle.
- *Shira,* milk and fruit (banana, grapes, guava, orange).
- Sandwiches of cheese or paneer, tomato and cucumber.
- *Chapati, usal* and carrot salad.

As you can see there are many more variations, which can be made from foods from the groups indicated. When the children eat with their friends and share their lunch with them at school, it improves their enjoyment of the meal. Such sharing may enlarge their food exposure and add variety.

There are some points, which must be remembered, in making a packed lunch, which is enjoyable. These are:

- Cool the preparation before packing to avoid spoilage.
- Pack food preparations, which taste good even when these are cold.

- Include some fresh vegetable or fruit, to help moisten the mouth.
- Pack the vegetable/fruit slices in a plastic bag, to retain fresh flavour and texture.
- Pack only as much as the child can eat happily, so that children learn to value food and do not waste it.

Between Meal Snacks

Some children may need a mid-morning and a mid-afternoon snack. A number of foods are normally available, these include fruits such as guavas, bananas, *amlas,* bor, etc. roasted legumes such as groundnuts, *chanas,* etc. These are available near school in addition to the snacks sold in the school canteen. If well chosen, these snacks can provide important nutrients in addition to calories. If the children buy candy, peppermints, soft drinks, ice fruit, they get mainly calories only. These foods reduce or dull the appetite, without meeting the body's need. Such foods supply only energy. Therefore, these foods are said to provide only "*empty calories*".

The Adolescent—12–16 years

This is a stage of rapid growth and intense activity. Individual variation is also great in this age group. A number of physical, emotional and mental changes occur in this period of life. Girls mature between 11 and 13 years of age, whereas the major changes occur in boys between 13 and 15 years.

It is normal for boys to eat a lot at this age, especially if they are fond of outdoor sports. The need to meet their nutritional needs through good planning cannot be overemphasised.

It may be noted from the table of recommended allowances that the need for all nutrients is increased at adolescence. Therefore, it is important to plan to supply sufficient amounts of proteins, minerals and vitamins in each meal.

Adolescence is the age of group activities. Therefore, if nutrition education is imparted as a group activity, it may help in improving eating habits.

Meeting Food Needs of Adolescents

The increased needs of this period can be met if increased amounts of foods listed in the daily guide are included in the diet. Boys may need to consume a lot of energy rich foods, in order to provide sufficient energy.

Girls may need to pay special attention to foods rich in protein, iron and other nutrients necessary for synthesis and regeneration of red blood cells. The girl's diet should include all foods listed in the food guide, with special attention to iron rich foods such as *dals,* leafy green vegetables, dried fruits and egg, liver and red meats may also be used if acceptable.

It is important for adolescents to gain appropriate weight for their height and body build. Any deviation from normal indicates some feeding problem, which must be identified and corrected with the help of a nutritionist or dietician. Checking a three day food intake record, may help in identifying the specific lack or excess and thus form the basis of a plan of action.

Diet During 17–21 years

Growth is usually slow in this stage of life. But there is certain degree of maturation of the body tissues, which is aided by good nutrition.

If the boys and girls are away in hostels, they tend to economise on food, especially if the food charges are collected on the basis of meals eaten.

A number of institutions (colleges/universities) provide accommodation and food at moderate cost to this age group; part of the establishment cost is paid as subsidy by the government to reduce food cost to the college students.

It is necessary to educate this group about the relationship between the food intake and body's needs to store up nutrients in preparation for the responsibilities of adulthood.

Nutrition for Middle Age Adults (40 – 60 yrs.)

Often the middle years are a stage of stability in life. Normally the person is efficient in one's profession, income is steady, the physical demands of caring for children are over. The basal metabolic rate starts decreasing from 30 years of age.

Thus the energy need decreases, but the need for other nutrients (proteins, minerals and vitamins) do not decrease.

As for adults, food selection is made according to the Daily Food Guide (Table 14.1). The number of servings included from various groups will be dependent on the body size and activity of the person. In general, the reduction in energy intake can be achieved by decreasing intake of sugar, sweets, oils and fats to ensure that the body weight is maintained at a desirable level. A sensible programme of regular exercise, such as walking and yoga can help to maintain optimum health.

Nutrition for Senior Citizen (60 + years)

The rate of aging varies from one person to another. There are several factors which affect the aging, which include heredity, the psycho-social and nutritional background and activity pattern. Due to these variations, no two people age in a similar manner.

One reassuring observation is that people, who keep physically and mentally active have been reported to retain their sense of smell and taste even in their eighties. Those who practise weight-lifting are able to retain their lean muscle mass and the density of their bones. If teeth are lost, well-fitting dentures permit enjoyment of foods of varying texture. Use of hearing aid helps those with hearing defects to maintain social contact. Lens implants after cataract surgery permit reading and free movement thus ensuring the ability to pursue intellectual interests.

Thus more senior citizens are found to be travelling and participating in social and community activities than they did before the development of technologies mentioned above.

How does one avoid potential problems?

Healthy eating habits throughout life helps to maintain physical well-being. Regular fitness programme of one's choice helps to prevent physical deterioration. Enjoyable social activities help to keep a happy frame of mind. A happy outlook, a regular practice of prayer and thankfulness are assets which ensure a happy life at all stages including late years.

Try to live life in a way that requires less use of medicines. If sleepy, try a short nap or meditation instead of taking stimulants like tea or coffee. If you suffer from constipation, try taking enough exercise with regular intake of fiber and water.

Nutritional Requirements: Normal nutritional needs remain the same throughout life. Good nutrition can speed recovery from illness and generally can improve the spirit and quality of life and even prolong life. It is necessary to know the extent to which aging has affected a person's physiological capabilities. The declines in physiological functions with aging of sedentary people are depicted in Figure 16.3.

Except for energy need, due to decrease in the metabolic rate (Table 16.7), the need for all the nutrients remains the same as before.

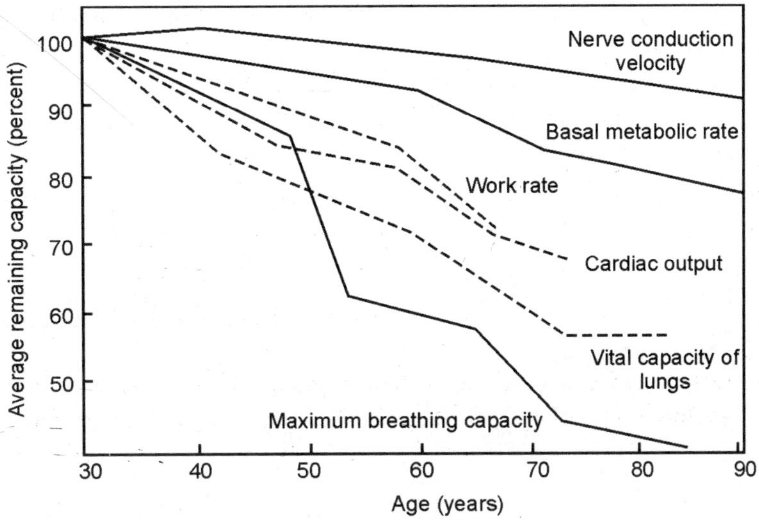

Figure 16.3: The declines in physiological functions with aging in sedentary people

Table 16.7: Variation in Energy Needs (Basal & Total) of Senior Citizen with Age

Age Yrs	*% Reduction in BMR(1) After 30 yrs*	*Male (60 kg)*		*Female (50 kg)*	
		Basal energy Need in kcal(2) (A)	*Total energy Need in kcal* (A) × 1.6	*Basal energy Need in kcal (2)* (A)	*Total energy Need in kcal* (A) × 1.6
30	100	1515	2424	1171	1874
31–40	3	1470	2352	1136	1818
41–50	3	1424	2279	1101	1762
51–60	7.5	1310	2096	1013	1621
61–70	7.5	1197	1915	925	1480
71–80	10	1045	1672	808	1293

1. Chaney Margaret S. **Nutrition,** 6 edn., p.66, Houghton Mifflin Co., Boston, USA, 1960.
2. ICMR Expert Group Report, 2000, **Nutrient Requirements & RDA for Indians**, NIN, Hyderabad.

The protein requirement remains at the average of 0.8 to 1.0 per kilogram. Vitamin requirements do not change after the age of 50 except for a slight decrease in the need for thiamin, riboflavin and niacin, which are proportional to the total energy intake (Table 16.7).

Food and Other Habits of Senior Citizens

Some food habits of older persons are nutritionally poor. These include excessive use of sago and potatoes in place of a meal on particular week days such as Monday, Tuesday, Thursday, Friday or Saturday; Ekadashi, Pradosh (biweekly) and Sankashti (monthly). Some may observe fast by taking drinks only such as tea, coffee, lemon sherbet and buttermilk. Loneliness may reduce the intake of proper meals. Proper meals may be substituted with snack foods such as toast, upma etc. They may think they have eaten, when they have not, due to forgetfulness. At times they may ask for meals when they have already eaten, annoying relatives and caretakers. They may reduce water intake to avoid having to use the bathroom in the night. This results in constipation.

Reduced movement to avoid falls and accidents affects circulation, digestion and muscle tone adversely.

If the diet intake is reduced to less than 1500kcal/day, a multi-vitamin tablet/capsule needs to be taken to meet the recommended allowances. Intake of a variety of nutrient dense foods should be encouraged. Intake of sufficient water is necessary to prevent constipation, to maintain urinary volume and to prevent dehydration. Poor or missing teeth may decrease intake of vegetable and protein foods. In such cases, blended vegetable and protein rich soups can be used.

Any adjustment in food habits must be carefully made in consultation with the person concerned.

Food Habits and the Elderly

Elderly persons crave for attention and are often duped into buying unnecessary food supplements and special foods. The sales person appears to be interested in their health and persuades them to buy expensive food supplements and special foods. Thus they spend money that could be used to buy ordinary foods recommended in the food guide, which could provide more nutrients at less cost.

In short, a basic plan for health promotion and disease prevention includes eating a proper diet that focuses on a variety of foods and moderation in food intake, exercising regularly, abstaining from smoking, limiting alcohol intake and limiting stress.

Study Questions

1. Why is breakfast an important meal? List the foods which are included in breakfast in your region. What nutrients do they provide? What modification could you make to improve it.
2. List a typical lunch/dinner menu in your home and its nutritional merits. Is there need for improvement? If not why not?
3. How will you guide your younger brother/sister to choose snacks in a snack bar? Explain the reasons for your advice.
4. Why is special emphasis laid on nutrition during pregnancy? Plan supplementary foods to meet the additional needs of pregnancy during the last trimester.
5. Discuss other problems encountered during pregnancy. How will you help a pregnant woman to overcome these.
6. Discuss the factors, which need attention to ensure successful lactation.
7. Compare and contrast the nutritional needs of a child in first year of life with those of an adult.
8. List the advantages of breast-feeding.
9. List the weaning foods used in your region. Indicate if these need modification, and the kind of modification needed.
10. Discuss how parents can help children to develop good food habits.
11. Write notes on: Empty calories, packed lunch.
12. List your own meal pattern. Discuss its merits and demerits.
13. What are the physiological functions which change with age? How does the change affect the nutritional intake of Senior Citizens (those above 60 years of age)?

CHAPTER 17

Indian Meal Patterns–Vegetarian and Non-Vegetarian

AS YOU may realise our meal pattern is affected by the kinds of foods available. For example, rice is grown in certain parts of our country and it forms the staple in those regions; similarly wheat, *jowar, bajra, makka* (corn) and ragi are used as staples, where these are the major crops. Secondly, the amounts and kinds of foods we eat is affected by the money that can be spent for food. Thirdly, our family's meal pattern is dictated by the geographic region, religion, community and family practices developed over several generations.

The *dals,* the vegetables and fruits, which we habitually include in our menu, are mainly those, which were a part of our regional meal pattern. Even when we move to other regions for work or business, we tend to retain a large part of our food heritage. For example, Punjabis residing in Bombay or Calcutta, retain their food pattern, which includes wheat *parantha, rajmah, palak,* and peas, etc. A Tamilian in similar situation would include, rice, *sambar* made from *tur dal* and vegetables such as ash gourd and amaranth. As you know, it makes little difference whether the leafy vegetable used is amaranth or *palak* from the nutritional point of view, for both provide pro-vitamin A in substantial amount. Thus the regional patterns can meet the nutritional needs of people, if sufficient food from each of the five groups is included; the particular food chosen from each group and the way it is prepared is a matter of individual choice.

In addition to these regional variations in food acceptance pattern, two major patterns are prevalent in the world—the vegetarian and the non-vegetarian dietary. Let us examine and understand how these affect our food choices and nutrition.

It is good to remember that in India, vegetarians include milk and milk products such as curds, *lassi, paneer, cheese,* buttermilk, etc., which are animal foods, in their diets; while the Indian non-vegetarians may exclude fish, eggs and meat from their menu on certain days of the week, such as Mondays, Thursdays and/or Saturdays; these factors need to be taken into account while examining these dietaries. Let us understand the historical basis of evolution of the Indian dietary before discussion of nutritional aspects.

Evolution of the Vegetarian Dietary Pattern[1]

Before the advent of Jainism, there appears to have been no restriction in the food acceptance of our people, except on an individual voluntary basis. The philosophy of non-violence, which was preached by the prophets of Jainism had a profound influence on the dietary practices of their followers. Jainism can be traced back to three centuries before the advent of Buddhism, i.e., 800 BC Mahavira Vardhamana, a Jain prophet and a contemporary of Bhagvan Gautama Buddha, was responsible for the spread of Jainism and its concept of abstinence from flesh foods. Emperor Ashoka the Great (about 264 BC), became an exponent of Budhhism. Not only did he become a vegetarian, but he refrained from hunting and banned it in his kingdom. One of the reasons for abstaining from flesh foods was the belief in the transmigration of souls between living beings, which, included animals. Thus Vegetarianism represents a conscious choice with respect to one's diet, which is quite different from foregoing meat because it is expensive. Thus it does not connote a dietary practice only, but is a way of life that has cultural and spiritual implications. Abstinence from meat, as a dietary discipline, is evident in most religious practices. For meat is avoided by certain Christian sects during Lent; Muslims avoid pork, and Hindus avoid meat during religious celebrations.

Pythagoras, the Greek philosopher, who was a contemporary of Gautama Buddha, believed in the transmigration of souls, and espoused the cause of vegetarianism. In fact, he is recognised as the founder of vegetarianism in Europe. The ethical aspects of non-violence seem to have appealed to some of the thinkers, such as, Sir Francis Bacon and George Bernard Shaw, and they became vegetarians. Thus the movement to popularise vegetarianism as a desirable dietary practice, started in the Western countries. Leonardo da Vinci, the Italian painter, Sir Issac Newton, the British physicist, John Wesley, the founder of the Methodist Church, Helena Blavatsky, the founder of the theosophical movement, and Mahatma Gandhi, the Indian leader, who practised non-violence, were some of the great protagonists of vegetarianism.

In the mid-nineteenth century, vegetarianism flourished under the leadership, of breakfast cereal developers Kellogg, Graham and Post, as well as writers such as Uptom Sinclair. In 1978, there were 9 to 10 million Americans, who were vegetarians, according to a Roper poll. In addition, there were 40 to 50 million people, who restricted the consumption of meat in the United States of America. This trend is observed in other Western countries also.

Vegetarian Dietary Patterns

The traditional Indian dietary consists of cereal preparations, such as rice, *chapati, roti,* as the main course, with preparations of *dal,* legumes, vegetables, *dahi/*buttermilk, as accompaniments to the staple food.

The word vegetarian is derived from the Latin root 'vigitore', meaning *giving strength and health.* According to the *Concise Oxford Dictionary,* a vegetarian is one, who uses or advocates the use of a diet of vegetable foods, usually with the addition of milk, eggs, to the exclusion of meat. A person, who includes an animal food such as milk in the diet, cannot be a vegetarian, in the strict sense of the word.

1. Mudambi, SR, and MV Rajgopal, *Nutrition,* 3(6), 373–78, 1987.

Thus the word vegetarian, as used for the traditional Indian dietary, is a misnomer; and creates unnecessary misunderstanding about its identity and nutritional quality.

In recent years, there has been an increase is the followers of vegetarian dietary pattern in the Western countries, as mentioned earlier. As a result; a number of variations of vegetarian dietary pattern have emerged. These fall into the following five groups:

(*a*) *Lactovegetarians* are those, who include milk and milk products, in addition to plant foods, such as cereals, *dals,* legumes, vegetables and fruits in their diet.

(*b*) *Ovolactovegetarians* include eggs, in addition to all the foods mentioned in (*a*) above.

(*c*) *Ovo-vegetarians* include eggs, in addition to the plant foods.

(*d*) *Fruitarians* include grains, nuts and fruits, *i.e.*, the parts of plants, which are obtained without destruction of the plant itself.

(*e*) *Vegans* include only plant foods in their diets, and abstain from all animal foods, even milk and milk products. This is comparatively a new population group, that has emerged from omnivores (who used to eat all plant and animal foods), in the Western countries.

In India, traditional vegetarians belong to the first group, the lacto vegetarians. The second group is comparatively a recent development.

As we may realise, it is possible for vegetarians to select foods from the basic five groups and meet their nutritional requirements.

Non-Vegetarian Dietary Patterns

It is good to remember that there are two distinct patterns of non-vegetarian diet observed around the world. The first is the Indian non-vegetarian pattern, which has a cereal preparation as a main course with fish, poultry or meat dish as an accompaniment, in addition to vegetables, *dal*/pulse preparation and salad. The fish or meat are served one to three times a week in the meal. The amount of fish, poultry or meat served in such a diet is naturally smaller than when these foods are served as the main course.

The second non-vegetarian pattern is that which is followed in the Western countries such as U.K., U.S.A., Canada and Europe, which has meat, fish or poultry dish as the main course, with preparation of cereals, vegetables, fruits, as accompaniments to the main protein course. In such a meal, the animal foods such as chicken, fish or meat roast form the main course in each meal and thus are eaten at least twice a day. Thus the total amount of animal protein consumed is several times that included by those, who follow the traditional Indian non-vegetarian meal pattern, though both are designated as non-vegetarian dietaries. This aspect needs to be remembered while assessing the nutritional adequacy of these meal patterns.

Nutritional Adequacy of Indian Diets

It has been proved in a number of studies that dietaries made up of predominantly plant foods, can be nutritionally adequate, if these are derived from natural foods belonging to the basic five groups, and meet the energy needs of the individual. As we know the Sherpas (in Himalayan expeditions), who follow a non-flesh dietary pattern, have demonstrated that their dietary is adequate to prepare them to endure the most severe stress that can be laid on the human body-extreme altitude, almost unbearable cold, supreme endurance and elephantine strength.

Like any other diet, the adequacy of the vegetarian diet depends on the individual food selection. In reviewing typical menus from various countries around the world, nutritionists found that a diet, which supplies 2500 calories, would contain 50 per cent more protein than needed by 98 per cent of the population. It is difficult to find a mixed vegetarian diet that will produce a negative nitrogen balance, unless a large part of it consists of sugar, jams, jellies and other essentially non-protein foods.

The myths about magical qualities of proteins, especially animal proteins, have been perpetuated for generations. It is important to take stock of the hard facts about overconsumption of proteins, especially in the form of animal foods.

Apart from the waste of money by overconsumption of animal proteins, the disposal of its metabolic waste products may overburden the kidneys and tax the body's circulatory functions, due to the high fat and cholesterol intake. Last but not the least, the obesity, observed in the population, due to the high energy intake associated with such a diet, is a predisposing factor in a number of diseases prevalent in the developed world. The major dietary risk to health in the U.S.A. and Europe comes from eating too much food and the wrong kind of food.

The dietary goals for the U.S.A. and U.K. have emphasised the need to reduce the animal foods, saturated fats and sugar in the diet, and increase the intake of whole grain unrefined cereals, vegetables and fruits in the diet. There are several advantages in such a shift in diet. Plant foods are high in complex carbohydrates, which according to the U.S. dietary goals, need to be increased to account for 55–60 per cent of the total energy intake. Animal foods such as meat, fish and eggs do not contain any carbohydrates. In addition, plant foods are good sources of fibre, which is needed for the maintenance of muscle tone. Most plant foods are low in calories, as they contain a low percentage of fat.

The nutritional needs of Indians are met, when they follow the traditional vegetarian or non-vegetarian dietary pattern. Please note that the staples in both Indian dietary patterns are cereals. The fish, meat or poultry are served as only a side dish in the Indian menu, while in the Western menu it is served as the main course. Therefore, those, who follow the traditional Indian non-vegetarian pattern, are likely to have very few health problems, resulting from excessive consumption of animal protein foods, such as degenerative diseases of heart, kidney and colon.

Several studies have been carried out to assess the efficacy of predominantly vegetarian diets for athletes and other sports persons and how these diets affect their performance. On the basis of these, a strict vegetarian diet is advocated for athletes and other sports—persons, for optimal endurance and athletic skills. It is reported that a high carbohydrate and low protein diet increases the stamina of bicycling athletes by 300 per cent, while skiiers fed high carbohydrate diet, were able to work about three times as long as on a very high fat diet. Thus the vegetarian diet is not only adequate to maintain good health, but is also appropriate for athletes, be they runners, bicyclists or cross-country skiiers.

Important Nutritional Aspects of our Dietary Pattern

There are several desirable practices in our meal pattern. It is important to understand the nutritional significance of these and ensure their retention. For example, we grind whole wheat and use the flour to prepare *chapaties, phulkas,* or *puri.* Thus we get all the minerals and vitamins present in the outer layers of the grain. If we substitute bread or other products made from *maida* (refind wheat flour), in our dietary in place of *chapati,* made from whole wheat flour, we would be deprived of iron, thiamin and niacin, present in the whole wheat flour. For example, bread, which is made from *maida,* contains a fifth of the vitamin thiamin, found in whole wheat flour. Therefore use of bread in place of *chapati* is not a desirable change from nutritional point of view. Similarly, we make *roti* or *bhakari* of flour made from whole *jowar, bajra, makka* or *ragi,* which is a good practice and must be retained.

In some parts of India, parboiled rice is used, which is an excellent practice, as it is richer in minerals and vitamins than raw milled rice. It is important to retain the use of parboiled rice.

In our traditional diet, a number of fermented foods are made, which not only add variety, but also important nutrients to our menu. For example, fermented foods, like *idli, dhokla,* curds, buttermilk and *lassi,* have higher amount of B-vitamins than the unfermented rice, *dal* and milk from which these are made. A word of caution, please remember that most of the instant mixes you buy for convenience, rely on chemical additives to leaven the product and therefore lack the nutritional improvement we get during fermentation in these foods, when these are made by the traditional process.

Another desirable practice is the use of germinated pulses in our traditional dietary. As you may know, during the germination of food, vitamin C is synthesised, thus improving the nutritional content of the food. Another practical benefit of germinated foods is that they need less time to cook and are easy to digest. In some regions, germinated pulse preparations are made for special occasions and shared. For example, in Maharashtra, germinated pulse *usal* is made and distributed to people on the fifth day after a baby is born; in Mysore and Tamil Nadu, *shunda*l, made from germinated *chana,* is given to ladies and children, during *Navaratri* as a benediction. During Chaitra Gauri *haldi-kumkum,* germinated bengal-gram is given as a gift to ladies and girls in Maharashtra. These practices emphasise the use of germinated foods and must be retained to ensure good nutrition.

If you observe the traditional menus for everyday meals as also for feasts, you will notice that leafy vegetables form an important part of it. For example, *sarson-ka-sag* (mustard greens) in Punjab, *aluchee bhaji* (colocaisa leaves) in Maharashtra and *keere sambar* (leafy vegetable soup) in Tamil Nadu are examples of use of leafy vegetables in daily meals. Besides this, a traditional menu for weddings in Maharashtra is not complete without a preparation of leafy vegetables, bengal gram *dal* and groundnuts. If we stop and examine our regional menus, we will find many examples of use of leafy vegetables in the menu. Retaining this rich food heritage will add to our eating pleasure, and ensure good nutrition.

In our regional menus we include a variety of salads, which we call *koshimbir, raita* or *bharta.* So use of a variety of salads also forms an important part of our traditional food pattern. We use curd, lemon juice, mango scraping, roasted groundnuts, soaked *dals* (such as *chana* and *mung*), coriander leaves, mint leaves, etc., as salad dressings, which add variety of flavours and improve the nutritive value of the product. It is perhaps not out of place to mention, that these salad dressing are not fatty like the French dressing or mayonnaise, which some of you may be tempted to use in their place in order to mimic the Western pattern.

Traditionally fruits form a very important part of our tropical food heritage, for we have some fruits in season all through the year. So you find that we use fruits as offerings in temple, and receive these as prasad (benediction). We give seasonal fruits as a gift to guests, especially ladies and children. Fruits are also the gift of choice, to be taken to sick relatives and friends, when we visit them in hospital or at home. As you have learnt the nutritional contribution of fruits in the dietary, you can appreciate the wisdom of retaining these traditional practices.

Study Questions

1. Trace the evolution of the vegetarian dietary pattern with particular reference to India.
2. List the various foods in a typical Indian vegetarian meal of your region. Explain how you would check whether it is nutritionally adequate.
3. What is the difference between the typical Indian and Western non-vegetarian diet?
4. List some of the desirable and undesirable practices in the meal pattern of your region.

PART - IV

Foods

CHAPTER 18

Food Selection, Purchase and Storage

FOOD SELECTION is the first step in ensuring good nutrition for the family. The daily food guide helps in deciding the kinds and amount of foods to be purchased.

Food Selection and Purchase

Selection of foods, from the available variety, is an important aspect of marketing. Intelligent selection of foods from the basic five groups is based on the knowledge of attributes of high quality foods.

How often we purchase food depends on its storage life. Foods are classified, on the basis of their stability during storage, into non-perishable, semi-perishable and perishable foods. Let us consider the criteria used for selection of various foods prior to purchase.

Non-perishable Foods

Non-perishable foods include whole grain cereals, whole and split pulses, nuts and oilseeds, sugar and jaggery.

Cereals and *dals* supply about 330 to 350 k calories per 100 g. There is a distinct difference in the amount of protein supplied by these, the cereals supply only 7 to 12 per cent protein, while the *dals* and whole pulses supply twice as much protein, viz., 17 to 25 per cent.

The criteria for selection of all these with the exception of sugar and jaggery are similar.

General Criteria of Selection: Whole grain cereals, *dals* and whole pulses (*mung, chawli, math, rajmah,* etc.) are selected on the basis of their appearance, feel, colour and variety. The grains are inspected for uniform size, cleanliness, soundness of grain, absence of broken pieces, freedom from insect infestation, absence of admixture with foreign seeds and trash, dirt, mud, stones and sand.

The grain can be chewed to detect the texture and flavour. Hollow, soft fibrous texture indicates deterioration in quality. Sour or rancid flavour and odour indicate spoilage during storage. Nuts and oilseeds must be free from any absorbed or rancid odour and flavour.

Cereals: Cereals, millets and their products are the staple foods in the Indian dietary. It is important that these be selected carefully as they supply a major part of our energy, protein, iron and thiamin needs.

Grain quality has two aspects. The first is physical quality, which refers to cleanliness, soundness of grain and freedom from foreign matter. The second is processing quality, which means suitability for use. For example, thin long grain rice, which does not clump after cooking, is considered suitable for making *pulao,* a particular type of wheat is required to prepare *puran poli,* etc. Let us consider the specific criteria for selection of these foods.

Wheat is selected on the basis of the quality aspects mentioned above. Whole wheat is ground for individual use by the families. Whole wheat flour is mainly used to prepare unleavened bread (*chapati, roti, parantha,* etc.) in India. In these preparations very little nutrient loss occurs. Normally consumers buy the variety that suits their needs in terms of performance. Not much information is available about the performance of various varieties in indigenous wheat preparations. Therefore, selection is based on the consumer's personal knowledge and experience.

Rice is available as milled, hand-pounded and parboiled varieties. The degree of milling and polishing affects the nutrient content. The parboiled rice and hand-pounded rice contain significant amounts of thiamin; highly polished milled rice has very little thiamin.

A number of grain types such as long, medium and short, are available. The selection is made depending on the intended use and price. For example, thin, long varieties are preferred for table use, medium and short varieties are used for preparations of rice made after grinding.

Indians prefer the individual grains of rice to retain their identify after cooking. Ageing appears to help develop this characteristic in the grain. It is observed that old grains absorb more than two times their volume of water during cooking, while new rice absorbs *only* two times their volume. It is difficult to judge the extent to which rice has aged, by its appearance, as no visual criteria of agening have been established, to guide the consumer.

Millets: Other grains include *bajra, jowar, ragi,* maize and other millets, which are used as a staple. The criteria for selection are the same as for all grains—soundness of grain, cleanliness, freedom from admixture with other grains and trash.

Most of these millets are ground and the whole grain flour is used to prepare unleavened bread (*roti*). As whole grain flour is used in most preparations, very little loss of nutrients occurs. It must be noted that *ragi* is an exceptionally good source of calcium, and *ragi* and *bajra* of iron.

Dals and Pulses: Tur, mung, chana, lentil and *urad,* are the most used varieties. These are selected according to the general criteria of selection indicated above. Freedom from moisture, during storage, is very important to avoid spoilage. The *dals,* which contain broken pieces, cost less than those, which do not. These less expensive ones can be used in preparations, which are made after grinding (wet or dry) such as *vadas, idli, dhokla, pakodas* etc.

Sugar is made from sugarcane in India. It is normally available in three main forms—granulated, powdered sugar and large crystals (*khadi sakhar*). Granulated sugar is the most commonly used sugar. Selection is made on the basis of cleanliness and absence of dirt and dust. Jaggery is also made from sugarcane in India. There are two main types. One is solid, light golden in colour, and the other is soft and dark in colour. Jaggery is selected for colour and consistency needed in terms of intended use. Dark variety is preferred for preparations such as *chikki,* while light coloured variety may be used in *payasam* (milk pudding or *kheer*).

Semi-perishable Foods

These include processed cereals and pulse products, roots and tubers, fats and oils.

Processed Cereals and Pulse Products

A number of processed products are made from cereals and pulses. These include wheat products, such as, cracked wheat, semolina (*rawa*), *atta, maida,* rice flakes, puffed rice (*murmura*), roasted *chana dal* (dale), *chana,* etc. These are made by grinding the grain to varying degrees of fineness (various particle sizes), by roasting the whole grain or by any other method. These processes increase the surface area of the product exposed to atmosphere, decrease the preparation time and also reduce the shelf-life of the products. While the whole grains have a shelf-life of a year or more, the shelf-life of these processed products may vary from two weeks to a few months.

Broken Wheat or Dalia is whole wheat coarsely ground into large particles. As the losses during milling are very little, it is a very nutritious food. Good quality is indicated by sweet taste and an absence of sour, mouldy odour and flavour. It spoils very quickly in storage, due to insect infestation. It can be cooked as such, made into *upma, shira* or porridge.

Semolina, Suji or Rawa is available in varied sizes. The fine grain varieties are used for preparation of *halwas,* while the large grain varieties are suitable for preparation of *upma, shira,* etc. These are selected on the basis of uniformity of size, freedom from oxidised or mouldy odour, grit or bran.

Maida is white finely extracted wheat flour. It is free from bran and has a lower content of protein, iron and B-vitamins. It has a lower shelf-life than semolina, as the large surface area permits faster rate of spoilage. Good quality *maida* is free from insect infestation, bad odours and lump formation.

Processed Rice Products

These include rice flakes and rice puffs. Rice flakes are made after soaking the paddy in hot water; parehing it by roasting and then flattening it by force while it is hot to form flakes. It retains a large part of the iron and B-vitamin of the aleurone layer. The roasting helps to toast the grain, resulting in partial cooking of the grain. It needs very little time to prepare and is used as a snack. It should be free from bran, broken particles, fragments of the seed coat, insects, stones, trash and bad odour.

Rice Puffs are another ready-to-eat rice product. It is selected for crispness, freedom from stones, seedcoats, sand and dirt.

Roasted chana dal and *chanas* are selected for crisp texture, sweet flavour and absence of flat flavour.

Roots and Tubers

These include potatoes, sweet potatoes, onions, tapioca (*cassava*), colocasia (*aravi*), yams and many lesser known varieties of roots and tubers. In general, these should be firm, heavy, free from bruises, spots, dirt and discolouration.

Potatoes are chosen according to the recipe to be made. These should be free from sprouts, heavy in relation to size, firm, with shallow eyes and without green discolouration. The varieties, which hold their form during cooking, are preferred in most preparations.

Onions—Select hard, well-shaped globes, with dry skins, free from spots and bruises.

Fats and Oils

A number of household fats are available in India. The choice depends on the food preparation in which the fat is to be used, the family needs, the food budget and regional preference.

Ghee is preferred for its delicate flavour, in preparation of sweets (*halwas* especially) and to serve with rice or snacks. Butter is used as a spread and in some baked products for the same reason.

Oil is normally used for seasoning vegetables, *dals* and as a frying medium. The choice of oil varies from one region to another, e.g., mustard oil is used in Bengal, coconut oil in Kerala, groundnut oil in Gujarat and gingelly (*til*) oil in Tamil Nadu.

A large amount of oil is marketed as unrefined or crude oil. Criteria for selection of crude oil are presence of the natural characteristic aroma, natural colour, clarity, freedom from admixture with other kinds of oils, freedom from solid particles and flat or rancid odour.

All the oils and fats supply energy irrespective of their source. Most of the vegetable oils supply poly unsaturated fatty acids (Table 18.1). The animals fats, ghee and butter, supply some vitamin A also. Some refined oils are fortified with vitamin A almost to the same level a cow's ghee (750 mcg or 2500 I.U. per 100 g). Refined oils have a longer shelf-line than unrefined oils of the same kind. As impurities are removed in refining, the smoke points[1] of refined oils during frying is higher than that of unrefined oils. Refined oils are used in bakery products (bread, biscuits, etc.) by large bakeries.

Hydrogenated fats (*vanaspati*) are also available for use in food preparation. These are manufactured from vegetable oils by the addition of molecular hydrogen to the double bonds in the unsaturated fatty acids in the presence of a catalyst. These are partially hydrogenated to obtain the physical characteristics desired in terms of texture and boiling point.

The product thus formed is more stable than the vegetable oil from which it is made. The process is designed to produce characteristics most desired in terms of use and consumer acceptance. In India, it is made as a substitute for ghee, and therefore its physical appearance and texture resembles ghee. It is also fortified with vitamin A to the same level as ghee (750 mcg or 2500 I.U. per 1001g) to protect the consumer. Hydrogenated fats have a higher smoke point than refined oils, and are used for frying bland foods. These are also used in pastries.

1. Smoke point is the temperature at which a fat or oil gives off a thin bluish smoke when heated.

Oils and fats are selected for colour, clarity, characteristic aroma and absence of bad odour (rancid), dirt, dust particles, etc., in the product.

Table 18.1: Polyunsaturated Fatty Acids (PUFA) in Oils & Fats[1]

Oil or Fat	*PUFA Content %*
Kardi oil (Safflower)	75
Soyabean oil	55
Cotton seed oil	50
Maize (Corn) oil	45
Til (Sesame or gingelly) oil	42
Groundnut oil	28
Mustard oil	25
Olive oil	10
Coconut oil	2
Vanaspati	6
Ghee (butterfat)	4

1. *Nutritive Value of Indian Foods,* p.149. ICMR; 197p.

Perishable Foods

Perishable foods include plant foods like fresh vegetables and fruits, and animals foods, such as milk, eggs, poultry, fish and meat.

Vegetables and fruits are good sources of vitamins, minerals and dietary fibre. Milk, eggs, flesh foods are good sources of proteins and B-vitamins. These foods are easily spoilt, if stored at room temperature, due to the action of enzymes and microorganisms.

One criterion for selection of perishable foods is that these must be fresh. In practice this means milk freshly drawn, fish freshly caught from a river or sea, meat soon after slaughter, eggs just laid, vegetables just harvested from the garden and fruits just picked from the tree.

As population increases, foods have to be purchased further away from the point of production. Knowledge of quality characteristics of foods may help you to select and purchase perishable foods.

Vegetables and Fruits

Vegetables and fruits make a meal attractive and enjoyable by the variety of colours, textures and flavours they contribute. Vegetables and fruits are the major source of $\beta-$carotene and vitamin C in the diet. In addition they supply varying amounts of minerals and other vitamins also.

Most fresh vegetables and fruits retain their freshness for a short time under ideal conditions of storage. Standards for selection of vegetables vary with the specific commodity. In general, freshness, uniformity of size, variety, colour, degree of ripeness and freedom from defects are the qualities most frequently sought. When purchasing, select fresh vegetables and fruits, which are firm, crisp, bright in colour, with no visible bruises or signs of decay and wilting.

At the peak of season, each vegetable and fruit has the highest nutrient content, flavour and is available at a reasonable price. It is therefore advisable to buy vegetables and fruits which are in season, as the quality is high and the price low.

Leafy Vegetables include all *sags* or *keerai* such as amaranth, *bathua,* coriander, fenugreek (*methi*), spinach (*palak*), colocasia leaves, mint and mustard. Dark green, leafy vegetables are good sources of minerals, iron and calcium, and vitamin A, C and some of the B-complex vitamins.

Select clean leafy vegetables, which are tender, crisp, brightly coloured and free from flowers, insects, mud and spots or holes in the leaves. In head vegetables, such as cabbage, the hard, heavy and compact heads free from bruises and worm injury are a good buy.

Other Vegetables include stems, fruit vegetables such as brinjals, cucumber, all gourds, pumpkin, ladies finger, pepper, tomatoes, pods such as cluster beans, french beans, immature seeds-corn, wal, *chawali* and peas, cauliflower and all other vegetables, which are not included in the groups leafy or roots and tubers.

Generally tender, firm, crisp, bright coloured vegetables free from worm injury, are selected and too mature, dry, wilted, shrunken, shrivelled discoloured vegetables are rejected. Small or medium-sized vegetables are likely to be more tender and less fibrous in texture than large and too mature ones. Each vegetables is selected according to the preparation in which it is to be used. For example, tomatoes used for salads need to be large and fleshy; small and medium-sized ones can be used in mixed vegetables or stews.

Fruits

Many fruits are used as vegetables, e.g., cucumber, tomatoes, etc. What we eat as fruit is normally seedbearing parts of plants, which consist of edible tissue, which is juicy, pulpy and sweet or sweet-sour in taste and mature seed or seeds enclosed in it. Most ripe fruits can be eaten as such. Fruits have delicate, delectable flavours and aroma and attractive colour and texture. Most fruits are enjoyed by all groups and at all times either as an appetiser, a snack or as a dessert. Fruits are important sources of minerals and vitamins. Deep orange-yellow varieties are important as sources of pro-vitamin A (beta-carotene). *Amla,* guavas, citrus fruits, pineapple, are rich sources of vitamin C. In purchasing fruits, it is necessary to learn to judge the appropriate size and colour for the kind and variety of fruit, as these are indicators of the high quality of the fruit and its maturity. As with vegetables, fresh fruits are best at the peak of the season, as the flavour and nutrient content is high and prices competitive.

Citrus Fruits: Select mature, firm, just ripe, thin skinned, heavy in relation to size fruit, which is free from blemishes, bruises, soft spots. Citrus fruits include oranges, sweet limes (*mausambi*), grape fruits, pomoloe, lemons, etc. These are sorted according to size and the price decreases with the size. These are sold per dozen or per basket, which contain two to six dozen of larger fruits and hundred of smaller fruits. In some markets lemons are sold by weight. Citrus fruits which are thin skinned, firm, and heavy in relation to size are preferred, as these are likely to contain more juice. Citrus fruits are valued for their taste and refreshing flavour and add to the appetising quality of fruit salads and fruit cocktails.

Bananas: A number of varieties—green, yellow and red are normally available throughout the year. Each one has its own characteristic flavour. Of these green ones are more common than the other two. The bunch is plucked when it starts ripening on the tree. It is better to purchase bananas which are free from bruises and slightly hard and then allow them to ripen at room temperature, as fully ripe fruit is easily bruised even as you carry it home from the market. Shelf-life of green bananas is very short after ripening. Ripe fruit does not store well in the refrigerator, as the sugar to starch conversion is favoured at low temperature.

Some varieties of yellow bananas (such as velachi) can be stored for two to three days after ripening and are not easily bruised, and are a good buy, when available.

Apples are now available throughout the year, as these are now held in cold storage. Good apples are firm, crisp, well coloured and heavy. Each variety has its own characteristic colour and shape. Apples become mealy, have less flavour and taste, when stored too long. Hence, it is advisable to buy apples only in season. The red and golden apples are suitable for serving as such, while small, tart fruits are suitable for making jelly, sauce and pies. Grapes should be plump, shiny, well coloured, firmly attached to stem, free from discolouration and bruises.

Remember not to, refrigerate bananas, pineapples, papayas and avocadoes, as these fruits undergo undesirable changes in texture and flavour at refrigerator temperature. Most other fruits keep well, when refrigerated.

Milk and Milk Products

Milk: Fresh milk has a slightly sweetish odour and flavour, is white in colour and has a faintly acid reaction to litmus. Stale milk has a sour odour and flavour. Fresh cow's and buffalo's milk is sold through home delivery or dairies. It is advisable to boil fresh milk before use.

Pasteurised Milk: In the larger cities, pasteurised milk is distributed by government, semi-government, co-operative or private agencies. The milk is pasteurised, bottled or put into plastic packets and sold. The price of the milk is indirectly related to the amount of fat present. Major part of the pasteurised, milk sold through Government channels is defatted to varying degrees. As the fat separated is sold after conversion to butter, it helps to reduce the price of the milk.

Butter: Butter is made from milk cream. It contains 11 to 16 per cent moisture. It has a delicate flavour and has a short shelf-life at room temperature. Processed butter keeps up to two weeks in the refrigerator. Home-made fresh butter contains more moisture and therefore has a shorter shelf-life than processed butter.

Paneer: Paneer is coagulated milk protein with high moisture content. It should be used immediately after purchase. It should be bought from clean hygienic dairies or made at home.

Khoya or Mava is prepared from milk by evaporation of water. Fresh *khoya* has a sweet delicate aroma and taste. Stale *khoya* has a rancid odour and a flat taste.

Eggs, Poultry, Fish and Meat

Eggs: A fresh egg has a small aircell, which can be observed against a light or a candle. Eggs are sorted according to size. Large eggs are preferred for table use. When eggs are used in preparation, size is not important and selection is made in terms of price in relation to size. It is advisable to purchase fresh, clean and unbroken eggs.

Poultry: In poultry, there is a relatively high proportion of waste from live weight to edible portion. Edible portion is only about 55 per cent of live weight. Selection is made on the basis of intended use of the poultry. Good quality poultry is full fleshed, meaty and has a good layer of fat. The skin is smooth, without tears and discolouration or pin feathers. Poultry which is dressed, should be properly refrigerated.

In a young bird, the skin and breast-bone are pliable, soft and tear easily. Older birds have hard calcified breast-bone and may have a lot of long hair. Weight is not necessarily related to the age of the bird. In young birds sex difference is not significant, but older male birds are less fatty and are inferior in flavour to female birds.

Fish: Fresh fish has firm flesh, a stiff body and tight scales. If you press the body, no indentation is left. If placed in water, fresh fish sinks; stale fish is flabby; has sunken and dull eyes, scales are easily brushed off, gills are not bright red and has a stale or sour odour. Select fresh fish, which have red gills and bright eyes. Be sure to purchase fish, which has been refrigerated or stored on ice, and is not slippery or slimy to touch.

Select fish according to intended use, e.g., whole fish or fillet for baking; steaks for boiling or frying. Frozen fish should be frozen solid when purchased, and should have no odour. It should be wrapped in water proof packaging material. It should be kept frozen until use.

Meat: Meat is selected on the basis of conformation or form, finish and quality.

Conformation or form refers to the shape or build of the animal. Good form consists of short, thick, compact build, with large muscles, which have high proportion of meat to bone. *Finish* indicates the amount and distribution of fat. An even layer of fat on the outside of the carcass and even distribution of fat in the lean part are indicators of a good finish. In good *quality* meat (*i*) lean meat is bright red in colour, when cut surface is exposed to air; (*ii*) it is fine grained and smooth to touch, (*iii*) the fat is firm, brittle and creamy white in colour.

Dark colour, coarse grain, low fat content uneven distribution and yellow-orange colour of fat and soft texture are indicators of poor quality meat. In India lamb and mutton are used widely. Lamb is sheep's flesh up to the age of one year. When the sheep is more than one year old, its flesh is called mutton.

Pork is flesh of pig. The best quality of pork has muscle that is grayish white to pink in young and deep rose in older animals. The flesh is firm and fine grained and the bones are soft and red. It has a minimum of fat. Lower quality pork is heavier and contains more fat. Pork could contain a parasitic roundworm of microscopic size which produces a disease called *trichinosis.* It is, therefore, recommended that pork be always well cooked before being eaten, as cooking at high temperatures destroys this organism.

Meat prices vary according to the cut, quality and kind. Selection is made according to the intended use in preparation. Generally, the amount of meat purchased is 60 g uncooked boneless meat per person and 100 g, if it contains bones. The meat should be bought from a clean and hygienic shop and should be free from bad odour. Meat should be refrigerated after slaughter, until it is sold. Slime on the surface of meat indicates deterioration.

Storage of Food

Proper storage of food, that is produced at home or purchased for the family is an important part of meeting the food needs of the family. It is necessary to decide about what to store and how to store after considering the space available and the shelf-life of the foods.

On the basis of their stability during storage, foods have been divided into *non-perishable, semi-perishable* and *perishable* foods. Table 18.2 gives a list of common foods classified according to their stability during storage at room temperature. It may be noted that cereals, *dals,* legumes, which have been dried to less than 13 per cent moisture are non-perishable if stored in a cool, dry place.

The foods, which can be stored for a week to a couple of months, at room temperature without the occurrence of undesirable changes in flavour and texture can be termed as semi-perishable foods.

These include, baked foods, roasted, popped or toasted cereals and legumes, ground flours and some fruits and vegetables. Most of the fresh fruits and vegetables, milk, meat, fish, poultry are perishable foods. Their storage life varies from a few hours to a few days, depending on their composition and temperature and humidity at which these are stored.

Usually cereals (e.g., wheat, rice), millets (*bajra*), corn (*makka*), *jowar* legumes, nuts, oilseeds, oil, sugar, salt, etc., are some of the foods, which can be bought in bulk and stored. The quantities stored by a family depends on size of the family and the space available for storage. It also depends on the marketing facilities available and the monetary and other resources of the family.

In rural areas, people store a year's supply of cereals, *dals,* ground-nuts, jaggery, sugar, spices, salt, tamarind, etc. There are several reasons for this practice. The best material is available in harvest season at a reasonable rate. After the season, the rate fluctuates considerably. Many articles are out of stock after the harvest season, or, if available, the quality is poor.

In large cities the trend is quite different. The storage space may be limited. Salaried persons find it easier to buy on a monthly or fortnightly basis. The marketing facilities are relatively stable and storing enough groceries for a fortnight or a month is adequate.

Table 18.2: Storage Life of Foods at 25°C

Food Group	*Non-perishable*	*Semi-perishable*	*Perishable*
I	*Dals,* split, legumes, whole, nuts and oilseeds, dry salted fish and meat	Flours of *dals,* roasted *dals,* roasted nuts and oil-seeds, eggs	Cooked *dals* and legumes, wet-ground mixes (e.g., *idli* mix) milk, fresh *dahi,* butter-milk, *khoya,* cheese, meat, poultry, fish
II (*a*) II (*b*)	Nil Pickled mango, pickled lemons and other citrus fruits	Nil Citrus fruits–oranges lemons, sweet limes, grape fruits	All foods in this group *Amla,* guava cashew apple, pineapple, tomato
III	Nil	Apples, apricots, pumpkin, ashgourd roots and tubers, yams, potatoes, onions	Peas, beans, brinjals, carrots
IV	Whole cereals and millets, dry cereal products	Biscuits, cakes, *rawa* (*suji*), cereal flours, rice flakes, popped cereals	Bread, *roti, chapati* rice or other cooked cereals
V	Sugar, Jaggery, hydrogenated fat, *vanaspati,* oil, ghee	*Mithais*	Butter, cream

Storage of Non-perishable Foods

Dals, whole legumes, most of the whole pulses, oilseeds, etc., can be cleaned to remove stones, sand and any other foreign matter and washed with water to remove any dust and dirt adhering to the grains. Then these may be dried in the sun. After drying, the food materials should be allowed to cool, before being put in containers for storage.

Usually dry foods are stored in tins, which have tight-fitting lids. Spices and *murrabbas* are stored in battles and pickles in glass, earthenware or porcelain containers.

Whatever the material of the container, it is important to wash it with hot water and soap and any matter adhering to it should be scrubbed with a brush or coconut fibre. Next it should be allowed to dry, preferably in the sun. If any wiping is necessary, it should be done with a *clean* cloth.

Convenient Arrangements: Some houses have a separate storeroom. Some have a closet like space attached to the kitchen for storage. Some build a large storage cupboard in the kitchen itself.

Some storerooms are fitted with wall cupboards and these are convenient for storage. Others have cement shelves. If neither arrangement is in existence, wooden shelves can be made, which work well for storage.

To facilitate cleaning of the floor, it is better to have the lowest shelf about six to eight inches above the floor. The heaviest containers should be placed on the lowest shelf. Wherever two rows are placed, taller containers should be kept at the back and the smaller ones in front, so that it is easy to reach both.

Using clean ladles to remove the food from the large containers helps in getting a known amount and avoids spilling.

It is good to keep a few blank cards in the storeroom and note the amounts bought and used with dates. This helps to get an accurate idea of the amounts used. It also gives a fair idea of overall nutrition of the family. An idea of the actual usage of articles helps in making a realistic budget. One added benefit is that any pilferage of food is quickly noticed.

In many city houses, there is no separate storeroom. So it is necessary to fit up storage shelves in the kitchen. In this situation, it is important to put the shelves as far away from the cooking area as possible, because cooking results in heating up the air around the stove (or any other cooking device—gas or sigree). This frequent increase in temperature encourages the growth of moths and weevils in the food. Also, when air is heated, the moisture from the air is condensed, making nearby objects damp. This, too, aids the growth of moths and weevils. Therefore, the storage shelves should be located in a cool and dry corner of the kitchen.

In most rural households, cereals are stored in earthenware containers or containers made of bamboo and plastered with mud or cow-dung. These are improvised storage structures made from indigenous materials. Cereals after harvest and drying are stored in these containers and covered with dried-hay or straws. These storage structures are however susceptible to attack by rodents and consequently some losses of stored foodgrains occur. Pulses, spices, tamarind, etc., are also usually stored in earthenware pots or jugs.

For bulk-storage of foodgrains usually maintained by wholesale traders. State Trading Corporations, Central Warehouses, Food Corporation of India, the foodgrains are stored in gunny-bags (jute bags) in piles in big godowns usually made rat-proof. These godowns are to be properly ventilated, periodically fumigated and kept free from water-logging to prevent dampening of stored commodities.

Storage of Semi-perishable Foods

When cereals, *dals* and legumes (including groundnuts) are subject to any processing such as grinding, roasting, baking or frying, their high quality storage life is reduced depending upon the storage temperature and relative humidity (presence of moisture in the air).

The flours, *suji,* rice flakes (*chewda*), roasted *dals,* etc., which have a moisture content less than 13 per cent are stored in the same manner as cereals and pulses described above. Flour and Semolina (*suji*) spoil faster than whole grain, because the insects can use these foods more easily. When rice flakes or popcorn is made some flavour compounds are formed, which are responsible for the characteristic flavour. These are slowly lost during storage, thus these products become less palatable, as the period of storage increases. It is therefore better to use such products within a few weeks of production to ensure high quality.

Apples, citrus fruits, some gourds and root vegetables keep well in a cool storeroom, cellar or basement. Suitable temperature for storage of these fruits and vegetables is around 15°C. Table 18.3 gives optimal temperatures and relative humidity for storage of raw foods.

Table 18.3: Optimal Temperature and Relative Humidity for Storage of Raw Foods

Product (foods)	*Temperature* (°C)	*Relative Humidity* %
Bananas	12–16	85–90
Beans, peppers	7	85–90
Cabbage, lettuce, carrots	0	90–95
Lemons	13–14	85–90
Melons	4–10	80–85
Nuts	0–02	65–70
Onions	0	70–75
Tomatoes (ripe)	4–10	85–90

Storage of Perishable Foods

Foods spoil due to the action of enzymes and microorganisms (moulds, yeasts and bacteria) in them. Actual spoilage is usually quite easily noticed by the presence of rancid odour flavour of fats (caused by oxidation), fermented odour of fruit or fruit juices due to yeast growth, or the appearance of mould growth on bread, *roti* or cooked rice. Slime on the surface of meats, or sour taste in bland foods may be caused by bacterial action.

Low temperatures retard spoilage and other changes in the quality of perishable foods (Figure 18.1). The action of enzymes and the growth of spoilage organisms is slowed down by low temperature storage. Perishable foods include most of the fresh vegetables and fruits and animal protein foods such as milk, eggs, meat, fish and poultry.

Vegetables and Fruits continue to respire after they are harvested. Harvesting disturbs the normal life processes, and vegetables start losing their vitality, turgidity and food value. The harvested vegetables continue to respire during transport and storage. This involves the using of oxygen, the metabolism of cell food materials, and the release of carbon dioxide, water and energy. Most of the energy is released in the form of heat. The process of respiration must be slowed during storage, by control of temperature and relative humidity.

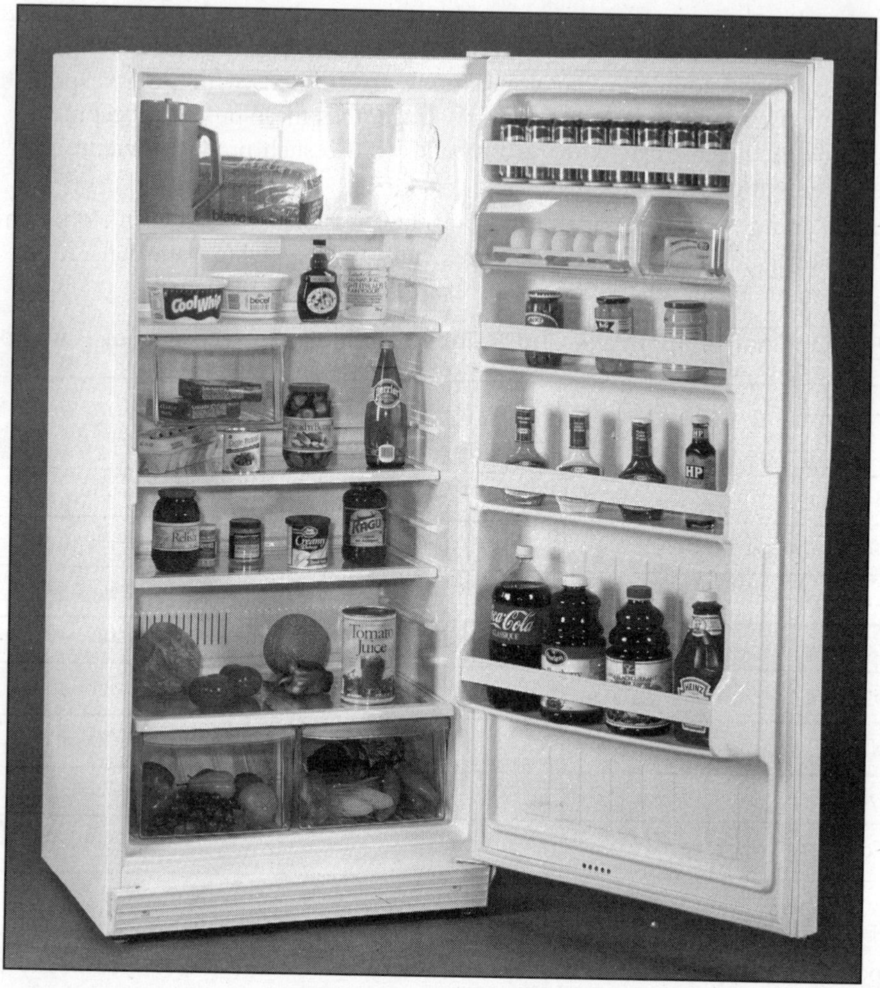

Figure 18.1: Refrigeration—a low temperature storage of perishable foods.

Plant (vegetable) tissues change during storage. These changes include loss of water, modification of the fibres, and change in the pectins. The loss of water is reduced by storing vegetables in an atmosphere of high relative humidity. Removing the tops of radishes, carrots and onions, reduces loss of moisture, due to decrease in surface area. Peas in pods keep better than when shelled. Peas and corn become less palatable during storage due to sugar being converted to starch. It is better to buy these vegetables only in the quantity needed for immediate use. Succulent vegetables should be kept cold in a dampened cloth or in a covered ventilated container. Roots and tubers may be stored in a cool, ventilated place the storage temperature being maintained between 3 and 10°C (38–50°F) — to keep sprouting to a minimum. Only sound vegetables should be selected and stored; even a few bruised tubers may contaminate the entire lot.

Leafy and other vegetables and fruits start ageing soon after harvest. The crispness and flavour of green leafy vegetables deteriorate as water evaporates from it. These changes related to ageing are retarded by low temperature storage.

Leafy and other vegetables tend to shrivel and become unpalatable when stored uncovered in the refrigerator. Most refrigerators provide at least one covered container called a 'crisper' for storage of vegetables and fruits. Use of plastic bags for storage of clean dry vegetables and fruits, retards the evaporation of moisture from them.

Milk: Deterioration starts soon after the collection of milk. It is necessary to retard the changes during storage, so that there is minimal loss of quality prior to the preparation and use. Some of the steps taken to ensure quality during storage of these foods are discussed here.

Milk is normally boiled in Indian homes, as soon as it is brought to the kitchen and stored in covered containers. Boiling destroys spoilage organisms and also the enzymes present in milk. Thus boiling helps to store milk in good condition for 12–24 hours, at room temperature. Milk is converted to curd by inoculating it with buttermilk containing lactics. The conversion to curd and buttermilk, helps to extend the storage period of milk by 24 hours. The storage life can be further extended by storage in the refrigerator. Butter and cheese are also perishable products of which the storage period can be extended to two weeks, by refrigeration.

Fish, Meat Poultry: Fresh fish, meat, poultry can be kept for short periods at temperatures just above freezing. Ground meat is more likely to spoil than roasts, chops, steaks, due to (i) the handling, (ii) exposure of larger surface to air, and (iii) equipments. Organ meats such as liver, kidney, brain are also more perishable than other cuts.

Oxidation of fats in meats produces off-flavours and oxidation of meat pigments causes discolouration. Both these are undesirable changes, which can be retarded by storing meat in the coldest part of the refrigerator. The fats in pork and poultry are more easily oxidised than others. Therefore, it is recommended that these meats be held for very short periods, prior to use.

Shell Eggs should be refrigerated promptly. Flavour and quality changes occur rapidly if eggs are held at room temperature, but very slowly at refrigerator temperature.

Study Questions and Activities

1. List the criteria for selection of:
   (*a*) Rice, wheat, *suji, maida.*
   (*b*) Green leafy vegetables.
   (*c*) Fruits.
2. List the foods, which are perishable. Discuss how to store these so as to retain nutrients.
3. What are the criteria in selection of oils and fats?
4. Discuss the statement "the period of storage of foods is related to the moisture content".
5. Discuss the factors that affect storage period of vegetables, fruits and eggs.
6. What precautions will you take while storing rice, wheat, *dal* and *maida*? What type of losses are likely to occur if these precautions are not taken?

CHAPTER 19

Food Preparation

Reasons for Cooking Foods
Quality of Food
Preliminary Treatment of Foods
- Seasoning

Food Preparation Techniques
Methods of Food Preparation
- Choice of Fuel

Medium of Food Preparation
- Water
- Steam
- Oil or Fat
- Air

Combination of Methods
Study Questions and Practical Activities

FOOD IS A complex mixture of many different chemical components. The study of food preparation involves understanding the changes that occur in these components during preparation as a result of their interaction with one another, with the medium of cooking, the temperature of cooking and the environment.

Food preparation is an important step in meeting the nutritional needs of the family. It is not enough that food be nutritious, it has to be pleasing in appearance and taste so that it is eaten. Good preparation is an important prerequisite of food acceptance. Therefore, it is important to acquire the ability to prepare and serve food, which is nutritious and acceptable to the family. The science of food preparation is based on the understanding of physical and chemical changes that occur in food during preparation.

This knowledge can be used to combine food ingredients in diverse ways to prepare innumerable combinations with delicate flavours, textures, and colour, which delight the senses. Thus food preparation is both a science and an art. Food preparation is very much a part of the culture of the region. Each region has its own methods of blending flavours to bring about acceptable combinations.

Reasons for Cooking Foods

Most foods are acceptable only when they are cooked. Except for some fruits and vegetables, most of the food we eat is cooked. Even the tea or coffee or milk we take in the morning and the bread we take with it involves some manner of cooking. For centuries we have nurtured this art of cooking. Let us see why we cook food.

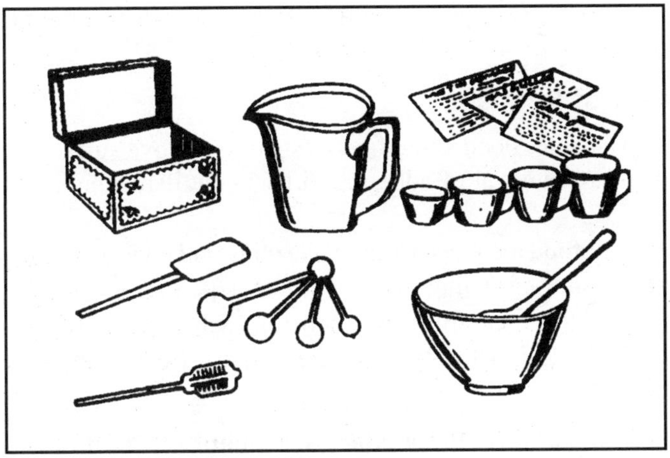

Figure 19.1: Food preparation.

One of the foremost reasons for cooking is that it improves taste. Cooking does improve the taste of as simple a food as rice. It also makes the food more palatable. The sight of a raw potato may not even attract a hungry person but the sight of potato chips allures us to sample a few even when we are not hungry. Thus cooking helps to enhance the taste and flavour of food and makes it more appetising.

A number of desirable changes occur in foods during cooking. For instance vegetables become soft. Starchy foods like cereals and *dals* take up water, swell and soften.

Food preparation is very much a part of the culture of the region. Each region has its own methods of blending flavours to bring about acceptable combinations. Spices and condiments are added to the food and the food is simmered until the flavours blend. Some foods are also seasoned with heated oil in which some of the spices are fried. These steps help to blend the flavours of the ingredients and thus enhance the acceptability of the product.

As cooking involves heating of foods, many microorganisms are destroyed, during the course of cooking. This renders the food safe for eating. For example, boiling milk results in killing pathogens like tubercle bacilli if these are present; spoilage organisms are also killed by heating milk. Therefore heated milk keeps longer than unheated milk. Some of the toxins present in the foods are rendered inactive at the cooking temperature. Thus cooking helps to remove heat-labile toxins.

Cooking food helps to provide unlimited variety in the menu. Thus with the same raw foods it is possible to provide innumerable dishes, which makes eating a pleasure.

Cooked food is easily chewed and swallowed. It is easily acted on by digestive juices. This makes its passage through the digestive tract smooth. In this manner, cooking improves the digestibility of food.

Quality of Food

The condition of the food when it is brought into the kitchen determines the nature of the final cooked product. Foods bought must be of good quality. Conditions of storage should be such that the quality does not deteriorate during storage. Vegetable that have been stored too long, milk and milk products that have deteriorated (i.e., *dahi* which is sour) and oils that are flat or rancid cannot improve in the preparation. This does not mean that one must buy the most expensive foods in the market. But it does mean that one must buy good quality food. Expensive foods need not necessarily be of good quality.

Preliminary Treatment of Foods

Only clean food is palatable. Food should be washed to remove surface dirt. Each food needs to be handled carefully to ensure removal of adhering dirt without damaging its form and structure, and causing loss of nutrients.

Preliminary treatment of food includes washing, cleaning, peeling, cutting, slicing, grating, soaking, germinating, fermenting, roasting, grinding or some other step.

These procedures have to be carefully planned for each food so that the natural flavour and texture are retained. Table 19.1 lists the type of preliminary treatments of various foods prior to preparation.

Table 19.1: Preliminary Treatment of Foods

Preliminary Treatment	*Foods*
Washing	Vegetables, fruits, whole grains
Peeling, cutting, slicing, grating, cubing	Vegetables and fruits
Pounding/milling/grinding	Cereals, legumes, spices, nuts
Soaking	Rice, *dals,* legumes
Fermenting	Cereals, *dals* and their mixtures
Germinating	Cereals and legumes
Roasting	Whole cereals, legumes, nuts, semolina, spices, etc.
Mixing	All ingredients in preparations
Kneading	Flours for breads, *chapatis, puri,* etc.

The pre-preparation steps mentioned above need to be carried out in such a manner that nutrient loss is minimised. For example, while washing rice and *dal* to remove external dirt, care must be taken not to scrub the grain, which may lead to unnecessary loss of water-soluble nutrients. Vegetables and fruits must be cut into even pieces, which are symmetrical and convey a sense of order. Some fruits darken on cutting and peeling, e.g., apples. It may not be necessary to peel these. It is advisable to cut such fruits just before use (Figure 19.2).

Vegetables and fruits need to be drained after washing, to reduce spoilage. Soaking rice, *dal* and whole legumes before cooking may result in reduced cooking time and improved texture.

In short, care and planning in preliminary handling is essential to prepare an acceptable finished product. Poor preliminary treatment cannot be corrected later.

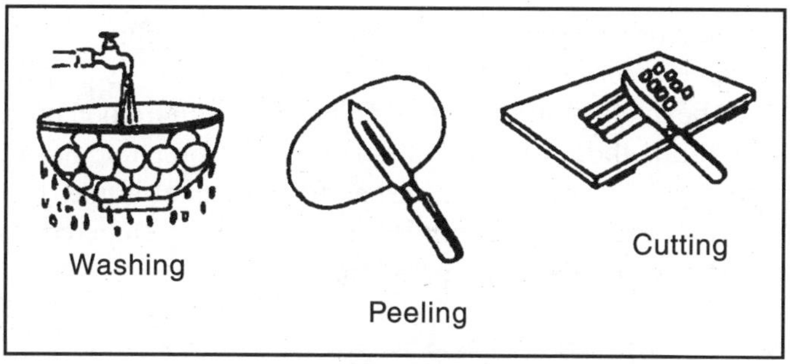

Figure 19.2: Steps in food preparation.

Seasoning

Some foods require no seasoning. Others are improved by addition of small amounts of seasoning materials. The purpose of seasoning is to enhance the flavour of the food and to make it more delectable. Seasoning should be used judiciously so that it blends with the food flavour and is not excessive.

Food Preparation Techniques

Good food preparation requires understanding of the composition and structure of food and the changes that take place during preparation. Basic principles must be observed for each group of food products to obtain good results. Skill in handling foods is acquired by applying knowledge of cooking principles. Some techniques are more difficult to master than others; e.g., making an attractive salad is easier than preparing vegetable cutlets.

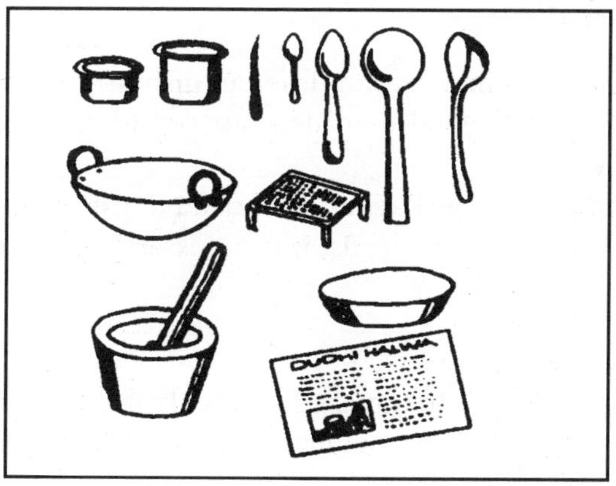

Figure 19.3: Utensils used in food preparation.

In addition *good equipment* used scientifically helps to achieve good results in food preparation (Figs. 19.1, 19.3, 19.4, 19.5, 19.6). Knowledge of the correct *recipe,* which indicates the proportion of various ingredients and the order and method of combining these helps to ensure a good product. As books which give basic proportions and recipes of Indian dishes are few, one has to record one's own recipes and improve or modify them to create variety.

The magic ingredient in food preparation is *imagination.* It is the ability to visualise the effect of change in ingredients on the recipe in terms of flavour, texture and colour. As in any other art, practice is essential but the practice must be intelligently directed. To be proficient in food preparation skills, one must make efforts to observe carefully those who are proficient in food preparation and get opportunities to handle food. The chance to organise and prepare dishes for parties at home, for the class and for friends help to develop one's skills and creative abilities. It must be remembered that foods are most palatable and nutritious when served soon after preparation.

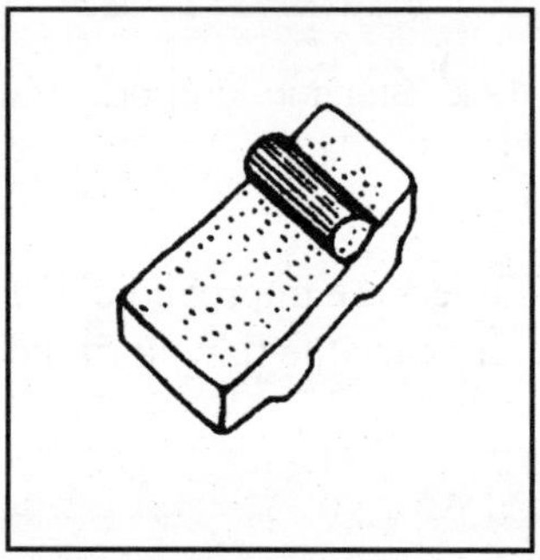

Figure 19.4: Grinding stone.

It is necessary to think of how the foods combine in terms of colour, flavour and texture. Pleasing combinations increase the appeal of a meal. Here again, one can make innumerable combinations from the same ingredients if one uses one's experience and imagination.

Methods of Food Preparation

Each food item can be prepared into several different dishes. The methods of cooking of these items, however, are not many. The method used depends on the kind of product desired and the ingredients available.

Desirable appearance, colour, texture, flavour, odour and moisture must be retained or produced in the course of preparation. To achieve these ends, it is necessary to understand the methods used in the preparation of food.

Choice of Fuel

Before we proceed with discussing the methods of cooking let us try to understand how heat energy, which is necessary for all forms of cooking, is produced. The heat for cooking is usually generated by the use of kerosene, gas, electricity, charcoal, wood or sawdust as fuel. The choice of fuel depends on the availability and the comparative cost of various fuels. Ease with which the fuel ignites and is put off and safety in use are also important considerations in the choice of fuel. Fuels, which can be converted into heat energy without production of offensive by-products and leave none or minimum residue, are preferred as they are economic and convenient to use.

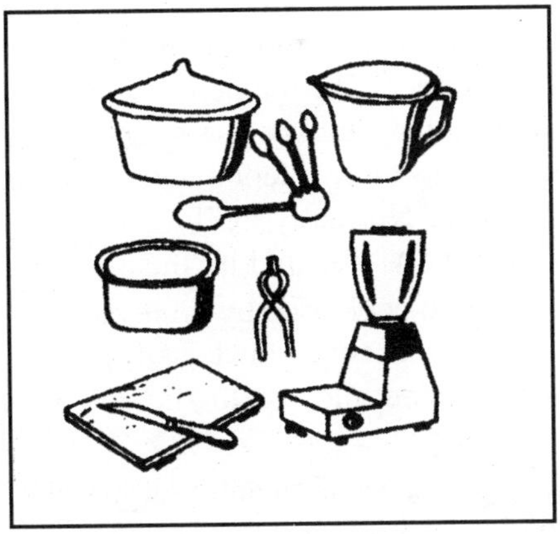

Figure 19.5: Food preparation equipment.

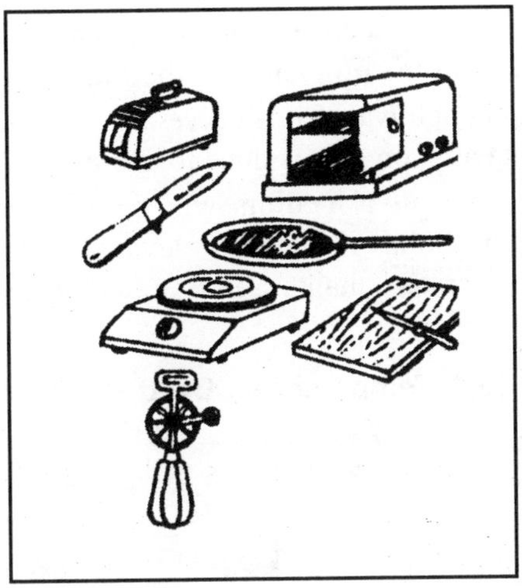

Figure 19.6: Food preparation equipment.

By these criteria the fuels may be listed in the order of preference thus cooking gas, electricity, kerosene, charcoal, sawdust and wood. In practice, two more factors may affect our choice, availability and cost.

Medium of Food Preparation

The methods of cooking can be classified on the basis of the medium used for heat transfer. The media normally used are water as such or in the form of steam, oil and air.

Water

Water is most commonly used medium of cooking. Boiling, simmering and stewing are methods in which moist heat is used. Many of the foods are cooked by using a combination of these methods.

Boiling: The food is washed, covered with an adequate quantity of water and heated to boiling. The intensity of heat is then reduced to keep the food simmering till done. The temperature of boiling water is usually 100°C and when it simmers, the temperature may range from 85 to 90°C. If the food is boiled continuously water is evaporated quickly, the structure and texture of the food product is affected adversely (damaged) and the loss of heat-labile nutrients is increased. The continuous boiling of food results in wastage of fuel also. Normally, boiling followed by simmering is used in food preparation. Soups and broths are normally prepared by this method.

Simmering and poaching are used to cook food by immersion in a liquid maintained at just below the boiling point (85°C–90°C) so that bubbles form slowly and collapse below the surface. As mentioned earlier, most foods are brought to boil and allowed to simmer till done. Milk preparations such as *Kadhi, Kheer* are prepared by simmering.

Stewing refers to simmering food in a small quantity of liquid. The temperature of stewing is the same as that of simmering. The food is stewed when the finished product is intended to contain a small amount of liquid. Most of the vegetables and meats are prepared by this method.

Foods cooked with water as the medium are heated by transfer of heat energy from the fuel through the container to the water. Water is heated both by conduction and convection currents. The time needed for cooking the food is thus dependent on the amount of food being cooked, the material, thickness and size of the container and the efficiency of the fuel used.

If the food is cooked in just enough water, it is necessary to reduce the heat, keep a watchful eye and remove the food from the stove as soon as it is done to avoid burning the bottom layer of the food.

The cooking of food with water as a medium will be affected by the quantity of dissolved substances in it because the boiling point of water is elevated in the presence of solutes. At high altitudes water boils at a lower temperature than at sea level and therefore cooking may take a longer time than at sea level.

Table 19.2: Temperatures Used for Cooking

Method of cooking	*Approximate temperature*
Simmering/stewing	95°–90°C
Boiling/steaming	100°C
Pressure cooking	110–112°C
Baking	110°C–205°C[1]
Deep fat frying	180–220°C

1. The temperature attained by the food is only about 43°C

Steam

Steaming of food also involves the use of moist heat. When food is cooked in water vapour with or without pressure it is said to be steamed. The water vapour is produced from water placed at the bottom of the pan. Some of the products that are prepared by steaming are *idli, khaman-dhokla, modak,* etc.

Pressure Cooking: When steam under pressure is used the method is known as *pressure cooking* and the equipment used is known as a pressure cooker. As the temperature is elevated quickly in the food cooked with steam under pressure, the cooking period is reduced as also the loss of heat-labile nutrients. In this method, heat is transferred from the steam to the food; the steam condenses on the cold food and heat is released. Condensation of the steam occurs until the food reaches the temperature of steam (100°C); then the condensation decreases and steam pressure is built-up in the pressure cooker, to the point desired. Rice, *dal*, some pieces of meat, potatoes and other roots and tubers, and various types of beans, and peas and some gourds are cooked in the pressure cooker.

Steam cooked foods are light, fluffy and easily digestible. As the period of cooking is reduced, the loss of heat-labile nutrients is minimised and there is saving of fuel and time. As the steaming of food does not need constant attention as in simmering or stewing, the time saved can be used for other activities such as preparing salad, *chapati* or dessert.

Oil or Fat

Oil or fat is used as a medium of cooking in pan-frying and deep fat frying. *Pan-frying* or *shallow frying* is the cooking of food in a lightly greased pan, e.g., *dosai, thalipeeth,* fried egg, pancake, *puda,* etc. The heat is transferred mainly by conduction to the food. Only a thin layer of mix or thin pieces of food are cooked in this manner. The food must be turned from one side to another to ensure complete cooking.

Deep fat frying is similar to boiling. The fat is heated by conduction of heat from the frying pan; the heat is then distributed by convection currents through the fat. The food is cooked very quickly by this method as the fats can be heated to much higher temperatures than boiling water. Therefore, it needs constant and careful attention. The temperature of frying varies from 180–220°C depending on the oil or fat used as a frying medium and food preparation being made. It is important to choose fats with high smoking temperature as the frying medium. Fats and oils should not be heated to the smoking point[1] as at this temperature the fat starts decomposing, and is not suitable for frying foods.

Frying imparts a special flavour and texture to the foods making it tender or crunchy. There is an increase in the energy value of the food when it is fried. The high temperature used destroys any pathogens present on the surface.

These foods are not digested quickly, due to the fat absorbed in frying. This method is not suitable for tough cuts of meat. It is used to make *puries, pakoras, samosas,* chips cutlets, etc.

Air (dry heat)

Methods in which air is used as a principal cooking medium include roasting, baking, broiling and grilling.

Roasting means to cook food by dry heat without covering it. Food is roasted or baked on heated metal, on stones or under hot coals, in hot ashes and/or in an oven.

Foods prepared by this method include *chapati, roti,* nan, and other unleavened breads, potatoes, sweet potatoes, other tubers, *jowar,* corn, paddy, groundnuts, cashewnuts, walnuts, pistachios, etc.

Baking is also cooking by dry heat in an oven or oven-like appliance, covered or uncovered containers may be used for baking. The food placed in the oven, to bake or roast may be partially

---

1. Smoking-point of fat is the temperature at which decomposition starts with emission of blue smoke, which is irritating.

cooked by dry heat, by the convection currents of hot dry air and conduction of heat from the container to the food and partially by moist heat. Hot sand baths are used in baking on top of the stove. In this improvised method, the baking dish is placed in the sand bath, which is then covered to prevent loss of heat. Bread, cakes, pies, pastries are examples of baked products. The temperatures attained in different methods are given in Table 19.2.

Broiling or *grilling* refers to cooking of food by exposing it to direct heat. The food is cooked in part by contact with the hot broiler (conduction) and partially due to the radiant heat energy. Grilled sandwiches are an example of this method of cooking.

Combination of Methods

Many food preparation are made by using a combination of methods. When we roast semolina before putting it in boiling water for preparing *upma* or season vegetables with oil and spices and then add water, two cooking media—air and water, fat and water are used. It may be noted that many food preparations are made by using more than one method of heat transfer.

Study Questions and Practical Activities

1. List the reasons for cooking food.
2. What are the preliminary steps in food preparation? What is the function of two of these in preparation of an acceptable food product?
3. Write notes on:
   (*i*) Simmering
   (*ii*) Stewing
   (*iii*) Steaming
   (*iv*) Pressure-cooking.
4. Discuss the advantages and disadvantages of using oil as a medium of cooking.
   Food Selection and Preparation
   Practical Work to include
   Methods of food preparation:
   (*i*) Cereals
   (*ii*) Pulses and legumes
   (*iii*) Vegetables and salads
   (*iv*) Fruit
   (*v*) Meat and eggs
   (*vi*) Milk
   (*vii*) Snacks
   (*viii*) Desserts.

Observe changes in colour, texture and flavour during and after preparation.

CHAPTER 20

Effect of Preparation on Food Components

A NUMBER OF changes occur in the food components as a result of preparation. It is necessary to understand and manipulate the changes to obtain an acceptable food product.

The major constituents of food are carbohydrates, proteins, fats and their derivatives and water. In addition, a number of inorganic mineral components and a diverse group of organic substances are present in very small amounts in foods. These include pigments, flavour components, vitamins, acids, enzymes, etc. Let us consider their properties and the changes that occur in these components during handling, cooking and processing.

Carbohydrates

Starch, sugars, pectins, gums, celluloses and hemicelluloses are the important carbohydrates found in foods.

Starches are the major component of cereals, millets, *dals,* roots, tubers, and sago. Starches are bland in taste, not readily soluble in cold water but absorb water when soaked in cold water. When starch granules are added to cold water, a temporary suspension is formed, the starch tends to settle out as soon as the mixture is allowed to stand.

When dry starch is mixed with warm or hot water, the part which comes in contact with water becomes sticky and the starch granules cling together in lumps. Heating does not help to separate the granules, because once formed the lumps stay intact. If one of these lumps is broken open, raw starch is found inside.

Lump formation can be prevented by mixing starch with a little cold water before introducing it into the hot water; roasting a little before addition of hot water or addition of a little fat, helps to separate the starch granules and allows them to gelatinise separately. The starches take up water, swell and burst on cooking. When a starch and water mixture is heated, it becomes translucent and forms a paste. This change is accompanied by a change in viscosity. This property is used when starch is used as a thickener in soups, starch puddings and other preparations. A gel is formed at a higher concentration of starch, e.g., puddings. The water is held in a physical bond by the starch. The change in texture, colour and physical state, which occurs when starch is heated in water, is known as gelatinisation of starch. In roots and tubers, the presence of starch, which absorbs the water during cooking, results in retention of size.

Sugars: About 5–11 per cent are present in ripe fruits, malted beverages and in milk. Sucrose the sugar we use in food preparations is one of the pure, manufactured (extracted) foods we use daily. It is manufactured from sugarcane or sugarbeet. Sugar is sweet and is usually used in foods for its sweetening power.

Sugar dissolves in water and when heated this solution easily forms a syrup. When the solution is supersaturated and cooked, crystallisation occurs. This is the process used to prepare sweets such as *laddus,* candies, etc.

When a high concentration of sugar is used it acts as a preservative by binding moisture, e.g., preserves such as *murrabbas,* jams and jellies. In the presence of acids, the sugar (sucrose) is partially hydrolysed to form glucose and fructose, which is known as *invert sugar,* which is more soluble than sucrose. If sugar is heated beyond its melting point it caramelises or browns. the caramel formed has a bitter, astringent flavour. Sugars are readily fermented by microorganisms, thus causing spoilage of food products containing it.

Pectins and gums are responsible for holding the plant cells together. These are found in fruits and vegetables in a very small amount. Pectins and gums form colloidal solution when extracted in hot water and contribute to the viscosity of the product to which they are added. Therefore, these are used as thickeners and stabilisers in food preparation and processing. Pectins form gels in the presence of an appropriate amount of sugar and acid, e.g., fruit jellies.

Celluloses and hemicelluloses, the fibrous parts of vegetables and fruits are not soluble in cold or hot water. These soften as the water trapped in their tissues is released and used in cooking or processing. Thus there is a decrease in volume, especially of leafy vegetables. Celluloses are not digested by man even after cooking but as it has the capacity to bind moisture, it is helpful in smooth movement of the food through the digestive tract.

Proteins

Egg, fish, poultry and meat are good examples of protein foods. In *dals* and legumes the presence of a large amount of starch (50-60 per cent) masks the reactions of proteins during preparation.

All proteins are first denatured and then coagulated by heat. The coagulation occurs between 65 and 90°C. The temperature of coagulation increases with the addition of other ingredients. For example, egg proteins coagulate at 65–70°C, but egg custard coagulates at 85–90°C. Cooking results in softening of proteins in foods such as eggs, fish, poultry, meat, as water is bound in the process of coagulation. If the coagulated protein is further heated, it loses moisture and becomes dry and rubbery. Therefore, it is important to monitor the temperature and time while preparing these foods. Proteins are precipitated by change of pH, e.g., addition of lemon juice to milk to prepare *paneer.* Proteins bind water, if the coagulation is gradual, e.g., addition of lactic inoculum results in the formation of solid curd from liquid milk.

Oils and Fats

Milk, eggs, meat, oilseeds are foods, which contain fat. When foods containing fat are heated, the fat has a tendency to separate from the food. For example, heating milk results in the fat layer floating on top, while in cooking meat fat is released as drippings. When milk is curdled to prepare curd, the cream layer is always on top of the curd.

Oilseeds are extracted to obtain pure oil, butter is clarified in the manufacture of ghee (butter fat). Oils and fats are used as a cooking medium. Since these have a higher boiling point than water, the food is cooked quicker in fat. Some fat is absorbed during frying, the amount absorbed depends on a number of factors such as the composition and consistency of the food being fried, the temperature used and the nature of the fat used for frying. Fried foods have a higher energy value as compared to the same foods prepared by other methods such as boiling or baking. Fats which are solid (congeal) at room temperature, soften on heating, but do not have a sharp melting-point. When heated beyond its boiling-point, a fat smokes (smoke point), then flashes (flash point) and lastly it catches fire (fire point). If the fat is heated for a long time, it browns and thickens. These changes are accompanied by changes in flavour, which may not be acceptable. Therefore effort should be made to minimise these in food preparation.

Fats and oils are used to prepare food emulsions with water and air. Stabilisers such as proteins, gums, starches, finely ground spices, in small amounts are used to stabilise these emulsions.

Fat has shortening power, i.e., its presence between (protein and starch) layers makes the product crunchy (e.g., baked goods); its presence in meats tenderises it.

Fats and oils become rancid by action of air (oxidised), water (hydrolysis) and enzymes. These changes must be minimised, so that the foods in which fat is used remain acceptable.

Minerals

There is no loss of minerals in the normal cooking procedures. If cooking water is discarded, some (a small fraction of) water-soluble minerals may be lost.

Vitamins

As we know thiamin and vitamin C are the two vitamins, which are most affected by cooking. The losses may occur due to dissolved nutrients being discarded and destruction due to exposure to heat in cooking. The amount lost depends on a number of factors.

Thiamin is partly lost in solution and is also destroyed by heat. Some thiamin loss occurs when rice and *dal* are scrubbed and washed repeatedly prior to cooking. Being soluble in water, if the cooking water is discarded some thiamin is lost. The losses of thiamin in normal cooking vary from 10 to 25 per cent.

Vitamin C is the most labile vitamin. It is water soluble, is easily oxidised and is also affected by heat. Washing vegetables after cutting, exposing cut vegetables to air for long periods before cooking and/or serving, result in the loss of a part of the vitamin C present. The average cooking or processing losses range from 30 to 35 per cent. Therefore, cooking procedures that minimise the loss of vitamin C result in conserving all other nutrients.

Pigments

Colour of food has much to do with its acceptance and enjoyment. Vegetables and fruits contribute a variety of colours to the dietary. The plant pigments chlorophyll (green leafy vegetables), carotenoids (yellow-orange carrots), flavonoids (white potatoes) and anthocyanins (red beetroot) are present singly or in combination in plant foods. These may be affected by the method of preparation. The soluble pigments such as anthocyanins may leach in the cooking water and changes may occur due to the effect of heat and pH (acidity). Table 20.1 summarises the properties of plant pigments, understanding these may help us in retaining the colour of vegetables and fruits. Other colour changes include the change in meat pigment during cooking.

When milk is heated slowly it browns a little due to the reaction of sugar, (lactose) with amino acids. This is a change which is accompanied by flavour changes, which are enjoyed when these are very slight; if excessive, these are not liked. Similarly caramelisation of sugar, slight browning of starch in roasting, bring about colour changes, which are liked when these are slight, but not when these are excessive and give the dark brown colour of burnt food.

Some colour changes, which occur during food preparation are undesirable and efforts are made to minimise these. For example, certain fruits and vegetables such as some varieties of apples and brinjals brown when cut surfaces are exposed to air. Efforts made to avoid exposure of the cut surfaces to air include-brinjals are cut into water, apples are covered with sugar and/or lime juice, fruit salad is served with custard.

Table 20.1: Properties of Plant Pigments

S.No.	*Food source*	*Name of pigment*	*Colour*	*Soluble in*	*Effect of prolonged heat*	*In presence of*	
						acid	*alkali*
1.	Rice Potato	Flavones Flavanols	White or Yellowish	Water	May darken	White	Yellow
2.	Beetroot	Anthocyanin	Red	Water	Little	Bright red	Reddish purple
3.	Leafy vegetables	Chlorophyll	Green	Fat	Olive green	Olive green	Intense green
4.	Carrot Mango Tomato	Carotene Xanthophyll Lycopene	Yellow-orange	Fat	May darken	No change	No change

Flavour Components

Sugars, mineral salts, organic acids and salts are the flavour components found in fruits and vegetables. In addition salt, sugar, acid, herbs and spices are used in food preparation to modify or enhance the natural flavour of foods during preparation.

Salt is the most widely used seasoning in food preparation. When used in pickles, it draws out the water from the fruit or vegetable and binds it in solution. Organic acids used in food preparation are lemon juice (citric acid), vinegar (acetic acid), tamarind extract (tartaric acid), and cocum extract. Tomato juice and mango pulp are also used in preparations for the acidity these contribute. Some of these extracts contribute thickness as well as acidity to the product. Some of the organic acids slow down bacterial action and therefore are used as preservatives in pickles. Lactic acid produced in milk, coagulates milk proteins to form curd and cheese. This change is accompanied by a change in flavour and texture.

Oxidants and antioxidants: When food is exposed to air, oxygen from the air acts as an oxidant, and changes occur that are mostly undesirable. For example when cut surfaces of vegetables and fruits are exposed to air, vitamin C is partially lost due to oxidation, the surfaces become brown in colour; fats and oils become flat and then rancid. the metals, copper and iron act as catalysts in such oxidations. therefore, these metals are not suitable for use in food preparation or processing.

Some natural substances such as vitamin E, lecithin, some sulphur-containing amino acids act as antioxidants. These inhibit or prevent oxidation of fats and oils and other substances during storage and preparation. For example, vitamin E is found in some oils and prevents rancidity in these.

Enzymes are organic catalysts and control a number of reaction in vegetables and fruits. Ripening of fruits as well as over-ripening is controlled by enzymes. When fruits and vegetables are cooked or exposed to heat, e.g., blanching of vegetables before freezing, enzymes are inactivated. Purified enzymes are used to modify texture of foods. For example, papain is used to tenderise meat and rennin is used to coagulate milk protein in cheese making.

Retention of Nutritive Value During Preparation

It is important that all efforts should be made to retain the nutritive value of foods, during preparation. Another important objective in food preparation is to make food that is enjoyed by those who eat it. It is important to ensure that while retaining the nutritive value of the food, palatability is not sacrificed. It's good to remember that the food can provide nutrients to the body only after it is eaten. For example, some loss of thiamin (a vitamin of the B-complex) occurs when beans are cooked. But as we do not relish uncooked beans, we do cook beans and try to take care in the preparation to ensure that the loss is minimal. Thus we cook beans in just enough water to avoid loss of nutrients in the cooking water. We cook beans for the minimum time required. We can reduce, cooking time by using a pressure cooker, if possible. We can prepare the food just before serving, so that reheating before serving, is avoided.

Some simple rules for retaining nutritive value and flavour are given below:

1. Wash vegetables before cutting.
2. Cut vegetables just before cooking and introduce cut vegetables into boiling water, if to be cooked in water.
3. Use just enough water for cooking, if the vegetables or other foods are to be served as such.
4. Cook foods until just done and serve immediately.

5. When preparing soups, the slowest cooking ingredient should be added first, followed by addition of other ingredients, which cook in shorter time. For example, meat needs longer time and hence can be cooked half-way before adding vegetables, which need much less time. This procedure helps to avoid overcooking of the vegetables.
6. Spices and other flavour ingredients should be added in the oil used for seasoning, as the flavour compounds which are soluble in fat, are thus easily dispersed in the preparation with the oil or fat.
7. Vegetables, salads should be prepared just before serving.
8. Use of acid foods, such as lime juice, tomatoes, vinegar or yogurt as dressings in salads prevents loss of vitamin C, because it is stable in acid medium.
9. Fruits are best eaten as they have been customarily eaten in tropics. Bananas are eaten right after peeling. Oranges are usually sucked after peeling. Grape fruit is usually peeled and eaten. Mangoes are sucked to get the juice. In this manner of eating, no loss of vitamin C occurs, as the fruit is not much exposed before eating.

Effects of Cooking on the Microbial Quality of Food

As cooking involves heating of foods, many microorganisms are destroyed during cooking. This renders the food safe for eating. For example, boiling milk results in killing pathogens like tubercle bacilli if these are present; spoilage organisms are also killed by heating milk. Therefore heated milk keeps longer than unheated milk. Some of the toxins present in the foods are rendered inactive at the cooking temperature. Thus cooking helps to destroy heat-labile toxins.

Study Questions

1. Discuss the changes that occur in starch during food preparation. Give examples to illustrate the changes you describe.
2. Write short notes on:
   (*a*) Invert sugar,
   (*b*) Pectin,
   (*c*) Smoke-point,
   (*d*) Plant pigments,
   (*e*) Caramel,
   (*f*) Flavour components.
3. List the changes that occur in proteins during food preparation with examples to illustrate the change.
4. Discuss the steps which help to retain nutrients during food preparation. Which are the nutrients easily lost during food preparation?
5. How will you prevent the nutrient losses from the following foodstuffs:
   (*a*) Green leafy vegetables,
   (*b*) Milk,
   (*c*) Meats and eggs,
   (*d*) Citrus fruits.

CHAPTER

21

Factors Affecting Food Acceptance

WE SPEND a number of hours each day to plan, purchase, prepare and enjoy food. A large part of our income is utilised to purchase food for the family. Therefore, it is important to understand personal preferences in food, for without attention to the sensory aspects of food, there can be no true enjoyment of it. Let us consider the factors which affect our food acceptance.

Colour in Food

Colour affects our acceptance of food. It is said we eat with our eyes, because the first impression of foods is formed by its appearance, which includes colour, shape and aroma. The initial attraction or rejection of food depends on its looks.

Most of our traditional or rejection of food depends on its looks. Most of our traditional colour concepts affect our reaction to food. For example, we associate orange-yellow colour with ripe mangoes, red colour with ripe tomatoes and green colour with leafy vegetables. A green orange or a light coloured tomato looks unripe or anaemic and does not attract us.

The colour of food is one way to judge its quality. For example, a green colour is associated with unripe fruit such as mango or orange, a brown banana is thought to be spoilt. In food purchase, colour is used as an important criteria of quality. For example, mature ripe alfonso mangoes have orange-yellow colour. However colour is not always a true indicator of quality. Some varieties of oranges have a green colour even when these are mature, while orange coloured fruit may have sections, which are not juicy.

It is observed that fruit preserves and vegetable pickles darken during storage. Such darkening is caused by oxidative changes. These changes can be minimised by reducing the oxygen in the top of the container by heat before sealing it. The presence of traces of metals such as iron, tin and copper, in foods also causes darkening and needs to be avoided.

Colour added to foods: Since colour affects food acceptance, it is added to food products during processing to improve its acceptance. Fruit preserves, cheese, butter, icecream, cakes, confections and candies are some of the food products that have such addition of colour. When we buy these products, it is important to select appropriate delicate colour, to ensure attractive, acceptable appearance.

Colouring materials used in foods belong to two groups—natural colouring material and synthetic coal-tar dyes. After extensive testing, it has been found that only some of the coal-tar dyes can be safely used in foods; and these have been certified. Some of these are used in carbonated beverages and fruit preserves.

Some of the natural colouring matters, which we use in food preparation, are turmeric and saffron. In addition to these, other natural colouring substances used in food preparations are annato, betain, caramel, carotene and chlorophyll.

Texture in Foods

Each food has a particular texture that we associate with it. Thus well-cooked rice is soft, potato wafers are crisp and cucumber slice has a crunchy texture. We learn about food texture very early in our eating experience.

A variety of qualities are included in texture, such as, crisp, soft, hard, sticky, elastic, tough, gummy or stringy. If there is change in the accepted, characteristic texture, we find the food unacceptable. Thus we reject tough beans, hard rice, lumpy *upma,* and fibrous vegetables, because their texture is unlike the texture we associate with these foods. On the other hand, we enjoy crisp toast, soft velvety *halwas,* flaky pastry and sticky *jalebi.* The textural qualities of food depend on the ingredients, their proportion, the manner in which these are combined and the method of preparation.

Cereals: Texture is developed with meticulous care in cereal preparations such as *chapati,* bread, and cakes. In preparation of *chapati,* we knead the dough and set it aside for a few minutes to obtain a soft velvet textured *chapati.* In preparation of bread, the dough is allowed to ferment after mixing with yeast, punched to ensure even, sponge-like structure. In making cakes, the sugar and fat are creamed, the flour is sifted to incorporate air, and mixed with the creamed sugar to obtain the desired structure, when baked.

Fruits and Vegetables: The texture of fruits and vegetables is determined by the cell wall. The cell wall is composed of polysaccharides. During maturation, ripening and preparation, there are changes in the amount and kinds of polysaccharides, which result in changes in the texture of vegetables and fruits. For example, when a fruit ripens, a large part of starch is broken down to sugars, resulting in softening of texture and change in flavour of the fruit. When a bean gets mature, the bean toughens and gets lignified, its texture becomes very hard and it needs more time to cook than the immature bean. There is a change in the taste also. Thus the texture of the food affects the time taken to cook or process it. It also affects its acceptability.

Meal: As you know the texture of meat depends on the part of the animal from which the cut is taken, the age of the animal and the method of preparation and the duration. The meat cuts with low content of connective tissue, can be cooked by dry methods, such as roasting or shallow frying. But meat cuts, which have a large amount of connective tissue, are prepared by use of moist methods of preparation, such as pressure-cooking, boiling or stewing, to make these cuts tender.

The texture of meat is very easily determined by the number of times one needs to chew and how hard one has to bite to cut the piece. If it takes long to chew the meat, it is a tough product. It is possible to improve the texture of meat by treating tough meat with chemical tenderisers. These help to break down the connective tissue partially and thus improve the texture of the product.

Flavour in Food

Flavour is the sum-total of the sensory impression formed, when we eat food. It includes the aroma, the taste and even the texture, and thus involves all our senses. It is the most important aspect of food, which decides our choices of food. While an appropriate colour and texture may induce us to *sample* a food, whether we will eat *more* of it, depends on its flavour. Thus flavour of food is as important a quality as its nutritional composition.

Food flavour is intimately related to food preparation practices. We like flavour of foods made in our home in our community and region, because these are familiar to us. Thus food flavour acceptance is intimately related to our dietary pattern. If our exposure to food flavours has been limited, it is not easy for us to adapt to new flavours, and we may not enjoy a variety of flavours.

Odour: The odour or smell of food influences our food acceptance. The aroma of ripe mango attracts us, while the smell of overripe fruit repels us. The substances, which are responsible for odour of food, are volatile, which means these evaporate and form vapours easily. The odours are carried by the air to our nose, and are transmitted by special nerves (olfactory nerves) to our brain. You can get the odour even before you eat the food; you also perceive the odour when you eat the food. The odour affects our acceptance of food, depending on whether it is liked or not. The primary odours are sweet or fragrant, sour or acid, burnt and rancid. You may have noticed that our sense of smell is far more acute than the sense of taste. Therefore anything that affects its function, impairs our enjoyment of food. For example, if you suffer from a cold, your sense of smell is impaired and you find that the food does not taste as good as when you are well. Similarly, the function of sensory organs is impaired with age, which results in decreased enjoyment of food by the aged persons.

Touch: The sense of touch contributes to our perception of food. It identifies the textural qualities of the food, such as softness and hardness. Similarly, we perceive the crisp, the crunchy or sticky texture by touching the food. When the touch conforms to the textural profile of the food in our memory, it enhances the anticipation and enjoyment of food. If it does not create a favourable image, we hesitate to taste the food. For example, a slimy touch indicates spoilage, be it a carrot or a bread slice.

Taste: Taste sensations are the sum-total of the sensations created by food when it is put in the mouth. The sensation of taste is perceived when the taste receptors (taste buds) are stimulated. The taste buds are located on the surface of the tongue. The food must be dissolved in liquid to enable us to perceive its taste. Hence we have to masticate dry foods such as roasted groundnuts mix these with saliva, so that we can taste these. We can perceive the taste of liquids, such as tea, *sherbet* or *lassi,* immediately, as these can stimulate the taste buds as soon as we drink these.

There are four primary taste sensations—sweet, sour, salty and bitter. The taste of the food is determined by its chemical composition. Sugars present in foods or added to foods are responsible for sweet taste, while salty taste is due to salts present in foods or added to food. Sour or acid taste is contributed mainly by organic acids found in foods (such as citric acid in limes), added to foods (such as tamarind extract added to *dal*) or developed in food (lactic acid formed when milk is made into curd).

Certain foods such as coffee beans and fenugreek have bitter taste, while breakdown of proteins produces substances, with bitter taste. The taste of most foods is a blend of these primary tastes.

The primary tastes can be modified by combination of the compounds responsible for these. For example, the sourness of lime can be reduced by addition of sugar; the bitterness of fenugreek is reduced by adding coconut and jaggery. Thus you find that a variety of steps can be taken to modify the flavour of natural foods. We can use flavouring substances, naturally present in foods or those synthesised in the factory, during food preparation and processing to improve acceptability and add variety to our diet.

Flavouring Substances

A variety of materials are used in food preparation and processing to enhance, blend and alter the natural flavours. Appropriate use of these can make a insipid dish into a highly palatable product. There is ample scope for creativity in use of flavouring substances in food preparation. A large variety of flavouring substances are used in Indian homes. These include salt, a variety of acidic substances, herbs and spices, and extracts of herbs and spices.

Salt: Salt is the most widely used condiment. It is one of the few pure chemicals used in food preparation. It is obtained by evaporation of sea water. It is used to season all food preparations except sweets. It is used in food preservation to make pickles, *chutneys* and sauces. Salt has the unique property of enhancing the flavour of herbs and spices in food preparations.

Acids: Lemon juice, tamarind, *cocum, amchur* and vinegar are the acid substances very commonly used in Indian homes. Lemon juice is used in salads and savoury preparations such as *upma, batatepohe, bhel,* etc. Tamarind is soaked and the acid extract thus obtained is used in *sambar, rasam, puliyore* (tamarind rice), and many other vegetable preparations in the southern parts of India. In western India, where *ratambi* (the fruit from which *cocum* is made) is available, *cocum* is used in food preparation. Vinegar is dilute acetic acid. It is used to flavour salads, pickles, and sauces. *Amchur,* made from raw mangoes, is also used in some preparations to impart acidic taste.

Herbs and Spices: India is known as the 'Home of Spices'. Spices and herbs form an indispensable part of our cultural food pattern. These impart a subtle flavour to foods. Their presence is evident by their irresistible aroma, which whets our appetite. They add zest to otherwise insipid foods. Hence these are the most important group of flavouring materials in the Indian cuisine.

Spices and herbs come from various parts of plants, such as the fruits, seeds, berries, roots, rhizomes, leaves, the bark, the floral parts, kernel, aril and exudate of bark. The flavour is due to small amounts of essential oils and organic acids present in the specific part of the plant. Each one of these has a characteristic component, which is responsible for its individual flavour. These are available as whole dried spices and as ground powders also. One problem associated with spices is adulteration. As these are expensive products, ground hulls, sawdust, and other waste materials are added to increase the bulk and thus increase profit margin. Microscopic and chemical tests can help to identify the adulterants.

Flavouring Extracts: Flavouring extracts are obtained from spices by extraction with alcohol, steam distillation or by expression in a press. These are normally solutions of the essential oils in alcohol. These are best stored in a cool place in tightly stoppered containers. As these are concentrated solutions of the flavour, very minute amount is needed to be added to impart the desired flavour. Some of the flavouring extracts available include ginger, cardamom, saffron, vanilla, orange, cinnamon, etc.

Many synthetic chemical compounds are now available in the market, which have a flavour similar to that of the natural extract. These are used extensively, because these are much cheaper than the natural flavouring extracts.

Use of Spices and Flavourings: These are added to the food normally towards the end of preparation. There is no set proportion, which is acceptable to all, as individual variation in the tolerance to these is very great.

Spices may be used in the whole or powdered form. Whole spices are usually added to hot oil as a seasoning, before being dispersed in the food preparation. Oil acts as a solvent for the flavour components present in the spices. Ground spices may be added to the food directly, e.g., pepper, jeera powder, spice mix, etc.

Herbs are normally cut and simmered in hot fat or oil to extract the, characteristic flavour before being added to the preparation. As prolonged cooking will cause loss of volatile components, it is advisable to add flavouring material towards the end of preparation. As you may know, these materials are very light and very small amount is needed to impart the flavour. For example, a teaspoonful *sambar podi* weighs only two grammes, and it is sufficient to flavour about 600 milliliters of *sambar.* Thus it amounts to only 1 part in 300, but its contribution to improving the palatability of the product is truly remarkable. In the use of flavouring materials it is good to remember that while a small addition is good, more of it may result in decreased acceptability of the food product. So you must practice moderation in use of these materials.

Study Questions

1. Discuss the texture of food with reference to cereals, fruit and meat.
2. What are the primary odours? Explain how these affect food acceptance.
3. List the various flavouring substances used in foods.
4. What are flavouring extracts and how are these prepared?

CHAPTER 22

Food Sanitation and Hygiene

FOOD SANITATION implies cleanliness in the producing, preparing, storing and serving of food and water. Food sanitation is an essential aspect of food preparation. It needs to be emphasised at every stage of food handling and preparation. Some of the items which need particular attention are:

(*i*) a safe and potable water supply,
(*ii*) selection of wholesome ingredients and
(*iii*) hygienic handling, during preparation and serving.

These steps prevent entry of spoilage and pathogenic organisms in the food.

In addition, all the equipment coming in contact with food should be scrupulously clean; the surroundings should be clean and there should be a proper and safe method for the disposal of waste. Inculcation of hygienic habits would help in preventing foods from being contaminated during handling.

Water

Water is essential in food preparation. It is used to wash food before cooking, it is used to act as a cooking medium, it is used to clean the containers of food before and after preparation and it is used also as the most important beverage. Therefore, it is essential that all water meant for drinking and cooking purposes should be free from pathogenic bacteria. Water used for making ice must also be potable. The ice may be used to cool foods or added to cold drinks. Thus it is important to ensure that the ice we sometimes buy be made from potable water. Some of the diseases, which can be spread by the use of contaminated water are cholera, typhoid, paratyphoid, bacillary dysentery and amoebic dysentery.

Potable Water

Water, which is free from pathogenic bacteria and is palatable, is known as potable water. The necessity of a potable water supply in the home and place of work can never be overemphasised. It is also important in institutions preparing, processing and serving food.

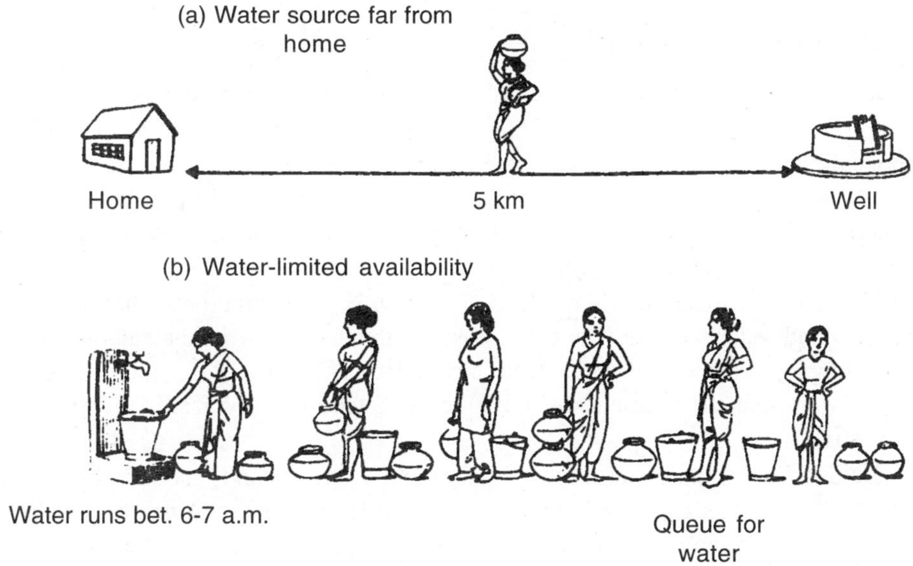

Figure 22.1: When water is scarce, sanitation suffers.
(a) Water sources far from home (b) Water—limited availability

Apart from the primary precaution to ensure that water be free from harmful bacteria, it is also necessary to make it palatable. For example, water may contain dissolved salts or minerals, which may give it a brackish taste. For specific uses such as chemical analyses water may have to be given special treatment with resins to remove dissolved impurities or salts. We will concern ourselves mainly with the treatment of water to render it safe for potable purposes.

In India, even though the necessity of using 'pure water' has been known for centuries[1], there was no safe and protected water supply up to 1949 for as much as 81 per cent of the population who stay mostly in the villages.

---

1. In some of the Sanskrit texts written around the year 2000 B.C., it has been stated that 'it is good to keep water in a copper vessel, to expose it to sunlight and to filter it in charcoal'. Similarly, another text says, 'Water should be purified by boiling over fire, by heating in the sun, or by dropping a heated iron in it and then allowing it to cool; or it may be purified by filtering through coarse sand gravel.'

The National Water Supply and Sanitation Programme was launched in 1954 as a part of the Health Plan to assist the States in their urban and rural water supply and sanitation schemes so as to provide adequate water supply and sanitation facilities in the whole country. By 1979, 2,108 towns had been provided with water benefiting an urban population of one hundred million people. 217 towns with a population of forty million people (about 36 per cent of the urban population) had been covered by partial sewerage system. Of the 5,76,000 villages it is estimated that more than two lakh problem villages remained to be covered with potable water supply as on April 1,1980. Efforts are being made to meet the water and sanitation needs of the entire country.[2]

Even today the average Indian, educated or uneducated, a villager or a city-dweller, is very particular about seeing that the vessels used for storage of water is not contaminated in the home. So it is not the use in the home but the source of the water supply which may be suspect.

Sources of Contamination of Water

The usual source of contamination of water is through the seepage of sewage.

Sewage can be a carrier of many pathogenic bacteria because many healthy persons may be 'carriers' of pathogenic bacteria without being affected themselves. Persons who are suffering from enteric diseases will also contribute to the presence of bacteria in sewage. The disposal of sewage is not paid much attention to, especially in the rural communities, where human excreta is deposited near shallow wells, ponds or even rivers; contamination from this source is widespread.

In cities, the huge influx of population, which results in rapid formation of hutment dwellings without proper sanitary and water facilities, develop into a health hazard. Sufficient water is not available usually at such dwellings and the use of water from any source is resorted to, sometimes even gutter water being used. It is not that the hutment dwellers are not aware of the hazards involved, but they have no other alternative.

There is no facility for drainage and the used water and sewage stand, encouraging breeding of mosquitoes and flies. These pests carry and spread pathogens from sewage to nearby localities, thus creating health problems. Exposed ready-to-eat foods sold in such localities may be contaminated by the flies.

Another difficulty experienced in cities with protected water supplies is the difficulty of maintaining a positive pressure in all pipelines. In cities many of the pipelines have become very old and unless there is a continuous flow of water into them with a positive pressure there is a possibility of seepage of bacteria, from sewage into water pipes. With limited supply of water available, in many Indian cities, all the pipes can never be holding water all the 24 hours. This is a problem, which does cause concern.

The effluents from many industries, which are at present mostly discharged into rivers are another source of contamination; this problem is assuming serious proportions. Many of these effluents use up much of the oxygen from the water with the result that fish and other aquatic animals are unable to survive.

Foul smell emanates from such streams, due to anaerobic decomposition (putrefaction) of dead fish, thus making the water unfit for human consumption.

Treatment of Water

It is thus essential that water used for potable purposes be free from pathogenic bacteria. The best precaution one can take is to prevent the source of water from contamination with sewage.

---

2. *Source: India, Reference Manual;* Ministry of Information, 1981.

In villages this can be done by constructing cement sides to deep wells to prevent bacteria from seeping through the soil and gaining entrance in the water. Well water which may be contaminated can be purified by the addition of bleaching powder. A simple and inexpensive gadget using this principle has been fabricated by the Central Public Health Engineering Research Institute. Bleaching powder on reaction with water releases chlorine which is capable of killing pathogenic organisms. In villages where there is no treated water, drinking water should preferably be boiled and then cooled. This would destroy all the pathogenic bacteria. Water used for cooking need not be boiled, as it would be boiled anyway during cooking. Water used for washing, cleaning need not be boiled as long as it is not foul smelling and does not contain any suspended impurities.

In cities and towns where it is necessary to supply a large population with water, effective methods have to be used for the purification of water. The source of water is usually a lake in which the water is allowed to stand. This results in most of the suspended impurities settling down. Further the action of sunlight and the paucity of food results in the destruction of bacteria. In the next stage, which may consist of a filtration through sand most of the bacteria are eliminated. As an added precaution, water supplies to cities are chlorinated. This may either be done by the addition of bleaching powder, or as is done in most of the cities, by the injection of liquid chlorine. To make sure that the bacteria which may have entered into the pipelines through seepage when there is no positive pressure, additional chlorination is resorted to at different locations during the transportation of water from the lake to city reservoirs. This is understandable when it is realised that the source of water may be 60 to 70 km away from the city. Water may be rendered potable by use of water filter in the home.

What you can do about pesticide residue

Pesticide residue can pose a serious problem in the diet. There are certain precautions which you can take to reduce dietary exposure to this hazard. These are:

1. Thoroughly rinse and scrub fruits and vegetables. Peel them if appropriate.
2. Remove outer leaves of leafy vegetables, such as cabbage and lettuce.
3. Trim fat from meat, poultry and fish; discard oils and fats in broths and drippings.
4. Throw back the big fish—the little ones have less time to take up and concentrate pesticides and other harmful residues.

Food

All vegetables and fruits either from bazar or grown in one's own farm would have to be cleaned, and prepared for either eating directly or cooking. The dirt or dust which we find on foods as we buy them can be carrier of spores of microorganisms. Therefore, all exposed food must be washed with clean water before use. Outer layers, skins of plant material contain thousands of microorganisms and must be washed thoroughly before use. If any parts of fruits and vegetables are bruised these should be trimmed to reduce contamination.

The skin, hair, feathers, intestines of animals harbour a number of microorganisms. It is, therefore, necessary to remove these, before animal products are prepared for human consumption.

Food Handling

Food comes into contact with human hands during harvesting, storage, preparation and service. It is important that food handlers be free from any communicable diseases—colds, any other respiratory ailment, cuts or boils, as they may be responsible for transferring these to the food thereby spreading the infection to persons consuming the food.

Human hair, nasal discharge, skin can also be source of microorganisms. Therefore, persons handling food, must wash hands with soap before starting preparation, and refrain from touching hair or wiping nose during food preparation.

Food sanitation is a way of life. It can never be overemphasised. A number of gastrointestinal disorders, such as diarrhoea, cholera and communicable diseases such as typhoid, septic sore throat, diphtheria, dysentery, etc., are communicated by use of contaminated water or food (Figure 22.2). Therefore, it is very important that sanitary handling of food and water is religiously adhered to.

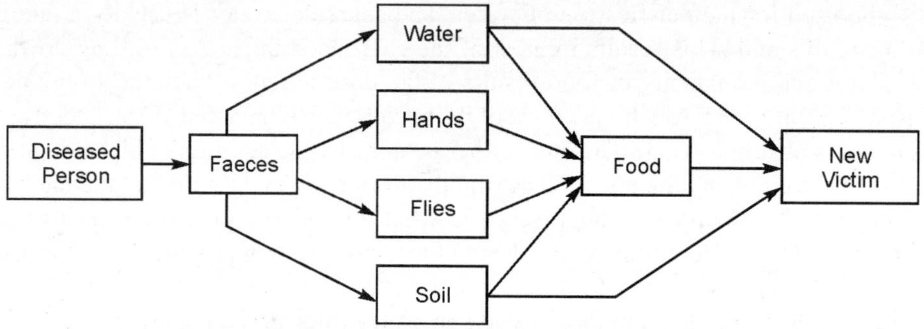

Figure 22.3: Spread of diseases through faecal contamination.

Food Contamination

Food may be contaminated if the:

1. Water used for washing or cleaning is not potable.
2. Soil adhering to foods grown close to ground is not completely removed.
3. Containers or utensils used for storage and preparation are not clean.
4. Personnel handling food have unhygienic habits.
5. Personnel handling food suffer from communicable diseases.

Equipment

It is necessary that all equipment coming in contact with food be kept clean. This includes knives, meat mincers, blenders, rolling pins, wooden boards, metal and porcelain dishes, utensils, etc. They should be scrubbed, cleaned with detergent and water and then rinsed with potable water. It is a good practice to see that such equipment are dipped in hot water at 80°C for at least 30 seconds or more and then allowed to drain dry. This sanitary step is especially important during epidemics such as infective hepatitis (infective jaundice), cholera, etc. Parts of blenders, mixers, etc., should be inspected after cleaning to ensure that there is no food material left over. If allowed to remain they could allow harmful microorganisms to grow and spoil the food. Equipment made of plastic and other such material which cannot withstand high temperatures need not be given the dip in hot water but should be given other treatments and then allowed to drain dry.

In villages it is a common practice to scrub utensils and dishes with ash and then rinse them with water. The utensils and dishes are then allowed to dry in the sun. The alkaline ash acts as a good agent for killing any microorganisms adhering to the utensils and a sanitary effect is produced by drying in the sun both because of heat and the ultraviolet rays.

Control of Insects and Rodents

One of the common insects contaminating foods is the housefly. These have minute hair on their legs and thus can be the carriers of harmful bacteria depending on where they come from. It is possible that they may carry faecal matter or other such sources of pathogenic bacteria and deposit it on the food.

Another insect which can also be a source of contamination in the same way as the housefly is the cockroach. These insects, which usually prefer darkness, have been known to cause diarrhoea and dysentery.

Apart from these two common ones, there are innumerable insects ranging from the larvae found in wheat and rice to locusts, which can cause serious damage to food.

Rodents, which include rats, mice and bandicoots, not only consume large quantities of food, thus contributing to the overall shortage of food in the country, but may also be the carriers of diseases such as plague.

The presence of insects, insect fragments, rodent excreta and other matter of insect and rodent origin (even though it may not necessarily be dangerous to health) is aesthetically resented by consumers. Health authorities condemn such food as unfit for consumption because it indicates poor practices of sanitation where the food was prepared.

It is thus essential that preventive measures be taken to exclude the entry of insects and rodents in the house, especially in the cooking and serving areas. This can be done by:

(*i*) Keeping the prepared food in cupboards with wire-netting.

(*ii*) Filling cracks, fissures in the walls and flooring which are usually the places where insects breed and multiply.

(*iii*) Covering drains, holes, etc., with wire gauze so as to prevent the entry of rodents.

Precautions such as these if taken in villages and small towns where people normally stay in independent homes would certainly prevent the entry of insects and rodents. In large cities, however, where each building may have many apartments, unless measures are taken by the whole community, there is always a danger of insects and rodents travelling from one apartment to another.

The control of insects and rodents can be carried out in several ways of which the most common one practised in the home is spraying or dusting with an insecticide. Fumigation may be resolved to in large godowns, factories, etc., as it destroys insects and rodents.

Sprays or dustings make use of chlorinated hydrocarbons (such as DDT, TDE, aldrin, dieldrin, etc.) and the organic phosphorus compounds (such as Parathion, Malathion, Systrex, etc.) as the active ingredient for killing the insect. Baits in which chemicals may be mixed with food are also successful in getting rid of pests. Examples of these are "Tygon" in which a chemical is mixed with sugar and a home-made mixture of boric powder and bengalgram *dal* flour, which when ingested by cockroaches results in their death. Warfrain may be mixed with food and used as a bait for the elimination of rodents.

It must be noted that insecticides are poisonous, and must be used in very small amounts only where needed. If used indiscriminately these are likely to enter our bodies and harm us after a period of time. It is important to store these out of reach of children and away from food, to prevent accidents.

Practical Rules for Good Sanitation

1. Tie hair neatly before starting food preparation. Use hair net or cap if necessary. Wash hands thoroughly with soap and water before starting preparation.
2. Wash fruits, vegetables, cereals and beans thoroughly before preparation with potable water. Boil milk in a clean container as soon as possible after receipt and keep covered. Bottles of milk need to be rinsed thoroughly with water and then washed with soap and water.
3. Use potable water in food preparation.
4. Boil water used for drinking or for preparation of cold beverages, if the purity of water is not guaranteed.
5. Utensils and equipment used for preparation should be scrupulously cleaned.
6. Cooked food should be stored covered, preferably in the container in which it is cooked.
7. Left over foods such as rice, vegetables, should be stored either in a refrigerator kept or in a pan of cold water. Reheating before use is advisable.

Study Questions

1. What is potable water? List the sources of contamination of water and how to prevent such contamination.
2. How does food get contaminated? List the steps to be taken to prevent contamination of food.
3. List effective means of control of household pests.

Laboratory Work

1. Cleaning of work surfaces, storage space and floors.
2. Demonstration on cleaning of equipment.
3. Labelling of containers and their proper storage.
4. Use of proper apron, hair-net or head cover, etc.
5. Expose sterile nutrient agar to various contaminants and observe the microbial growth.
6. Show slides of microorganisms causing food infection.
7. Make visual charts to emphasise Rules of Sanitation.
8. Visit municipal quality control laboratory if possible.
9. Simple tests to detect adulterants in various foods.

CHAPTER

23

Food and Environment

It is important to use environmentally sound technologies for improving the quantity and quality of food. To understand how this can be done let us first study in brief what environmental hazards we are facing at present.

Global Warming

Increase in the carbon dioxide in the atmosphere has caused shrinkage of the ozone layer of stratosphere. With the weakening of the protective ozone layer, the world temperature has shown a gradual increase. This increase in temperature can have deleterious effects on several fronts. Some of them are listed below.

Melting of Glaciers: Glaciers from the Himalayas supply most of the water to perennial rivers such as the Ganges, Indus, Yamuna and Brahmaputra. It is estimated that 70 per cent of the water in the Ganges is of glacier origin. These glaciers are melting very fast due to elevation of atmospheric temperature. If corrective measures are not taken to arrest the rise in environmental temperature, the

Ganges would become a seasonal river having water only during the monsoon. About 4070 lac people dependent on the water from the Ganges would become impoverished. The same pattern would hold good for the other rivers dependent on glacier water.

Lowering of Crop Yield: In Phillipines, the scientists reported that the pollination of rice falls from 100 per cent at 34 degrees Celsius to near zero at 40 degrees Centigrade, leading to crop failure. It has been observed by the International Rice Research Institute in Manila that a 1 degree rise in temperature could lower the yield of rice by 10 per cent. In India, a 2 degree rise in temperature depressed the yield of wheat from 8 to 38 per cent in a ten state study.

Rethinking Land Productivity: The grain yield rose only 1.2 per cent annually from 1990 to 2007, due to shortage of irrigation water. Now to raise crop productivity, one must plant crops more tolerant to drought and cold. Where soil moisture permits, productivity can be increased by planting two crops per year, as is done in northern India (rice and wheat) and China (wheat and corn). In U.S., wheat is cultivated in winter and soyabeans in summer.

In Africa, grain and legume are planted together. As the legume leaves provide nitrogen to the soil, it fertilizes it and the grain yield doubles in a few years.

In China, shifting the land tenure to farmers has resulted in improved yields.

Water Wastage and How to Avoid it

At present except for a few countries, a lot of water is wasted. Efficient use of water by using drip irrigation in agriculture can help reduce loss of a lot of water in irrigation. Drip irrigation methods cuts water use by half with minimal evaporation losses. It is labour intensive and water efficient. So it is well suited to India, which has a surplus of labour and shortage of water.

It takes about 1000 tons of water to produce 1 ton of grain. New varieties of grain should be developed which use less water.

Raising water Productivity: Water shortage reduces food production. Hence, the world must raise water productivity.

Worldwide, roughly 1,000 tons water is used to produce one ton grain. Hence 70 per cent of world water is used for irrigation. Thus raising irrigation efficiency is central to raising water efficiency.

New Environmentally Sound Technologies in the Food Processing Industry

A good deal of development on new, environmentally sound food processing technology has come about as a result of dedicated research and development on the part of governmental, non-governmental and industrial laboratories, primarily in response to strengthened environmental protection in the developed countries. Table 23.1 presents a list of types of technology that have in particular been the focus of such endeavours during the past two decades.

Table 23.1: Environmentally Sound Technologies of Primary Interest in The Food Processing Industry

Advanced water treatment technology	Use of wastewater technology based on new membrane technology.
Innovative sensors and process control	Use of advanced techniques to gain better in-line control specific processing operations thus reducing waste, increasing productivity and improving product quality.
Modern packaging material and techniques	Using less packaging material in absolute terms and a move towards more environmentally-friendly packaged products.
Food disinfection and irradiation	Use of radiation rather than chemicals to destroy or limit the propagation of pathogenic micro-organisms.
New materials in FPI operations	The use of new materials in the construction of equipment as well as in the extraction of vegetable oils, essences and flavours, provides the industry with superior tools for lowering emissions and improving product quality.
Biotechnology applications	Use of new biotechnology in FPI operations and in waste water treatment.
Innovative design and validation methods	Use of advanced computer software and high speed computing in the design and modeling of industrial operations, resulting in time and resource savings.
Innovative processing methods	Use of pulsed electrical, ultras-high pressure and up-to-date steam pasteurization techniques may also be reflected in reduced fuel utilization and longer shelf-life.

Source: "Food Online by J.E.Stratton, M.S., Dept. of Food Science and Technology. University of Nebraska.

The usage of irrigation water never reaches 100 per cent, as some water evaporates, some percolates downward and some water runs off. Irrigation water analysis shows that efficiency is:

In India, Mexico, Pakistan and Phillipines – 25 to 40 %,
In Malaysia and Morocco – 40 to 45 %,
In Israel, Japan and Taiwan – 50 to 60 %.

Large-scale drip systems using plastic lines that save water have become popular. These systems can pay for themselves in one year. By reducing water costs and raising yields, they can raise incomes of small farmers.

In many countries farmers' associations assume the responsibility for water management and do a better job than a distant government agency. Institutional shifts, specifically moving the responsibility for managing irrigation systems from government to water users associations improves water management and cuts costs. Mexico is a leader in this area. 80 per cent of Mexico's farms irrigations systems are managed by such water users associations.

A higher water price affects all water users, encouraging investment in more water-efficient irrigation technologies, industrial processes and household appliances.

Shift to more water-efficient crops boosts water productivity. Rice crop needs more water, hence it is being phased out around Beijing. In Egypt, wheat production is favoured in place of rice.

In the United States, annual consumption of grain as food and feed averages 800 kilogrammes per person. A modest reduction in the consumption of meat, milk and eggs could easily cut grain use per person by 100 kilogrammes. Such a reduction by 300 million Americans, would cut irrigation water use by 30 billion tons.

Recycling urban water supplies is another way to increase water availability.

Reducing urban water use: One-time use of water is obsolete due to water shortages. City water, contaminated with human and industrial wastes is discharged into rivers and lakes. If permeates aquifers, making water (surface and underground), unsafe for drinking. Waste water drained in the sea destroys life there, forming about 200 dead zones in coastal regions of oceans. This system is expensive and water-intensive, and is a major source of disease and death. Sunita Narayan of the Centre for Science & Environment, New Delhi, India, says that 'with this system, both our rivers and children are dying.'

Water shortage and ignorance, claims about two million lives worldwide; a third of those claimed by hunger and malnutrition.

In cities, reusing the same water continuously, is the most effective single step to raise water productivity. In this system, only a small fraction of water is lost to evaporation. Thus, water management in the cities can be efficient.

Some industries, such as paper and pulp, industrial laundries, etc. are developing 'closed-loop' systems, reusing all the waste water internally. Only small amounts of fresh water are needed to make up for water used up. The technologies they develop can be used in urban water recycling.

The use of water in the home can be reduced by using efficient appliances, e.g., showers and toilets, which use half or less water.

Producing Protein More Efficiently

Both land and water productivity can be increased by producing animal protein more efficiently. About 740 million tons of world grain harvest is used to produce animal protein. Even a small gain in efficiency can save a large quantity of grain.

Consumption of animal foods has increased from 1950 to 2007. Therefore, efficiency of conversion of grains to animal protein is important; it varies with animal species. Cattle in feed lots need 7 kilograms grains to produce one kg. gain in live weight; it needs three kilogrammes grains to produce a kg. of pork, 2 kilogrammes to produce a kg of poultry, and less than 2 kg, grains to produce a kg. of herbivorous species of fish. Both land and water are used efficiently, as the demand shifts to more grain-efficient foods.

The world pork production overtook beef production in 1979 and the trend continues. Poultry production grew rapidly worldwide to 83 million tons in 2006. Worldwide the herbivorous fish output expanded more than 9% a year since 1995. The growth potential for efficient animal protein lies here.

Fish polyculture is widely practiced in both China and India; it has increased production by 50%. In U.S. fish farming is concentrated in Mississippi in the South.

Mounting pressures on land and water has led to development of new animal protein production systems. For example, India today is the world's leading producer of milk and dairy products, with fourfold increase since 1970.

The remarkable thing is, India has built this largest dairy industry almost entirely on roughage such as wheat straw, rice straw, corn stalks and grass gathered from the roadside. In four provinces of China, where there is double cropping of winter wheat and corn, villagers feed the straw and cornstalks to cattle and convert roughage into animal protein (beef). The use of crop residues to produce milk in India and beef in China, lets farmers reap a second harvest from the original grain crop, thus boosting both land and water productivity. These new protein models, evolved in India and China, can be adopted in other countries.

In agriculture we often look at how climate affects the food supply, but not at how what we eat affects climate. It is heartening to know that a plant-based diet requires roughly one-fourth as much energy as a diet rich in red meat. Thus shifting from a diet rich in red meat to a plant-based diet cuts greenhouse gas emissions considerably.

Hence, the inclusion of soybean meal in feed rations to convert grain into animal protein efficiently, the shift by consumers to more grain-efficient forms of animal protein, and the movement of consumers down the food chain, can reduce the demand for land, water and fertilizer. This reduces carbon emissions and thus helps to stabilize climate as well. Such systems can pay for themselves in one year. By reducing water costs and raising yields, they can raise incomes of small farm.

Food Processing: Large quantities of water can be recovered in the food processing industry by using new technologies to treat and recycle waste water. The use of membrane technology to effect separation for recycling waste water with new synthetic membranes which use less energy for the removal of waste materials has reduced costs and increased the efficiency of the dairy industry by enabling the production of several new products.

Collapse of Fisheries: Overfishing has resulted in the complete depletion of certain varieties of fish leading to the closure of several fishery industries. The collapse of the cod fishery industry in the North Atlantic coast of the U.S. and Canada resulting in loss of jobs to a large body of persons employed in this industry is a good example.

In recent years, the creation of marine parks has been gaining momentum. It will result in following gains: (1) Fish will live longer, grow larger and produce more offsprings, (2) There will be increase in annual catch, which will increase its availability in diet, and (3) it will create more than a million jobs.

Several scientists have noted that within a year or two of establishing marine reserves, the fish population density increased by 91 per cent, average fish size by 31 per cent and species diversity by 20 per cent.

Two other measures are required to protect fish. One is to reduce nutrient flows from fertilizer runoff and draining untreated sewage in the sea, that create 200 or more dead zones near sea shores. The second is to eliminate $22 billion, which is given as subsidy to fishers, this amount can be used to create a network of marine reserves instead.

Some of the measures, which can be undertaken to save the environment in agriculture and the food industry are explained briefly below.

Use of New Environmentally Sound Technologies in the Food Industry

Some of the new technologies which are environmentally sound are:

1. Grow grains, which need less water for growing.
2. Reduced tilling or no-tilling in agriculture, to reduce energy expenditure in agriculture and reduction in loss of top soil.
3. Two or more crops per year, to reduce water use and increase yields per hectare.
4. Use of modern packaging materials and techniques which use less packaging material and thus save on raw material.
5. Use of new materials in the construction of equipment and the extraction of vegetable oils, essences lowers emission of volatile products and improves product quality.
6. Use of biotechnology in food processing operations and in waste water treatment.
7. Use of advanced computer software and high speed computing in the design of various industrial operations, which results in time and resource savings.
8. Using new methods of steam pasteurisation reduce fuel use and increased shelf-life.

Efficient Land Use for Growing Foodgrains

Forty years ago, North India produced only wheat. By using earlier maturing and high yielding wheats, wheat can be harvested in time and high yielding varieties of rice planted in the same acreage. This is being practiced in the whole of Haryana, Punjab and parts of U.P. The wheat yield of 3 tons and rice yield of 2 tons combine to give 5 tons per hectare boosting the production of foodgrains per hectare.

New Animal Production Systems

There is lot of pressure on land and water in developing countries. These countries have evolved new animal production systems. These are based on use of roughage rather than grain for feeding animals. A shining example of the success of this system is the phenomenal increase in milk production in India. Since 1970, India's milk production has increased to more than four-fold. In 1997, India overtook the United States to become the world's leading producer of milk and dairy products. At present India's per capita availability of milk is one cup per person. Thirty years ago it was less than half a cup per person.

China has had success in increasing beef production by feeding crop residues with small amounts of urea.

The use of crop residues to produce milk in India and beef in China has allowed farmers to reap a second harvest, boosting land and water productivity.

Protein can be produced more efficiently by encouraging the growth of poultry and fish farming. With cattle in feedlots, 7 kg of grain is needed to obtain 1 kg gain in weight. For pork it is 3 kg. Grain per kg weight gain. For poultry it is 2 and for herbivorous fish it is less than 2.

Changing patterns in food habits: People who consume plenty of meat such as Americans and Canadians can improve their health by moving down the food chain. This would reduce the pressure on the land, for those like Indians, who live lower on the food chain, inclusion of some animal products such as milk, fish and poultry would improve health and increase life expectancy.

Action on Many Fronts

The principal threat to food security today is climate change from burning of fossil fuels. It is necessary to minimize cropwithering heat waves, to prevent the melting of glaciers that feed Asia's major rivers during dry season, and prevent the ice melting that would inundate the river deltas and floodplains that produce much of the Asian rice harvest.

We must use water very responsibly and efficiently.

Choice of Convenience Foods

Eating prepared foods is now a fact of today's fast paced life. Almost any snack, bread, dessert, vegetable or meat dish can now be bought already prepared and packaged. One can also get a prepackaged breakfast, lunch and dinner either frozen or in tetra packs. Today one can eat all three to four meals of the day by using these prepared foods, which require little or no cooking.

While convenient, these prepared foods are generally not the healthiest items to be included in your diet. To ensure that these convenience foods remain tasty till they are eaten, large amounts of additives are added such as sugar, fat, salt, natural and artificial preservatives, food colours, etc. Generally they do not contain many vitamins, minerals and fiber.

However, you can lessen the unhealthful effects of these convenience foods by following these four simple guidelines when choosing these:

1. Check the list of ingredients: The ingredients should be less than 10 listed on the can or package. Avoid prepared foods with too many ingredients (e.g., chemical names you do not understand).
2. Check the percentage of calories from the fat per serving (you can check this by dividing the calories from fat by the total number of calories per serving and multiplying it by 100). Avoid foods when the percentage of calories coming from the fat is greater than 20 to 25%.
3. Follow this by looking at the types of fat. Try and avoid foods when most of the fat is saturated or hydrogenated/partially hydrogenated fat like vanaspati.
4. Finally check the sodium content. Avoid packaged foods with high amounts of sodium. A rule of thumb would be that the food should not contain more than 20% of your daily allowance of sodium (about 500 mg). If you have hypertension you may need to choose prepared foods with lower sodium or salt content.

Some tips on using and heating prepared foods: Try to use prepared foods as side dishes to supplement foods you have already prepared from basic ingredients at home. This will allow you to taste different foods that you may not prepare at home but reduce the amounts of prepared foods you eat.

Avoid heating prepared food in its plastic container. Transfer the food to suitable container and then heat it. This will prevent the plasticizers (possible cancer causing endocrine disruptors) present in the container from leaching into the food.

In Defense of Food Environment

In his book **'In Defense of Food',** Michael Pollan has made very important observation about food and environment.

One of his observation is that food certified organic is usually well grown in healthy soil. Now there is research which supports the hypothesis that soils rich in organic matter produce more nutritious food. Recently well-controlled comparisons of crops grown organically and conventionally have found appreciably higher levels of antioxidants, flavonoids, vitamins and other nutrients in several of the organic crops. Ideally you want to look for food that is organic and local.

He advises **to eat food, not too much and mostly plants.** He advocates, like Lester Brown, to grow your own foods. He writes, 'The food you grow yourself is fresher than any you buy. The garden offers a great many solutions to the whole problem of eating well'.

He thinks of the relationship between the plants and soil, between the grower and the plants he/she tends. The food reveals itself for what it is: a web of relationships among a great many living beings, some of them human, some not, but each of them dependent on the other, and all of them ultimately rooted in soil and nourished by sunlight.

Thus, the quality of food and its nutrient content is affected by the grower, seeds, the soil, the sunlight — in short the whole environment.

Study Questions

1. How can you avoid water wastage?
2. List four environmentally sound technologies.
3. How is protein produced efficiently?
4. List guidelines to choose efficiently.
5. What does Michael Pollan say "In Defense of Food"? List three of his points.

PART - V

Diet Therapy

CHAPTER 24

Adaptation of Normal Diet for Changing Needs

Normal Diet

Normal diet is modified to feed young children, elderly members and sick members of the family. The planning of diet whether normal, soft or liquid has the same basic objective—to maintain, or restore the good health of the person through a proper diet. The modifications are based on the changed needs of the individual, due to age or sickness. Figure 24.1 depicts changes in consistency of diet to suit varying needs.

Normal Diet forms the basis of all modifications of diets for age and sickness; but due attention must be paid to nutritional needs of the individual. Normal diet is planned according to the recommended daily dietary intakes, which are designed to meet the needs of all healthy persons and may not meet the needs of sick persons. The nutritional requirements depend on the activity, the increased or decreased demands for certain nutrients, which need to be considered in planning the diet.

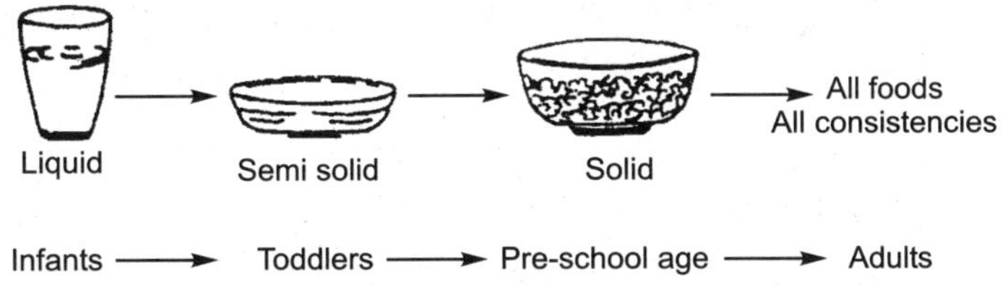

Figure 24.1: Changes in consistency of diet.

The plan given in Table 24.1 for a normal diet may be adapted to suit different cultural or socio-economic circumstances.

Table 24.1: Normal Diet

Food Group	*Foods to be Included*	*Amount*
1.	Rice *Chapati/Roti* *Upma/Shira/Pohe* Bread. etc.	6 or more servings
2.	Milk *Dal* Egg/Fish/Meat, if acceptable	2-3 Servings 2 or more servings 1 or more servings
3(*a*) 3(*b*)	Leafy vegetables Citrus or other vitamin-C rich fruits	1 or more servings 1 or more servings
4.	Other vegetables, fruits and roots, tubers	3 or more servings
5.	Oil Sugar/Butter/*Ghee/Vanaspati*	15 g or more As required to meet energy needs

Modifications of Normal Diet: The normal diet may be modified to:

1. Provide change in consistency, e.g., soft and fluid diets;
2. Provide foods bland in flavour;
3. Modify intervals of feeding;
4. Increase or decrease energy content;
5. Increase or decrease other nutrients, e.g., protein;
6. Increase or decrease fibre.

Liquid and Soft Diets

The type of modification relates to the condition and need of the individual concerned. The selection of foods is made on the same principles as the normal diet, using the daily food guide.

Mechanical Soft Diet: Many people, including infants, need soft diet because they have no teeth. Therefore, the only change made is in the consistency of the foods served. No restriction is placed on food selection. This diet is sometimes described as *mechanically soft diet.*

The following changes in the normal diet will meet the needs of individuals without teeth:

- Rice and other cereals to be served soft-cooked.
- *Chapati/roti/*bread—soft breads are substituted for hard, crusty preparations.
- *Dal* and whole pulses must be cooked thoroughly.
- Eggs—boiled or scrambled.
- Meat/fish should be ground or minced finely.
- Cooked vegetables may be used.

- Most raw vegetables are omitted, except tomatoes, finely chopped cucumber, lettuce, coriander, and mint (*pudina*). *Chutney* may be acceptable.
- Raw fruits, which are juicy and soft can be included—banana, mango (non-fibrous varieties), oranges, *musambi,* grape fruit, soft berries, jack fruit (soft variety), all melons, grapes, with soft skins, soft pear, peaches, apricots, plums (minus skins), etc.
- Apples may be served after cooking or baking.
- Tough skins, stones, fibres should be removed from fruits and vegetables, e.g., apple skin, potato skin, etc.
- Nuts and dried fruits need to be finely ground, when used.

Soft Diet: It is a step between the full liquid and the normal diet. It is served to persons suffering from acute infections, gastrointestinal disturbances or persons recovering from surgery. The diet consists of simple soft foods, which are easy to chew and easy to digest. Harsh fibre, fatty or highly spiced foods are avoided. It is nutritionally adequate, when planned according to the Daily Food Guide. The soft diet includes:

- Soft cooked rice, soft *chapati* and bread—6 servings or more
- Milk, *dahi* (curd), buttermilk, paneer, soft cheese—2-3 servings
- *Dals,* well-cooked—2-3 servings
- Eggs poached, boiled, trader ground meat, fish and poultry—1-3 servings
- Vegetables and fruits made up of
    1. Green leafy vegetables cooked and strained—2-3 servings
    2. Citrus fruits or juice or mango (non-fibrous varieties)—2-3 servings
- Other vegetables and fruits, not mentioned above, such as:
    1. Other vegetables—tender, chopped and cooked—2-3 servings
    2. Other fruits—banana or cooked fruits without skin or seeds—2-3 servings.

Additional foods such as butter, soups, soft desserts (such as *kheer/payasam*) and more of the above foods can be included to meet the nutritional needs.

The following foods are avoided:

- Legumes (whole).
- Egg (fried).
- Meat, tough, salted, smoked fish or meat.
- Vegetables and fruits raw, except those mentioned above; strongly flavoured ones.
- Bread and cereals coarse, with bran, whole-grain preparations and fatty recipes.
- Soups—fatty or highly seasoned.
- Fats—fried foods, e.g., potato chips.
- Miscellaneous: hot spices, pickles, nuts, etc.

Liquid Diets or full fluid diets are prepared for persons suffering from fevers, persons who have just undergone an operation or whenever a person is unable to tolerate solid foods. The adequacy of such a diet will depend on the types of liquids permitted.

Full fluid diet is served to persons, who are very ill and cannot chew or swallow solid food. It includes all foods, which are liquid at 37°C. To avoid difficulty in swallowing, fibrous foods and irritating spices are not included in this diet. The period of use of this diet depends on the condition of the patient. As the nutrient content is diluted, the interval between feeds is reduced and the number of feeds is increased to six or more.

The protein content of the diet can be increased by adding skimmed milk powder in the soups and beverages. Cooked, mashed *dal* can be used to prepare soups. Strained, ground meat or fish can be added to broths.

The energy content of the diet can be increased by adding (a) cream to milk, (b) butter/oil to cereal gruels and *dal* soups, (c) glucose to juices, milk, (d) using cream in desserts.

The following foods can be included in the full fluid diet:

- Milk—1 litre
- Eggs—2 (in custard or in eggnog)
- *Dal,* well-cooked—25–50 g
- Meat/fish cooked and strained—25-50 g
- Cereal strained—1/2 cup (100 g) cooked as gruel
- Vegetables—1/4 cup cooked, strained or puree for soup
- Fruit juices—1 cup, citrus and other strained juices
- Tomato or vegetable juices—1/2 cup
- Butter
- Sugar
- *Kheer,* icecream, gelatin dessert, custard
- Soups—broth
- Tea, coffee, soft drinks
- Flavourings, salt.

Clear fluid diet is given when a person is unable to tolerate food, due to nausea, vomiting, gas-formation, diarrhoea, or extreme lack of appetite. This diet is given for a day or two, until the patient is able to take a more liberal liquid diet.

As the name indicates the diet consists of clear liquids such as tea with lemon and sugar, coffee, cereal extracts (extract of puffed cereals also), strained fruit juices, carbonated beverages, *dal* extract, fat-free broth, etc. The amount is restricted to 30 to 60 ml per hour in the beginning and gradually increased. This diet replaces the fluids lost by the body, thus preventing dehydration.

Recent trend is to help the patient to progress from clear liquid to liquid to soft to mechanically soft to normal diet as quickly as possible. Therefore, the inadequacy of the first stage of diet may not affect the patient's health adversely, as he is encouraged to get through this stage in a day or two.

Study Questions

1. (*a*) What are the modifications made in normal diet?

   (*b*) List the foods to be included in soft diet.
2. What foods are included in liquid diet? Indicate the predominant nutrients supplied by each.

Practical Work

Plan and prepare diets for person suffering from

Diarrhoea; Dysentery; Fever; Constipation.

CHAPTER 25

Principles of Diet Therapy and Therapeutic Nutrition

Introduction

The best doctors in the world are:

"Doctor Diet, Doctor Quiet and Doctor Merryman" – Jonathan Swift.

Diet Therapy is use of appropriate foods as a tool in the recovery from illness. In most illnesses, the patient's diet complements the medical or surgical treatment. The rate of recovery thus is determined by the patient's acceptance and intake of the diet prescribed. In certain ailments such as obesity and **diabetes mellitus** modified diet is the most important input to help the patient's recovery.

All **therapeutic diets** are modifications of the normal diet made in order to meet the altered needs resulting from disease. As you may have noted in Chapter 14, the normal diet is planned to meet the recommended dietary allowances (RDA), using the basic five food groups.

Therapeutic diet is planned to meet or exceed the dietary allowances of a normal person as the aim of diet therapy is to maintain health and help the patient to regain nutritional wellbeing.

In certain ailments it may be necessary to restrict intake of calories (as in weight reduction diets) or sodium (as in heart ailment).

Food Acceptance in Illness

Illness leads to poor food acceptance due to:

(*i*) Reduced desire or interest in food due to lack of appetite, gastrointestinal disturbances or discomfort after eating.

(*ii*) Reduced appetite due to inactivity.

(*iii*) Reduced appetite due to some drugs.

In addition a patient in hospital faces a number of stressors. These include:

(*i*) Altered time of eating and rest as compared to home.

(*ii*) A lot of questions are asked; some of these are very personal.

(*iii*) Movements to various laboratories for investigations or tests.

(*iv*) A lot of waiting for tests to be done.

(*v*) Fear of tests and their results.

(*vi*) Hospital staff, who monitor the patient, may intrude on privacy.

(*vii*) Other patients in the ward or room may cause anxiety.

To counteract these stressors, a relative, a nurse or a case manager is needed to monitor the patient's care.

In this stressful situation, **the only comfort for the patient may be food**.

Illness Affects Nutrition

The nutrient needs and their use in the body may be affected by illness. The patient does not have appetite, may have pain and/or vomiting. This may result in insufficient food intake. Nutrient absorption may be poor due to severe diarrhoea, which may lead to loss of weight, malnutrition and even dehydration.

The patient may face problems such as poor appetite, too much or too little food served etc. Therapeutic diets may be bland, less salty, poor in texture and choice. Food acceptance of modified diets can be a problem. These problems need to be anticipated and resolved with the patient.

The patient may feel relief if the appetite is satisfied, meals are attractive, colourful and include some well-prepared favourite foods.

In fever, the metabolic rate is increased and so the need for all nutrients (calories, proteins, vitamins) is increased. Nutrient utilization is adversely affected in metabolic diseases.

The patient's lack of movement (due to confinement to bed or wheelchair) for many days increases loss of nitrogen and calcium from the body. These are some of the problems that need attention and solution.

Nutritional Assessment in the Clinical Setting

Nutritional assessment is used to decide the nutritional status of the patient. Nutritional assessment includes anthropometric, clinical, dietary and laboratory measurements.

Anthropometric measurements include height, weight, BMI (body mass index), triceps skinfold and sometimes other skinfolds.

Body Mass Index (BMI), It is calculated from height-weight data and is an indicator of the body fat content. Standards of BMI have been developed for use in judging the health status of the person. (Table 25.1)

$$BMI = Wt.\ in\ kg\ /\ Ht.\ in\ metre^2$$

Table 25.1: BMI in Adults (Men and Women)

Adults	*BMI*
Normal	19–24
Obesity – Grade I	25–29
Obesity – Grade II	30–40
Obesity – Grade III	>40

Skinfold measurements help to assess the energy reserves in the form of fat. An average of three of these values are used to compare with a set of normal values.

Midarm Circumference (MC) gives an indication of body protein reserves and helps to detect protein malnutrition.

Clinical Assessment includes examination of eyes, teeth, gums, tongue, skin and hair to observe symptoms of nutritional deficiency. It is quick, but subjective and not specific.

Dietary Assessment is an essential basis for dietary counselling. There are several methods used, which include 24 hour recall, food frequency list, a food diary, diet history and observations at meal times. These help in evaluation of the food intake to detect possible deficiencies.

Laboratory Assessment involves whole blood, blood serum and blood plasma analysis; sometimes urine analysis is done to determine the level or the excretion rate of the nutrients or their metabolites.

Dietary Counselling is intended to produce a desirable change in the food behaviour. Preventive health care, especially dietary care, can reduce the risks of patients developing chronic diseases. Its success depends on the trust and active involvement of the patient.

It has been observed that malnourished patients take longer to recover. Hence, nutritional assessment should be a routine part of all patients' care.

All patients do not need in-depth assessment. A simple method of clinical observation helps to detect those **at-risk** of malnutrition. Only patients at risk need to undergo comprehensive nutritional assessment.

Nutrition history and clinical evaluation can help to identify individuals who are at risk nutritionally (Table 25.2).

When the nature, extent and cause of the problems are determined, on the basis of clinical observations, a plan of nutritional care can be made.

Table 25.2: Clinical Observations Suggesting Malnutrition

1.	Recent loss of 10% or more of usual body weight.
2.	Restricted oral intake of nutrients for 10 days or more (e.g. clear liquid diet or IV infusions of simple solutions only)
3.	Protracted nutrient losses as a result of (*a*) Nausea, vomiting, diarrhoea, malabsorption syndromes (*b*) Surgical removal of portions of gastrointestinal tract. (*c*) Draining fluids, abscesses, wounds, burns. (*d*) Renal dialysis
4.	Increased metabolic needs due to (*a*) Fever, (*b*) Recent surgery or trauma, (*c*) Extensive burns, infections
5.	Chronic disease or impaired function of a major organ system.
6.	Use of drugs with antinutrient properties
7.	Excessive intake of alcohol
8.	Faddism and other personal problems

Latrogenic Malnutrition

Patients who are hospitalised for 2 weeks or longer are at risk of developing **iatrogenic** (doctor or hospital induced) **malnutrition** due to some of the factors mentioned above. These include insufficient food (hence nutrient) intake, stress, blood loss due to tests and surgery. For such patients, as also others, nutritional assessment and nutritional care are imperative.

Planning of Therapeutic Diets

The energy and protein needs need to be determined to ensure proper nutritional care of a malnourished patient.

Energy Needs: The energy intake has to meet the basal plus activity needs of the patient, taking into account the patient's need for – repletion, maintenance or weight loss. The **resting energy expenditure (REE)** can be measured with a portable equipment, which measures volumes of oxygen (VO_2) consumed and carbon dioxide expired (VCO_2). The REE is **increased** in patient suffering from burns, fevers, infection, fractures, trauma etc. and **lowered** in malnutrition.

The resting energy expenditure (REE) can also be determined using the classic Harris-Benedict equation derived from indirect calorimetry measurements, using the weight, height and age of the patient.

Harris-Benedict Equation

Women: REE (kcal) = 655.1 + 9.56W + 1.85H - 4.68A

Men: REE (kcal) = 66.5 + 13.75W + 5.0H - 6.78A

where A = Age in years, W = Weight in kgs, H = Height in cms

Protein Needs: Loss of nitrogen is increased by stress. If the losses in urine are measured, the protein intake can be increased to make up for the loss. When the loss is unknown, protein intake can be proportional to energy intake, as indicated below:

Calorie : Nitrogen ratio in Severe stress is — 150 : 1 to 100 : 1

For example, if a stressed patient needs 2400 kcalories, his N-need is–

2400 kcal = N(g) × 150 = 16.0 g N per day

Protein Needs = 16.0 × 6.25 = 100g per day

Therapeutic Diets

Food is an integral part of patient care and is a **major** contributor in his/her recovery. Therefore, careful selection of foods, their preparation and ensuring that these are consumed by the patient is an important part of the therapy. The medical personnel are responsible for diagnosis and indicating the kind of modifications to be made in the normal diet in view of the condition of the patient. The diet section staff use this information to plan the patient's diet.

There are **three aspects** of the diets prescribed. The first refers to the **composition** of the diet. Thus it indicates modification in the components of the diet. For example, low calorie diet, indicates that the energy content of the diet is reduced. However, it is important to include a specific amount intended to guide the user (such as 1200 or 1500 calorie diet).

Second aspect refers to the **consistency** of the diet. Thus you have normal diet, liquid diet (further classified into clear-liquid, full-liquid diet), soft diet, soft fiber-restricted diet, pureed diet, etc.

Thirdly, it is important to indicate the **manner and route** of feeding the diet, such as by mouth, by nasogastric tube, gastrostomy tube etc., depending on the condition of the patient.

Types of Diets

Normal Hospital Diet

Normal diet is the most commonly used diet in the hospitals. It plays a very important part in the patient's recovery. It aims to meet the recommended dietary allowances of nutrients through a planned diet. There are no restrictions involved in food planning, but the food plan is balanced to avoid over- or under-nutrition. In the hospitals, there is choice of menu based on normal food acceptance patterns of the patients. Thus in India, the hospitals serve vegetarian and non-vegetarian diet. There may be some choice of foods in the menu, which helps to retain a feeling of control in the patient. Table 24.1 gives foods included in the normal diet.

Modifications of Normal Diet

The normal diet is modified to form various diets according to the needs of the patient. These include various liquid and soft diets, which have been discussed in chapter 24.

Liquid Diets are further divided into **Clear-liquid Diet** and **Full-liquid Diet**. The details of foods included in liquid diets are given in Chapter 24.

Clear-liquid Diet or Clear-fluid Diet includes drinks such as tea, coffee, clear fruit juices, coconut water, sherbets, extracts of dal, rice, popped cereals, fat-free broth, carbonated drinks. Milk is not included, as it is not a clear liquid. Feeds are offered in small portions of about 20-25 ml every hour or two and the volume is increased gradually as the condition of the patient improves.

Liquid diet helps to maintain liquid and electrolyte balance, relieve thirst and stimulate the digestion system to function, after an operation or disturbance in the system due to infection. If the fluids are chosen well, the diet can provide 200-500 kcal, some sodium, potassium and ascorbic acid. It does not meet the requirement of most nutrients and is given only for a day or two during a transient phase before moving on to soft and then full diet.

A clear-liquid diet is given:

(*a*) for a patient suffering from nausea, vomiting or loss of appetite (anorexia).

(*b*) during acute stage of diarrhea

(*c*) post-operative first stage,

(*d*) after tube or parenteral feeding before resuming oral feeding.

Full-liquid Diet: In full liquid diet, foods included are –liquids and foods which are liquid at body temperature. It can provide adequate nutrition, with the exception of iron. As the nutrient-density is not high, six or more feedings are given. Skim milk powder is added to increase the protein content of the diet. This increases the lactose content of the diet and therefore, it should not be given to persons with low lactase activity. This diet has high calcium and fat content and is low in fiber. The foods which can be included in full-liquid diet are listed in Chapter 24.

Table 25.3: Daily Food Allowances for the Full Liquid Diet

Daily Food Plan	*Description*
I Cereal Group 1 or more servings	One half cup strained, cooked cereal contains about 80 calories, 2 g protein, iron and the B complex vitamins. Combine with milk in gruels and soups.
II Protein Group	
1 ¼ liter fluid cow's milk	One and quarter liter fluid cow's milk contains about 40 g protein and 820 calories, 2.5 g calcium, day's need of vitamin A and B vitamins.
¼ C skimmed milk powder (SMP)	If ¼ C skimmed milk powder is added to cow's milk, about 8 g protein and 80 calories will be added. This can be used in beverages, gruels, eggnog, custard, ice cream and kheer.
Dal - 50 g	Dal – 50 g, cooked and diluted contains 11g protein and 170 calories. It is valuable source of iron and vitamin B complex.
Eggs - 2 nos	Two eggs contain 12 g protein and 170 calories. It is a valuable source of iron, vitamin A and B complex. It can be served as eggnog, egg custard or egg flip.

(*Contd...*)

Daily Food Plan	*Description*
Meat	Meat 30 g, served as thick broth, contains about 6 g protein and 75 calories. Liver is an excellent source of iron, vitamin A and B complex. It can be served combined with broth as soup. Dal, egg and meat may be interchanged.
III & IV Vegetable and Fruits Group	The puree or juice of spinach, carrots, tomato, french beans may be used to serve as soups. Normally, mild-flavoured vegetables are served. Other vegetable purees or juices may be served if accepted by the patient. Calories from these are negligible. Amla, citrus (musumbi, orange etc.) and tomato and papaya juice or puree provide an important source of vitamin C. One cup of citrus juices provides 80 calories.1 C tomato juice provides less than 40 calories.
V Fats and Sweets 6 teaspoons, butter, ghee, oil. 8 to 10 teaspoons sugar	Eight teaspoons sugar contributes about 160 to 200 calories and serve as sweeteners for eggnog, gruel, tea, coffee, cocoa. Six teaspoons of butter, ghee, oil provide about 250 to 270 calories. These serve as flavorings for soups, gruels and desserts.

A daily food plan for full-liquid diet, is indicated in Table 25.3. Food allowances and sample menu for full-liquid diet for ovo-lact vegetarians is presented in Table 25.4.

Full-liquid diet is prescribed for patients: (*i*) post-operatively after clear-liquid diet phase, (*ii*) in acute infections of short duration, (*iii*) in acute gastrointestinal upset, after clear-liquid diet phase, and (*iv*) in situations when patient is unable to chew food.

Soft Diet: Soft diet is used after full-liquid diet and before moving on to a normal diet. It is nutritionally adequate. Foods included are those, which are easy to mix with saliva, swallow and digest. Exclude foods, which contain harsh fiber, strong flavours and too much fat. Food allowances for soft diet are given in Table 25.5. The calories and protein content of soft (low fiber) diet is given in Table 25.6.

Soft diets include several variations such as mechanically soft diet, pureed diet and fiber-restricted soft diet.

Table 25.4: Food Allowances & Sample Menu for Full Liquid Diet (1875 kcal, 70g protein)

Food Group	*Foods*	*Amount*	*Menu Plan*
I	Cereal, strained	25 g	**Breakfast-** Musumbi juice
II	Milk	200 g	Strained cereal (rava) with
	SMP	25 g	butter, hot milk and sugar
	Eggs 2 nos.	100 g	Coffee with milk and sugar
III	Spinach	150 g	**Mid-morning-** Egg custard (soft)
	Beans (strained)	50 g	Musumbi juice
	Carrots	75 g	**Lunch-** Dal – spinach soup, Tomato juice
	Tomatoes	75 g	Ice-cream, vanilla, Milk
IV	Musumbi 2 nos.	250 g	**Mid-afternoon-** Papaya,
	Papaya	100 g	milk shake, watermelon
	Watermelon	100 g	**Dinner-** Beans – dal soup, Egg nog,
V	Sugar	50 g	Carrot kheer
	Ghee, Butter	30 g	**Night**: High protein, High calorie
			Beverage: Milk +SMP+Sugar+flavour

Mechanically Soft Diet: In this diet the modification of normal diet is in texture only. The method of preparation and the seasonings used are not restricted. This is also called **Dental Soft Diet,** as it is prescribed for those who cannot chew, due to absence or removal of teeth or ill-fitting dentures.

Pureed Diets: Pureed diets include foods, which are smooth, soft and need hardly any chewing. These are good for patients who have difficulty in swallowing. All foods (except those that are already soft or smooth) are blended or pureed in a mixer. Liquids are added to get the consistency needed by the patient. To increase calories, fat and/or sugars are added.

Soft Fiber-Restricted Diet: Indigestible carbohydrates are excluded from this diet. Indigestible fibers include those which make up cell wall of plants (such as cellulose, hemicellulose, lignin, pectic substances, gums and mucin). The amount of indigestible carbohydrates in the diet can be reduced by using:

(*a*) refined cereals and breads
(*b*) immature vegetables
(*c*) fruits without skins and seeds and
(*d*) cooked vegetables and fruits

While cooking, both peptic substances and cellulose are disintegrated, hence cooked vegetables and fruits are used. To reduce indigestible carbohydrates, pureed vegetables and fruits or only the juice of vegetables and fruits is used.

Recent trend is a more liberal one as patients prefer and are happier with soft cooked immature vegetables than with pureed ones. Use of a wider variety of fruits and vegetables, including some raw fruits is the trend now. For example, peeled apples, pears, peaches, apricots and bananas are often recommended to be used.

A description of the daily food allowances and sample menu for soft fiber-restricted diet is presented in Table 25.7. Appropriate adaptations in this plan can be made to meet individual requirements.

Table 25.5: Food Allowances for Soft Diet

I.	**Cereal** servings 6 to 12 - Soft chapati, mashed bhakri/roti, bread, biscuits are included but not crackers and hard breads. *Idli, khandwa, khandpoli*, ragi balls, *sandane*, etc., are included to provide the servings needed
II.	**Dal** 2S, **Milk** 2S, **Eggs** 1S, **Meat-fish-poultry** – 1S
III and IV	**Vegetables and fruits** 3 to 4 servings Vegetables cooked to soft texture, and can be cut, grated or diced, e.g. finely cut tomatoes, lettuce, etc. Soft fruits such as banana, *musumbi* or orange sections, grapes, cut pear, apple, melons, berries can be eaten raw. All canned and frozen fruits are permitted.
V	**Sugars, Fats and Oils:** All desserts from normal diet which are easily assimilated by patients are allowed such as kheer, payasam, puran poli, kaju barfi, shira, rasgulla, gulab-jam, cakes, puddings, etc.; **avoid those containing nuts.**

Table 25.6: Calories and Protein Content of Soft Low-Fiber Diet

Food Group	*Food*	*Amt.*	*Cal.*	*Prot*
I	Bread 9s	180 g	450	14
	Cereal, refined	20 g	70	2
II	Milk, whole cow's	1 litre	670	32
	S.M.P	50 g	180	19
	Dal, mung	50 g	170	12
	Eggs 2 nos. (1)	100 g	170	13
III	Vegetables, leafy			
	Spinach	100 g	30	2
	Fruit juice, musumbi	120 g	50	1
IV	Vegetables-other			
	French beans, cooked	100 g	30	2
	Potato cooked	100 g	100	2
	Fruit other			
	Cooked apple	100 g	60	—
Total			2000	99
V	Fat (2) + Oil (2)	20 g	180	—
	Sugar	30 g	120	—
	Total		2300	99

(1) Part of egg and dal may be substituted with fish, meat or poultry.

(2) 10 g butter.

Some of the aspects that affect food acceptability include connective tissue, strong flavour and the amount of stimulant present.

Table 25.7: Food Allowances and Sample Menu for Soft Fiber-Restricted Diet

	Food Allowances	*Sample Menu*
I.	Cereal foods: Well-cooked, soft rice, chapati, Idli, porridge (rawa), kheer, bread, bhakari, Senvaya, noodles, macaroni, spaghetti	**Breakfast** Rawa porridge Toast/chapati + butter
II	Dal, well-cooked, like varan, soup	Egg, scrambled
	Milk, cow's, curd, buttermilk, soft cheese	Milk, sugar
	Eggs- All preparations, except fried	Tea/coffee + milk + sugar
	Meat- fish- poultry – very tender, minced or ground, baked, roasted or stewed	**Lunch** Rice
III	Vegetables: tender greens, cooked and blended	Chapati
IV	If not tender, strained cooked vegetables, cooked tender beets, carrots, peas, pumpkin, squash and other gourds, without seeds and skin	Dal Vegetable
	Fruits: banana, papaya, citrus fruits without membrane, chiku, water melon, mango, cooked apples. Pears, peaches, apricots – all without skins; all juices	Salad, Dahi **Supper** Similar to lunch
V	Sugars: syrup, honey, jelly, sugar candy (without nuts and fruits), molasses. Use in moderation	
	Fats: cream, butter, ghee, vegetable oils. Use in moderation	
	In addition one can include – Beverages – all,	
	Desserts: mithai without nuts and dry fruits, kheer – rice, rawa, senvaya etc. Plain cakes, biscuits, custard, ice-cream, sherbet, puddings	
	Miscellaneous: salt, seasonings & spices in moderation	

Connective Tissue: The texture of meat, tender or less tender is mainly decided by the amount of connective tissue present. The amount of connective tissue in meat depends on the age of the animal and how much the muscle is exercised. The acceptance of meat preparations can be improved by cooking. Meat may be made tender by using moist heat and lower temperature cookery.

Flavour: Strong flavoured vegetables such as onions, leeks, radishes, dried beans and cabbage family vegetables (brussel sprouts, cauliflower, broccoli, turnips) are normally omitted. But there is individual variation in patients' acceptance of these. Hence, the individual patient's preference needs to be considered in this matter.

The effects of spices on the digestive system have been studied. It is found that cinnamon, allspice, thyme, sage, mace, paprika and caraway, used to flavour foods, do not have harmful effect. But black pepper, chilli pepper, cloves, mustard seed and perhaps nutmeg are considered gastric irritants and best avoided.

Beverages: Both tea and coffee are stimulating beverages. When these are used in the diet, one needs to know how to prepare these to avoid undesirable side effects on the other components.

A mild cup of tea (from ½ tsp dried leaves) contains about 0.05g caffeine, but quick infusion extracts most of the caffeine, but not the tannins. As tannins precipitate proteins, a quick infusion is recommended for use in the diet.

Coffee contains an average of 1.25% caffeine. A cup of strong coffee contains about 0.1g of caffeine. Besides caffeine, coffee contains chlorogenic acid, which differs from tannins in that it does not precipitate proteins and is not astringent. Cocoa contains 31% carbohydrate, 9% protein and 10% fat. It contains about 1.5% theobromine and a trace of caffeine, both being stimulants.

Nutrient Content: In the past, it was common practice to put more emphasis on "foods to avoid" and less on "foods to eat". It led to this group of diets being one of the hazards of hospitalization, resulting in nutritional deficiency and delay in recovery. Such deficiency can be avoided by proper selection and use of correct amount of foods in the diet.

Foods from the first four groups may be used in amounts enough to meet or exceed RDAs. This is very important for persons, who have been ill for sometime, and may have suffered due to undue dietary restrictions. In addition, the disease itself may increase nutritional needs to ensure healing of tissue or to make up for poor absorption. Such extra needs would justify increased intake of foods from all the food groups. For example, if this diet is used to reduce gastric acidity, additional amounts of protein containing foods such as milk need to be taken. The protein content of milk can be increased by addition of skimmed milk powder to it. The number of meals may be increased to six or more feedings per day, to buffer the acid produced in the stomach.

The amount of protein foods, citrus juice and other foods need to be increased to exceed the amounts suggested for a normal individual. As personal needs vary, special adaptations can be made to suit the person.

A description of the daily food allowances and sample menu pattern is presented in Table 25.7. Appropriate adaptations can be made in this plan to meet individual requirements.

Tube Feeding

If a patient whose gastrointestinal tract is working, cannot take sufficient food orally, tube feeding is resorted to. Tube feeding is given in the following conditions –

(*i*) Babies who have low birth weight and cannot suck
(*ii*) Those who are undernourished and cannot take or retain food taken orally
(*iii*) Persistent anorexia patients, who need forced feeding
(*iv*) After certain types of surgery
(*v*) Patients with severe malabsorption
(*vi*) Patients who cannot absorb or digest food
(*vii*) Semiconscious or unconscious patients or any other condition which prevents intake of sufficient food.

Since the feed must be formulated to meet the nutritional needs of the patient, it is also called **formula feed**. It is important that the formula should be such that it is well tolerated. Many types of formulas can be made or purchased to serve the needs of the patient. The foods fed by tube may be :

(*i*) Natural liquid foods
(*ii*) Raw or cooked foods blended to liquid form, or
(*iii*) Commercially made special formulated diets.

Composition

The form of proteins in the formula can be intact proteins (milk, egg) or protein hydrolysates containing peptides and amino acids. When the patient has normal enzymatic digestive function (absorption) intact proteins are included in the formula. But if there is severe lack of enzyme or malabsorption, protein hydrolysates are used in the formula.

Carbohydrate is in the form of polymers of glucose, which are easily broken and absorbed. Starch or disaccharides (sucrose or lactose0 may also be used. Lactose is avoided in many ready-made formulas because in some problems of absorption, lactose is not tolerated.

Fats used in the formulas are vegetable oils, butter, lecithin, mono- and diglycerides and medium chain triglycerides (MCT). Formulas are fortified with vitamins and minerals to ensure adequate nutrition.

Formulas normally provide 1kcal/ml. Formulas are likely to be low in fiber, unless enriched with fiber.

Osmolality

The number and size of particles per kg of water is called **Osmolality** This is an important factor in deciding patient tolerance. **Isotonic** formulas as the word indicates, have the same osmolality as body fluids and are well tolerated. Hyper-osmoler formulas (with higher osmolality) may cause rapid movement of fluid and electrolytes across the cell wall, if these are introduced in the intestine.

Any formula which has a high level of electrolytes has high osmolality. Thus glucose and sucrose have higher osmolality than complex carbohydrates; free amino acids have higher osmolality than intact proteins; fat has little effect. It is good to remember that carbohydrates have the greatest influence on osmolality, because they are digested very rapidly.

Types of Formulas

Names of formulas indicate their components and their nutritional make-up. Thus **Balanced Complete Formulas** are made from ordinary foods or baby foods by blending these. These can be made at home or in hospital.

A milk-based formula is prepared from cow's, toned or skim milk with addition of pasteurised eggs, a source of carbohydrate and supplements of vitamins.

Lactose-free formulas are made for lactose-sensitive patients.

Specialty formulas are made for specific conditions, with the needed adjustments in nutrient content. For example, high fat and low carbohydrate formulas are made for pulmonary conditions; for phenylketonuria, a formula low or devoid of phenylalanine is given. In trauma or liver disease, a formula low in aromatic amino acids and high in branched chain amino acids is given.

The mode of administration of formula is decided taking patient's condition and the period for which tube feed is to be given. For short term feeding nasogastric tube is used.

When there is injury to the esophagus or for long term tube feeding, a gastrostomy tube may be surgically inserted into the stomach. This route is not suitable for patients with unchecked vomiting or where gastric emptying is disturbed. A jejunostomy tube may be used when the stomach must be bypassed.

The feeding can be continuous or intermittent. Intermittent feeding permits patient to move about.

Like all other diets, diluted formulas are fed in the beginning and gradually concentration is increased to full strength. The rate of feeding is begun slowly and then increased gradually. This decreases the possibility of diarrhea. The patient's bed (head side) is raised while feeding, to reduce chance of air block.

Home Tube Feeding

Long term tube feeding can be given at home, with guidance from the health care team. The care-provider needs to be given instructions about how to maintain sanitation and hygiene in handling feeds and the equipment used.

Parenteral Nutrition

In parenteral feeding, the nutrient preparations are given directly into a vein. When a patient is likely to be dehydrated and needs quick reversal of the condition, a 5% dextrose solution in water (DSW) is usually given by a peripheral vein (also known as IV drip) to provide fluids and some energy (calories). Electrolyte solutions can also be given by this mode. In some conditions the higher dextrose concentrations with amino acids and lipids are given.

Total Parenteral Nutrition (TPN)

TPN is used only when it is not possible to use enteral route and the patient is hypermetabolic or debilitated. Before giving TPN, a thorough nutritional and metabolic assessment of the patient is done. The blood levels of various nutrients are monitored frequently during TPN and the solution adjusted, if needed.

Composition of Solutions: Crystalline amino acids are used to meet protein needs, so that the composition can be controlled to meet patient's needs. Dextrose solutions (hypertonic) provide carbohydrates as energy source and ensure amino acid sparing action. For patients with lung problems, high dextrose load causes difficulty in breathing. For such patients part of the carbohydrate is replaced with fat, to prevent this problem.

Emulsions of safflower or soy oil are given separately, to meet part of the energy needs and to provide essential fatty acids.. As lipid emulsions are isotonic, these are given by central or peripheral vein. Other nutrients (vitamins, minerals and other electrolytes) are given in solution or by injection.

TPN solutions being hypertonic are introduced into a large central vein where the solution gets diluted quickly in the high rate of blood flow.

The patient should be helped to return to oral feeding as soon as feasible, as TPN is expensive and can lead to a number of complications, if not given properly.

Home Care of Patients

The family could be guided to take care of the patient's nutrition at home. Thus over 25 per cent of nursing home residents could be taken care of at home. There is a need to set up home health care services to reduce the need for institutional care.

Study Questions

1. List the problems which affect food acceptance in illness
2. Write notes on anthropometric measurements, iatrogenic malnutrition and three aspects of therapeutic diets.
3. List foods which can be included in soft-fibre-restricted diet.
4. When is tube feeding given?
5. Write short notes on: osmolarity, parenteral feeding.

CHAPTER 26

Nutrition in Infections, Fever and Lung Diseases

Introduction
Infections
Fever; Diet
Tuberculosis: Body's Metabolic Response, Diet
Asthma, Chronic Bronchitis and Emphysema
Nutritional Status, Treatment, Diet Therapy, Plan of Mealtimes

Introduction

The invasion of the body by a pathogen results in infections, fever, lung and other diseases. The nutritional needs of the body are increased to resist the pathogen, to recoup the losses incurred metabolically and rebuild the cells damaged by the invader. Hence, a high protein diet is indicated.

Infections

Infection occurs when a pathogen gains entry into the body in sufficient numbers or multiplies in the body and causes injury at a particular site. Depending on **where** the pathogen attacks, different types of illnesses develop. If a pathogen enters through the nose or mouth, and multiplies in that region, ailments of throat or bronchi occur. If pathogens enter the lungs, it can injure them. If pathogens are swallowed with water, milk or food, gastrointestinal symptoms such as nausea, vomiting, cramps and diarrhea frequently result. If the pathogens enter through cut skin, infections such as boils, skin ulcers or other inflammations occur.

The severity of the infection depends on the number of pathogens in the body and the body's ability to fight the infection. The ability of the body to resist infection is called **immunity**. Natural immunity is the sum-total of the defenses in the body which enables the body to resist infection under normal conditions. These defenses include –

- intact skin and mucous membranes, which bar entrance of microorganisms
- tissue fluids and blood, which contain cells and other substances which engulf and destroy foreign objects, and

- the normally harmless population of bacteria and viruses found in the body, which prevent the growth of harmful bacteria and viruses.

All these processes of normal immunity depend on proper nutrition, physical fitness and environmental conditions. When this natural immunity is depressed by poor nutritional status and other conditions, a person may develop infections. If the person is in poor nutritional state, an attack of common infectious diseases can endanger life itself.

A patient who is in poor nutritional status needs nutrient supplements.

In severe infections, nutritional status is affected in an adverse manner. Thus the food intake and absorption are reduced, while nutrient excretion is increased, metabolic rate also increases. Nutrients are diverted to minimize effect of infection and resist damage to tissues. Higher nutrient intake must be planned to ensure tissue repair and to make up for excretory losses.

Infection involves protein breakdown and hence there is an increased need for dietary proteins. The first goal is to identify and destroy the pathogen causing infection. The antibiotics, which are given to control the infection, may cause gastrointestinal disturbances which need to be taken into account in the diet management.

Fever

Fever often accompanies infection. The patient may have chills due to fever and may complain of feeling cold. But all fevers are not a result of infection, and elevation in body temperature is not fever. Thus, there is elevation of body temperature in heat stroke, as the body is unable to eliminate heat.

Infection affects protein catabolism (breakdown), often decreases food intake and increases nutrient loss through vomiting and/or diarrhea. Enteric (intestinal) infections, as in typhoid, interfere with absorption and reduce nutrient utilization. Fever, which often accompanies infection, increases energy needs of the body (about 7% per degree Fahrenheit) above normal temperature.

Fever may be acute and of short duration as in colds, intermittent as in malaria or chronic as in tuberculosis.

Diet: The dietary treatment varies with the kind of fever and its duration. When fever is acute and of short duration, the most important aspect is to feed sufficient fluids and electrolytes to make up for the losses from the body. As appetite is usually poor, frequent small feeds of liquid and soft foods need to be given to ensure adequate intake. As the condition improves, the size of the feed is increased to meet nutritional needs.

The critical problem is protein breakdown, which occurs in infection. A high protein, high calorie diet is prescribed (Table 26.1). Liquid and soft foods need to be fed often to ensure sufficient food intake as appetite is poor. Food allowances for such a diet are indicated in Table 26.2.

The drugs given (antipyretics) help to bring the temperature to normal. Most of the drugs contain ingredients to relieve pain also. The medication is taken with food to minimise gastric irritation.

Tuberculosis

In India, tuberculosis is a major cause of illness and death. According to one estimate, one in four Indians is infected by T.B.

Table 26.1: High Protein High Calorie Diet

Protein 75 g; Kcal 2,500				*Protein 110 g; Kcal 3,000*			
Food	*Amt/Serving*	*Protein*	*Kcal*	*Food*	*Amt/Serving*	*Protein*	*Kcal*
Milk, toned	800 ml	26	535	Milk,toned	1000 ml	32	670
Egg	1 no	6	75	Egg	1 no	6	75
Cheese/ Paneer/meat	2 S	9	133	Cheese/ Paneer/meat	4 S	18	265
Dal	2 S	11	170	Dal	3 S	17	255
Cereals,	6 S	15	510	Cereals,	12 S	30	1,020
Breads	9 S	22	165	Breads			
Vegetables	3-4 S	5	100	Vegetables	3-4 S	5	100
Fruits	3 S	3	180	Fruits	3 S	3	180
Ghee Butter/oil	9 S	0	405	Ghee Butter/oil	9 S	0	225
Sugar Jam etc.	10 S	0	200	Sugar Jam etc.	10 S	0	200
Total		75	2,508	Total		111	2,990

Tuberculosis is caused by the bacteria *Mycobacterium tuberculosis.* It is transmitted through the cough or sneeze of an infected person, when it gets sprayed into the air. Most people who breathe in the bacteria do not get infected. In those, who do not get infected even after inhaling the bacteria, the microorganisms may remain dormant as their immune system triggers activation of macrophages, which engulf the bacteria. About 10 per cent of those infected develop tuberculosis some time in their life, when the natural immunity is lowered.

In tuberculosis, lungs are the most frequently affected part, but other organs may be attacked sometimes. Tuberculosis (T.B.) is accompanied by cough, sneezing, fever and tissue wastage. In acute form, the fever is high and the symptoms are similar to pneumonia. Low grade fever is typical of the chronic form.

Body's Metabolic Response: Ability to utilise fat is reduced, hence muscle protein losses are increased. As available nitrogen is used to synthesize immune bodies, considerable protein wasting occurs with loss of body weight.

Diet: A high protein, high calorie diet is prescribed. It must provide sufficient energy i.e., about 2500-3000 calories and 75-100 g protein (Table 26.2). A sample menu and foods included are given in Table 26.3. In addition, if there has been lung haemorrhage, iron supplement with large intake of vitamin C is needed. As carotenes are not utilised well, preformed vitamin A must be included in the diet. In addition, vitamin A and vitamin B_6 supplements must also be given.

Isoniazid, a drug, which is prescribed for T.B., is a Vitamin B_6 antagonist. Hence, vitamin B_6 supplements must be given to avoid its deficiency.

Table 26.2: Food Allowances for High Calorie, High Protein Diet

Protein – 75 to 110 g and Kcal 2,500 to 3,100

Group	*Foods*	*No. of Servings, amount*
I	Cereals, breads	6 – 12 S (150 – 300 g)
II	Milk, toned/cow's Egg SMP/Cheese/Paneer/Meat Dal	800 – 1000 ml 2 no 50 – 100 g 2 – 3 S (50 – 75 g)
III and IV	Vegetables Fruits	3 – 4 S 1 S leafy vegetable 1 S raw (salad) 2 S other + root vegetable 3 – one of these citrus
V	Ghee, Butter, Oil Sugar, jam, murabbas, Desserts such as kheer, pudding, Custard, shreekhand etc.	5 – 10 S 10 S

Table 26.3: A Sample Menu– Foods Included in 80-100 g Protein Diet

Breakfast Orange Eggs, scrambled Milk toned – 1 C Bread/toast Butter Murabba Tea with milk, sugar **Mid morning** 1 C lassi & banana **Afternoon pm Snack** Milk 1 C Egg sandwich Tea	**Lunch** Rice Chapati Dal Usal Vegetable, beans "potato" Salad – tomato Dahi ½ C **Dinner** Bhakari Rice Dal L. vegetable Papad Fruit Salad

The drugs used in treatment may have adverse reactions, which need to be treated promptly. One of the problems in the control of tuberculosis is the fact that patients tend to neglect medication, as soon as they feel a little better. This leads to its recurrence. Education of patients about the need for **prolonged treatment and monitoring** until complete recovery is an important part of the control of tuberculosis.

It is very important to take the drug and diet treatment consistently until the patient is **fully back to normal health**. Failure to do so results in recurrence of the disease; the **resistant bacteria, which cause the second attack, are hardy and hard to treat.**

Asthma, Chronic Bronchitis and Emphysema

Asthma, chronic bronchitis and emphysema are grouped together as **Chronic Obstructive Pulmonary Disease (COPD).** The group has a common characteristic, which is air-flow reduction or obstruction. A lot of attention is given to its pathophysiology, but the nutrition aspect of treatment does not receive adequate attention.

There are about 300 million air-sacs (alveoli) in the lungs. **The symptoms of injury are noticed only after 60 per cent of these air sacs are affected**. The symptoms and possible causes of COPD are given in Table 26.4.

A very large number of Indians suffer from these ailments. A large percentage of annual deaths from chronic bronchitis and emphysema are due to excessive smoking cigarettes or *bidis.*

Table 26.4: Characteristics of COPD

Disease	*Symptoms*
Asthma	increased response of trachea and bronchi to stimuli, airways reduced, swelling of airway wall, excess mucus, wheezing, coughing, difficulty in breathing.
Chronic bronchitis	excess mucus, inflamed airways, hyperactive bronchi, difficulty in breathing out
Emphysema	reduced lung surface area, destruction of air sacs and air spaces in lungs, wheezing, chronic cough, chest shape distorted to barrel shape due to overwork and over-inflation of muscles

Nutritional Status: Nutritional status is poor and weight loss is noted. Breathing difficulties do not permit normal eating. The sputum formed affects tastes adversely. Due to insufficient oxygen supply, peristalsis is reduced resulting in poor appetite. In addition, the drugs given to improve breathing cause gastric irritation. In severe cases, the low oxygen supply and side effects of drugs may lead to ulcer formation in the stomach in about 20-25% of the patients.

Treatment: Avoidance of predisposing factors is an important part of cure. Dust allergy is one of the most common causes of asthma. The mites present in dust which have been found to be the cause, have to be removed by frequent washing of bed sheets and pillow covers, wet wiping of floors and fans and vacuum cleaning the books, papers and other articles, which the patient has to handle in daily life. It is essential part of the treatment.

Diet Therapy: The first aim in diet therapy is to prevent malnutrition or correct it if it has occurred. The **energy needs increase many fold** in comparison to normal needs of a person of comparable age and size. In extreme COPD cases, the energy used for breathing can be **10 times** that of the normal rate.

Energy: Energy needs need to be met; but intake must be monitored to match the oxygen available. Thus one can avoid production of excess carbon dioxide which may cause acidosis. These patients have limited ability to excrete carbon dioxide, so diet must contain foods with low respiratory quotient (RQ). RQ of fats is 0.7, proteins 0.8 and carbohydrates 1.0. So non-protein calories can be provided by high fat to carbohydrate ratio, which will decrease carbon dioxide production. Such formulas are available to treat severe cases.

Plan of Meal Times: Rest before meals helps to improve intake of food. Slow, deep breathing and relaxation practice helps eating. It also helps to avoid swallowing air, which can disrupt flow of food. Eating small meals slowly, wearing loose garments, not lying down, bending over or exercising soon after meals are helpful. Small frequent meals helps to reduce anorexia and decrease pressure on stomach due to fullness. It permits free movement of diaphragm and decreases fatigue.

Some drugs used to dilate bronchi have caffeine – like side effects, so caffeine should be avoided by patients on such days. To avoid undesirable side effects, it is advisable to take medicines with food.

Study Questions

1. What is infection? What is natural immunity?
2. How do you plan a diet for a patient suffering from tuberculosis?
3. Describe symptoms and treatment of chronic obstructive lung disease.

CHAPTER 27

Nutrition in Diseases of the Gastrointestinal Tract

Introduction

The gastrointestinal tract is involved in transforming the food eaten into energy to meet the body's needs for its sustenance and function. Anything that affects its function disturbs this process and leads to disease.

The gastrointestinal tract consists of **esophagus** (food tube), **stomach** (mixes food and forms chyme), **small intestine** (small diameter tube 20 ft. long, consisting of the **duodenum, the jejunum and the ileum**) and **large intestine** (large diameter tube which includes **cecum, colon, rectum and anal canal**).

The food is ground in the stomach into tiny particles. The stomach secretes mucous to protect the lining of the gastrointestinal tract. In addition, it also secretes hydrochloric acid and several enzymes and readies the food for digestion by changing it into semifluid chyme. The pancreas secrete pancreatic juice into the duodenum to facilitate the digestion of the food in the small intestine. Food products carried by blood vessels from the walls of the digestive tube are delivered to the liver, the largest organ in the digestive system (Figure 27.1).

The dietary factors associated with ailments of the gastrointestinal tract (G.I.) are:

(*i*) Acidity, (*ii*) inadequate fiber, (*iii*) fat, (*iv*) substances such as gluten in wheat and (*v*) lactose.

One more substance - alcohol – does affect the health of the G.I. tract adversely. But it is not a food, nor it is a dietary essential.

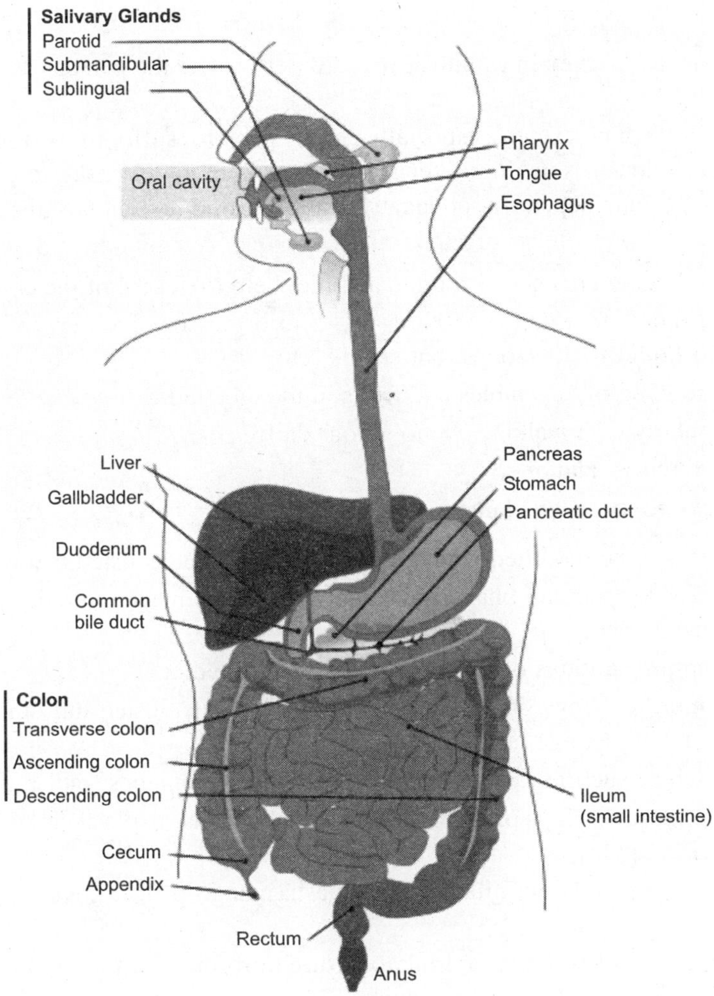

Figure 27.1 The gastrointestinal tract

General Aspects of Digestion

Food and Gastric Acidity : Foods normally have a pH of 5 to 7, while the pH of acid (hydrochloric) secreted in gastric juices in the stomach **is less than 2**. The pH of citrus fruits and other acid tasting foods is about 3.5 or more. **Therefore, no food is acid enough to change the acidity of the stomach contents**. This is very important information and needs to be given to patients who suffer from acidity, so that they will not avoid vitamin C rich foods and develop vitamin C deficiency.

Protein-rich foods neutralise gastric acid. Milk is therefore the food of choice used to treat acidity. Its neutralising effect lasts for half to two hours. Fat reduces acid production and decreases motility. Hence, addition of cream to milk was used to treat peptic ulcer. But the use needs to be moderated to avoid the risk of atherosclerosis due to the saturated fats in cream.

Stimulants increase the production of gastric acid. Hence these need to be avoided by persons suffering from acidity. The stimulants to be avoided include tea, coffee, alcohol, tobacco, meat extracts in soups and gravies and spices – chilli powder, black pepper, mustard seeds, nutmeg.

Constipation

According to a research survey in Mumbai, over 70 per cent of the persons studied complained of constipation.

Persons, who have little or no exercise especially elderly persons, suffer from **atonic constipation**. They limit their food selection to soft, low-fiber foods; they limit fluid intake to prevent urination, especially at night. They become dependent on laxatives and yet find no relief, as the causative factors are not eliminated.

Treatment: The following changes in routine and diet help to get rid of the constipation:

(*i*) Increase fluid intake to 1200 to 1500ml. *i.e.*, 5 to 6 glasses of water in addition to other beverages and liquid foods (soups, buttermilk, etc.)

(*ii*) Include 200 to 250g of vegetables and fruits in the diet and

(*iii*) Exercise regularly e.g., walking ¾ to 1 hour daily,

(*iv*) Do fitness exercises, and/or

(*v*) *Suryanamasksars* or *yoga* daily.

Diet: Their diet needs to be modified gradually to high fiber diet as listed below :

1. Eat whole wheat chapati and bhakari as major part of the meal and reduce intake of white bread and polished rice
2. Include cooked preparations of germinated pulses in the diet.
3. Take two or more servings of cooked vegetables such as cluster and other beans, gourds (snake, ridge, bitter, sponge, etc.)
4. Eat raw vegetables such as cabbage, carrot, cucumber, tomatoes, radish etc.
5. Include two or more servings of fruits such as amla, banana, papaya, chiku, guava, melons, jackfruit, berries, apples, etc.
6. Take beverages such as buttermilk, lemon squash, mango panhe, kokum drink, to increase fluid intake.
7. Drink 5 to 6 glasses of water, as a drink to ensure movement of food in the digestive tract and smooth elimination of waste products.

The changes in the diet must be introduced gradually to avoid feeling of bloating or cramping due to the changes.

Diarrhoea

Diarrhoea is one of the most common G.I. tract ailments. It is still the second most common cause of death in childhood, killing over 1.5 million children in India alone.

The occurrence of diarrhoea indicates that there is contamination of food and water with virus and bacteria from human faeces. In diarrhoea, the stools are liquid or semisolid and large volumes of these are passed frequently. There is also vomiting, cramps and abdominal pain. The food passes through the gastrointestinal tract so rapidly that its digestion and absorption is reduced. The fecal matter moves through the colon so fast that water and electrolytes are not reabsorbed.

Frequent and/or prolonged attacks result in loss of fluids, electrolytes, minerals, vitamins, proteins, fats, carbohydrates and as a result there is loss of body weight. This leads to dehydration.

Therapy: The first step is to identify the cause and remove it. If diarrhea is severe and dehydration has set in (eyes sunken, skin loose and inelastic, passing reduced amounts of dark urine), fluids and electrolytes may be first given intravenously to let the gastrointestinal tract to rest. This is followed by feeding fluids, with gradual move to oral rehydration therapy and later to a very low residue diet. (Tables 27.1 and 27.2)

Table 27.1: WHO Formula for Oral Rehydration Solution (ORS)

Sodium chloride	3.5 g	Dissolve in one liter
Sodium bicarbonate	2.5 g	boiled, cooled water. **Do not boil after dissolving**
Potassium chloride	1.5 g	**these ingredients in water**
Glucose	20.0 g	

Directions for use of ORS:

1. Use a clean cup and spoon.
2. For infants, use a dropper. Babies who are breastfed, should continue to be breastfed in addition to **ORS.**
3. Let the patient **sip the liquid** from the spoon, **not drink it.**
4. Feed one cup for each stool passed.
5. Even if the patient vomits, in the first couple of hours continue to feed ORS in small sips.

Table 27.2: Foods Allowed and Avoided in Low Residue Diet

Foods Allowed	*Foods Avoided*
Buttermilk, (2 C only)	Whole milk
Dal soup and soft cooked dal	
Eggs (all but fried)	Legumes, nuts, fried foods,
Soups and soup broth	Fibrous meat
Vegetable juices and cooked or pureed mild-flavoured vegetables, dudhi, pumpkin	Vegetable and fruit fiber
Fruit juices, banana, apple sauce, Fruit pulp (papaya, melons etc.)	Pickles, preserves
Coconut water	
Refined breads, soft cooked rice, noodles, chapati, etc.	Coarse cereals and breads Whole grain breads
Kheer, jelly, custard, biscuits, plain cakes	
Tea, coffee if allowed	

If oral rehydration mixture is not available, use a home-made one containing sugar (40 g), and salt (3.5 g) per liter supplemented with potassium rich foods such as coconut water, lemon juice, banana, mashed papaya, mashed plantains, etc.

Low Residue Diet

Oral rehydration therapy is followed by a very low residue diet in cases of severe diarrhea. The low residue diet of less than 10 g of fiber a day reduces the normal work of the intestines by restricting the amount of dietary fiber and reducing food residue. Food residue is the bulk in colon that includes undigested food, intestinal secretions, bacteria and cells shed from the intestinal lining. The foods allowed and foods avoided in low residue soft diet are listed in Table 27.2. It consists mainly of liquids such as buttermilk, dal soup, broth, vegetable and fruit juices, coconut water, etc., some soft foods such as soft cooked dal, cooked eggs, pureed mild-flavoured vegetables, apple sauce, fruit pulsp, refined breads, soft cooked rice, custards, kheers, etc., can gradually be added to improve the nutrient content, as the condition of the patient improves and appetite slowly recovers.

The patient needs to progress from liquid diet, soft diet to normal diet gradually. Contamination of food must be prevented to avoid recurrence of diarrhea.

Food Tolerance

Food tolerance is highly an individual reaction to intake of various foods. Some persons suffer from heartburn, flatulence and distention of abdomen, when they consume certain foods. Tolerance to such foods is highly an individual reaction and needs to be treated as such. The foods mentioned as cause of the discomfort include dry beans and split dals of redgram, bengal gram and sometimes black gram. Among the vegetables, strong flavoured ones containing sulfur compounds such as cabbage, cauliflower, leeks, onions, radishes and turnips are mentioned. Some persons cannot tolerate even cucumbers and watermelon. It is important to record the diet history of the patients, including their perceived food tolerance, before preparing a diet plan for treating them.

Persons, who are nervous, tense, too worried, insecure, feeling neglected and/or anxious, tend to suffer from gastrointestinal ailments. Their emotions affect the function of the digestive tract adversely. Other factors noted are:

(*i*) irregular eating hours,

(*ii*) quick gulping down of food and hence poor mastication,

(*iii*) lack of rest and

(*iv*) lack of rational schedule.

Luckily, there is a wide choice of foods available in each food group and it is possible to plan a nutritionally adequate diet, using foods, which are well tolerated by the patient.

In view of the above, in treating patients suffering from gastrointestinal ailments, diet plan needs to be individualized.

In addition to a diet plan, the persons need to be helped to modify their thinking to accept their duties rationally, plan their day's schedule of work and food intake. Stress should be reduced. They need to be guided to have regular times for meals, a short period before and after eating for relaxation and sufficient time for each meal to permit eating slowly.

Study Questions

1. List foods included in the treatment of acidity.
2. List the changes in routine and diet which help to treat constipation.
3. What is ORS? How is it given?
4. List foods to be avoided in low residue diet.
5. What are the factors which affect food tolerance?

CHAPTER

28

Nutrition in Diseases of Liver, Gallbladder and Pancreas

Introduction

The liver is the largest organ in the body, which plays a vital role, performing many complex functions essential for life. Liver serves as our body's internal chemical power plant. The health of the liver is a major factor in the quality of our life.

Functions of Liver

Some important functions of liver are:

- to convert carbohydrates in the food to stored energy and chemicals necessary for life and growth.
- to manufacture proteins, metabolise proteins, absorb fat products and make them available as fuel; produce bile, essential for the digestion of fats and stored in the gall bladder.
- to store iron, copper and other minerals for use in the metabolism.
- to ensure storage, absorption and function of fat soluble vitamins A, D, E and K and their precursors.
- to act as filter to remove alcohol and toxic substances from the blood and convert them to substances that can be excreted from the body.
- to process drugs and medications absorbed from the digestive system, enabling the body to use them effectively and dispose of them.

Thus, the liver manufactures proteins, processes carbohydrates, absorbs fat products and makes them available as fuel. The liver serves as a storehouse of vitamins and minerals and processes iron for the blood system. It dispatches sugars to tissues to burn to provide energy. Lastly, it detoxifies any poison that may enter the bloodstream and renders it harmless. Gall bladder is the store of a number of essential chemicals in digestion including bile (Figure 28.1).

A number of reactions in the metabolism of proteins, carbohydrates and fats take place in the liver. Iron, copper and other minerals are stored in the liver. Important reactions which ensure storage and function of fat soluble vitamins A, D, K and their precursors take place in the liver. Liver is also involved in detoxification of harmful substances (including poison) and alcohol metabolism.

As much as 85-90% of the blood that leaves the stomach and intestines carries important nutrients to the liver, where these are converted into substances the body can use. Carbohydrates or sugars are stored as glycogen in the liver and are released as energy between meals or when the body's energy demands are high. In this way, the liver helps to regulate the blood sugar level and prevent hypoglycemia or low blood sugar. This enables us to keep an even level of energy throughout the day.

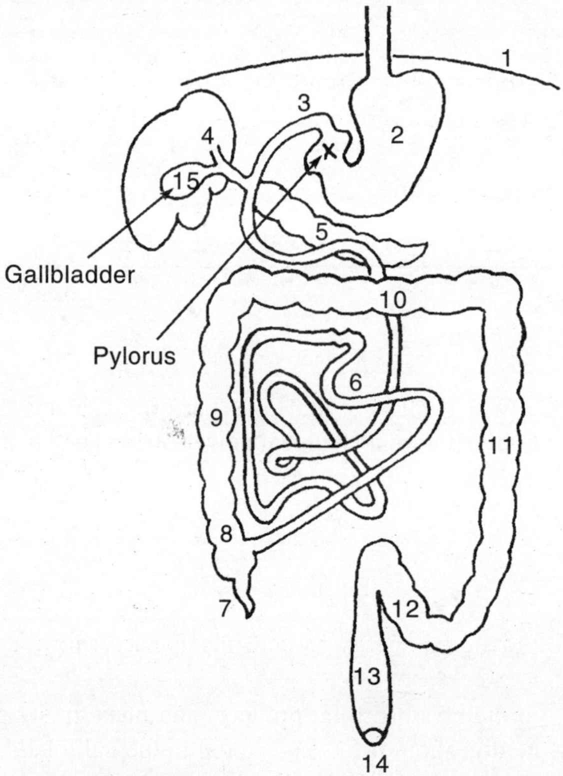

1. Diaphragm
2. Stomach
3. Duodeunum
4. Liver
5. Pancreas
6. Small intestines
7. Vermiform appendix
8. Cecum
9. Ascending colon
10. Transverse colon
11. Descending colon
12. Signmoid colon
13. Rectum
14. Gallbladder

Figure 28.1: The G.I. tract showing liver(4), Gallbladder and pancreas(5)

Liver and biliary system diseases are caused by infections (virus, bacteria and parasites), toxic chemicals, alcohol intake, poor nutrition and metabolic disorders.

Any injury to liver disturbs the body's capacity to use food nutrients and has a devastating effect on the well being of the person.

Jaundice

Jaundice is characterised by yellow colour of skin and tissues. In jaundice, the blood levels of bile pigments are high. This is a frequent sign of liver and biliary tract diseases.

Therapy: The primary aim is to protect the liver from further stress and help it to function as normally as feasible. Therefore, a nutritionally adequate diet is basic to avoid permanent damage.

Diet: The modification of diet is based on:

(*a*) Generous intake of good quality protein to regenerate tissues and prevent fatty infiltration

(*b*) High carbohydrate intake to spare protein and synthesis of glycogen

(*c*) A moderate fat restriction

(*d*) providing vitamin supplements and

(*e*) ensuring sodium restriction, if there is edema.

Hepatitis

In this disease, liver is inflamed and degeneration may have occurred. There are four types of hepatitis - A, B, C and D. In all these, the symptoms are similar. The symptoms are loss of appetite, nausea, abdominal pain, vomitting, diarrhea, fever and loss of weight. Jaundice follows, if these symptoms are not treated promptly by diet modification.

Diet: In hepatitis the main therapy consists of nutritionally adequate diet and bed rest. The aim is to ensure recovery of damaged tissues and to prevent further damage.

In the early stages, parenteral fluids or tube feeding may be necessary, if nausea and vomitting is severe. Interferon therapy may be useful in the beginning.

Appetite is normally poor. So it is crucial that meals are attractive, small and frequent – 5 to 6 meals at regular intervals are suggested. It is advisable to follow the tips given below :

- Give a full liquid diet in six small feeds, as soon as the patient is able to eat (refer to Tables 25.3 & 25.4, Chapter 25).
- Follow it by a soft fiber-restricted diet (please refer to Chapter 25, Table 25. 7) and then a normal diet.
- A high calorie, high protein diet is given (Table 26.2), if there is extensive weight loss.
- A low fat diet is given in the beginning and gradually move is made towards normal fat intake as the biliary tract obstruction is cured.
- Adequate calorie supply and glycogen synthesis are ensured by giving a high carbohydrate diet.
- Vegetables with strong flavours, spicy foods, as also rich desserts are avoided as these may affect food tolerance adversely. In this aspect, the patient's personal reactions are important.

Cirrhosis

Many chronic liver diseases are associated with malnutrition. One of the most common of these is cirrhosis. In cirrhosis, the damaged liver cells are replaced by fibrous scar tissue, which disrupts the liver's important functions. Cirrhosis occurs as a result of excessive alcohol intake (most common), common viral hepatitis, obstruction of the bile ducts, and exposure to certain drugs or toxic substances. It is also found in highly malnourished children.

Liver cirrhosis is a chronic disease in which there is considerable damage to its cells, with infiltration by fats and fibrosis.

Symptoms are similar to other liver conditions, mentioned already. These include loss of appetite, nausea, vomiting and weight loss, giving an emaciated appearance. Diet alone does not contribute to the development of this disease. Well nourished people, for example, who drink large amounts of alcohol, are also susceptible to it. If neglected, liver failure may follow.

Diet: Patients with cirrhosis require a balanced diet providing 2,000 to 3,000 calories a day to allow the liver cells to regenerate. Thus the diet recommended is a normal high calorie, adequate protein diet with vitamin and mineral supplements. Too much protein will result in an increased amount of ammonia in the blood, too little protein can reduce healing of liver.

There are a number of complications of cirrhosis which can be helped through a modified diet.

Persons with cirrhosis often experience an uncomfortable buildup of fluid in the abdomen (ascites), or a swelling of the feet, legs or back (edema). Both conditions occur due to hypertension that is increased pressure in the veins entering the liver. Since sodium (salt) encourages the body to retain water, patients with fluid retention need to reduce their sodium intake. Therefore sodium in the diet needs to be restricted to 500 – 700 mg per day. This level of sodium is achieved by ensuring that there is no addition of salt to foods and avoidance of sodium rich foods such as papads, pickles, baked foods containing baking powder or other sodium salts as leavening agents.

Patients with damaged esophagus may need to avoid stimulants (tea, coffee), irritants (spices, tobacco) and fiber.

Small frequent feedings of a full liquid diet, followed by a very low residue and then by a soft fiber-restricted diet may help the patient to recover.

Other liver diseases in which diet changes aid recovery include **cholestasis** and **steatorrhoea.** In this condition the bile cannot flow into the small intestine to aid in the digestion of fats. As a result, fat is not absorbed**.** Backup of bile in the liver is called cholestasis. In this condition fat is not absorbed and is excreted in large amounts in the feces. It is noticed when feces become pale-coloured and foul-smelling. This condition is called steatorrhea. The loss of fat calories may result in weight loss too.

To alleviate this condition special fat substitutes need to be used, which are les dependent on bile for their intestinal absorption. These include special fat substitutes such as medium chain triglycerides and safflower oil. Patients suffering from steatorrhea may also need to use water soluble form of vitamins A, D, E and K, as they may have difficulty absorbing fat soluble forms of these vitamins. As excess vitamin A is toxic to the liver, such substitution needs to be carried out under the guidance of a physician.

Hepatic Failure

Hepatic failure is also known as enlarged liver disease.

Liver function is severely reduced due to reduction in the number of functional liver cells. This affects a number of reactions such as:

(*a*) Conversion of ammonia to urea is disturbed, accumulated ammonia is toxic to the central nervous system.

(*b*) The breakdown of aromatic amino acids is reduced (phenylalanine, tyrosine and tryptophan) and these accumulate in the blood.

(*c*) Branched chain amino acids (leucine, isoleucine and valine) are broken in peripheral muscle for energy and their blood level decreases.

The neurological and neuromuscular abnormalities may lead to coma; if not treated, it may lead to death.

Diet: The main principle is to reduce protein intake to minimise ammonia production. This can be done as follows:

(*a*) **Protein free to low protein diet** – 20 to 30g is given for a few days. As improvement occurs, protein intake is increased by 5 to 10 g every few days, until the intake reaches 40 to 50 per day. The protein profile can be improved by ensuring intake of branched chain aminoacids, orally, enterally or parenterally.

(*b*) to prevent tissue breakdown, 1500 – 2000 kcal are provided in the form of carbohydrates and fat.

(*c*) Patients, who are unable to take nourishment orally, tube feeding or parenteral nutrition is given.

The bacterial growth, which results in ammonia production, is controlled by medication.

In extreme conditions, when liver damage is irreparable, liver transplant is made.

Diseases of the Gall Bladder

Bile produced in the liver is concentrated and stored in the gall bladder. Stones or inflammation of gall bladder obstructs the flow of bile. Fat digestion is impaired for want of bile and there is pain in the is abdomen, nausea and vomitting.

Diet Therapy:

(*a*) Obese persons are found more likely to suffer from gall bladder disease. Hence losing excess weight and maintaining normal weight is suggested for those who are susceptible to this condition.

(*b*) To ensure the contraction of the gall bladder and hence the pain, fat intake needs to be reduced.

(*c*) During acute attack, no food is given to rest the system. Gradually the patient is given clear fluids followed by soft fiber-restricted low fat (20 – 30g) diet.

(*d*) Secondary bile acids may be given to dissolve small stones present. Ultra sound shock waves are used to shatter the stones.

As a last resort, gall bladder maybe removed by laproscopic surgery.

After surgery, a low fat diet is given to permit healing.

Diseases of the Pancreas

Pancreatic Insufficiency (inadequate pancreatic enzyme production)

Pancreatic diseases include acute and chronic pancreatitis. The symptoms are inflammation, edema and self digestion of the pancreas by its enzymes due to blockage.

The digestion of starch, fats and protein is reduced and these are excreted resulting in malnutrition. Absorption of fat soluble vitamins is also reduced. In severe cases, there is necrosis and risk to life due to failure of cardiac, renal and/or respiratory systems.

Diet Modifications: The main aim is to stop pancreatic secretions and let pancreas rest. Therefore the patient is given nothing orally and total parenteral nutrition is given. Hydrochloric acid production is decreased.

When the patient stabilises, oral feeding with clear liquids is started, followed by soft fiber – restricted and later by high protein, high carbohydrate and moderate fat diet. It is divided into six small meals and given by using the foods allowed. Water-soluble forms of fat soluble vitamins are given as supplements. Pancreatic enzymes may also be given.

Cystic Fibrosis

Cystic fibrosis is a genetic disease in children. One in 2000 babies born alive may suffer from it. In this disease, the pancreatic and bile ducts, intestines and bronchi are obstructed by a thick secretion of exocrine gland, thus preventing their normal function.

Symptoms vary according to the systems affected and the extent to which they vary. When thick mucosa in the lungs affects the bronchi, there is dryness and coughing; respiratory infections occur often. When pancreas are blocked, enzymic digestion is disturbed and the undigested, foul smelling food (carbohydrate, fats) excreted in stools frequently. Other systems are affected as a secondary outcome. These include liver, intestine, heart, kidney and reproductive system.

Diet Therapy: A great breakthrough in treatment is the recent development of enteric, pancreatic enzymes microspheres , coated with a pH sensitive substance that will not dissolve until it reaches the small intestine. These are taken with meals and snacks to improve digestion of food. The nutrient needs may increase in this condition. For example, energy needs may be 50 to 100 per cent and protein 50 per cent above the recommended dietary allowances. If tolerated, 30 or more per cent of the energy needs may be given in the form of fat. Water soluble form of vitamin supplement and mineral supplements are given. Extra salt may be needed in hot weather and during heavy physical activity.

Good diet and bed rest are the main therapy. The aim is to recoup tissues damaged due to the disease.

Study Questions

1. List the functions of the liver.
2. Write short notes on: Jaundice, hepatitis, diet for cirrhosis patient, steatorrhea.
3. List metabolic changes which occur in hepatic failure
4. List the changes to be made in diet to treat gall bladder disease.
5. What is cystic fibrosis? How is it treated?

CHAPTER

Nutrition in Diabetes Mellitus

29

Introduction

Diabetes mellitus, commonly known as diabetes, is one of the most serious diseases affecting humanity. Its incidence has increased alarmingly and it affects 18 million Indians as reported in the Journal of the Diabetic Association of India in 1999.

Studies indicate that there may be just as many undetected diabetics and twice as many may be on the verge of getting it. Undetected and hence untreated diabetes is one of the main causes of further complications such as loss of limbs due to impairment of nerves and loss of vision due to retinal detachment.

Diabetes is a chronic, degenerative disease that affects the way body uses food. In normal digestion, body converts sugars, starches and other substances into glucose, which is carried by the blood to every cell in the body. The glucose is used with the help of insulin (a hormone made in the pancreas) to produce energy for every action– of our body.

Diabetics are unable to produce insulin, make too little or are unable to use it.

Diabetes is not a disease, which **can be cured. It can only be kept under control** by the patient with the help of the nutritionist assisted by the physician. If not kept under control, a number of complications occur. These include:

(*a*) loss of sensation in peripheral nerves, resulting in injury, infection and amputation of lower extremities.

(*b*) Eye disorders leading to blindness

(*c*) Thickening of arteries and

(*d*) Kidney dysfunction.

Proper care of diabetes is essential to **prevent** or at least **reduce incidence** of complications. It is vital that the patients learn all about the disorder and its management, for health care in diabetes is basically **self-care.**

A **proper nutrition plan** is the foundation of successful diabetes management. Control of diabetes rests on three factors: **diet, exercise and insulin.**

Symptoms and Diagnosis

As diabetes develops, the person complains of excessive thirst (polydipsia), increases frequency and amount of urine and feels very hungry. Young patients lose weight, while older patients may be overweight. The presence of sugar in the urine and above normal blood sugar level are clinical symptoms of diabetes. A fasting blood sugar level of 120 mg/dl or higher on two different days indicates that the person suffers from diabetes.

Classification of Types of Diabetes Mellitus

There are three types of diabetes mellitus:

Type I is Insulin Dependent Diabetes Mellitus (**IDDM**) – About 10 to 20 per cent of known cases of diabetes are of Type I. There is no insulin or insufficient insulin to regulate blood glucose, because the beta cells are destroyed or are very few. The reason for the destruction of the beta cells can be an auto immune reaction, viral infection, genetic aberration and/or stress.

It may occur at any age but a large number of patients are young. Most of the diabetic cases occurring before 20 years of age are Type I. The disorder starts abruptly with typical symptoms mentioned above.

Type II is **Non-Insulin-Dependent–Diabetes Mellitus (NIDDM)**: 80 to 90 per cent known cases are of type II. In these, insulin receptor response is decreased while insulin production may be normal, increased or decreased. Sudden shock, trauma or tragic event in the family, heredity and excess body weight are contributory factors. Most patients are obese. Most cases occur during the mid-thirties or mid-forties. The onset is gradual and the ailment is detected during a routine medical check-up. If the diet is suitably modified and regular exercise is taken, these persons do not need insulin except during stressful days.

Other types of **Diabetes Mellitus**: A **third** type of diabetes occurs in association with certain conditions. These include chronic pancreatitis or as a corollary to intake of some medications such as glucocorticoids, antihypertensives, etc. In this type the plasma glucose levels are higher than normal, but lower than those indicative of diabetes.

Gestational diabetes occurs in some women during pregnancy. Diet modification as indicated for type II diabetes helps to correct the glucose intolerance during pregnancy. The blood glucose returns to normal after delivery; but many of these women develop diabetes mellitus in later years.

Nutritional Care: is the cornerstone of **diabetic therapy**.

Energy needs are same as for other individuals. The aim is to attain and then maintain a healthy weight for the body size and type. If an obese patient loses weight, it leads to improved glucose tolerance. Ideally 55 – 70 per cent calories should be mainly from complex carbohydrates. The aim is to control blood glucose and lipid levels.

Fibre: It is observed that substituting highly refined carbohydrates in the diet with foods, containing complex carbohydrates and fibre, benefits both type I and type II **diabetics**. Such diets improve glucose tolerance control, often decreases insulin requirements and tends to lower serum cholesterol and triglyceride values. It also helps to control weight and lower blood pressure.

Intake of fruits is beneficial for diabetics. The soluble fibres (pectin, gums, hemicelluloses) present in fruits increase transit time, slow glucose absorption and lower serum cholesterol. Fibre content of common foods is given in Table 29.1.

Fenugreek seeds, recommended as addition to diabetic diet in ancient medical system, are valuable due to their high content of mucilaginous and total fibre. It also contains an alkaloid (trigonelline), which is known to lower blood sugar level.

Table 29.1: Fibre Content of Common Foods (Per Serving)

Food	*Serving Size*	*Fibre/Serving EP*
Guava, red gram tender	50 g	2.6 – 3.1
Cluster beans, peas	50 g	1.6 – 2.0
French beans	50 g	0.9 – 1.5
Grapes, chiku, seetaphal	50 g	0.9 – 1.5
Legumes, chawli, mung, vatana	25 g	0.9 – 1.1
Fruits: Banana, apples, papaya	50 g	0.4 – 0.6
Whole wheat, jowar, bajra	25 g	0.3- 0.5
Carrots, beetroot, suran, potato, onion	50 g	0.2 – 0.6
Dry spices	1 g	0.2 – 0.3

Lipids: In diabetic diet, the total fat should be 20 to 30 per cent of the total energy. Of these saturated fats contribute about a fourth (7–10%), monounsaturated half (10–13%) and polyunsaturated about a fourth (8–10%) of the total energy. Cholesterol content of the diet should be less than 300 mg per day.

In a 2000 calorie diet, the calories from fat would thus be 400 to 600, which amounts to about 45 to 65 grammes of fat in the diet, a third of it is taken in hidden form. Hidden fat as we have seen in chapter 5, occurs in foods such as milk, ***dahi,*** nuts, oilseeds, eggs and meat. Hidden fats content of diet varies, but is estimated to provide about a third or more of the total fat in the diet. Thus, the visible fat intake in the diet as butter, ghee and oil used in food preparation can be 30 to 40 grammes. In order to control the saturated fat intake, the amounts of animal foods such as ghee, butter, cheese, eggs and meats must be monitored to provide less than 15 grammes of the total fat intake.

Proteins: The recommended amount of protein is 0.8 g/kg of ideal body weight. Adolescent children, pregnant or nursing mothers need increased intake up to 15 to 20 per cent of total energy.

Sweeteners: Use of artificial sweeteners in reasonable amounts is acceptable to control total calorie intake.

Sodium: A moderate sodium intake of 1 gram/1,000 calories is recommended, because many diabetics are hypertensive or have hypertension. Foods containing sodium such as pickles, papads, and baked foods containing baking powder should be avoided.

Vitamins and Minerals: Requirements are similar to those of other individuals. There is no need for supplements.

Alcohol: Alcohol is not a food and its use places an additional burden on the system. Its use is not advisable especially when oral hypoglycemic agents are to be taken as part of the therapy.

How do we translate the above guidelines into a diabetic diet prescription?

Suppose, the diabetic person is 50 years old, who is involved in light activity.

His healthy weight is 55 kg.

Total energy needed: 55 × 30 = 1,650 calories

Proteins: 0.8 g/kg or 0.8 × 55 = 44.0 g, rounded to 45 g.

45 × 4 = 180 calories from proteins (11%).

Fats: 28% or 16.50 × 28 = 462 calories/9 = 51g fat

CHO: 1650 – (180 + 462) = 1008/4 = 252 g (61%)

Diet Plan: The diabetic has to follow the diet plan through the rest of her/his life. Hence, the meal plan should be based on her/his normal schedule, meal pattern, food acceptance, food preparation methods and facilities available. It should also take into account the cultural – religious factors. Meal plans should be realistic, attractive and flexible, within the limits of the diet prescriptions. Meals should be as similar to the family meals as possible.

Meal Distribution: It is important to distribute the carbohydrate foods in the meals through out the day. Avoid taking too high amount of carbohydrates at any one meal. The type I diabetics need three meals and two or three snacks each day. As these persons use insulin, the carbohydrate intake should coincide with the action time of the insulin used.

Type II diabetics or NIDDM patients, who do not need insulin, can take the three large meals at 7-8 am, 12-1 noon and 7-8 pm; in addition a snack at 4-5 pm and a fruit after supper may be eaten around 10 pm before retiring.

Exchange Lists: The patient must study the food exchange lists available for planning diabetic diets (Table 29.2). Plan the menu by dividing the food exchanges into various meals according to the patient's need and choice. A sample menu for a 50 g protein diet is given in Table 29.3.

Sample menu can be distributed according to the needs of the patient and whether the patient is type I or type II diabetic.

It is important to include minimum number of servings of basic food groups. Ensure that you include whole grain cereal preparations (chapatis, bhakari/roti, whole wheat preparations, etc.), three to four servings of vegetables, two of fruits (one being vitamin C rich) and four to five servings of protein foods.

Table 29.2: Veg. and Non-veg. Diet Plan for Using Exchange List

Exchange list	*No. of Exchanges*	*Vegetarian*			*Exchanges No*	*Non-Vegetarian*		
		CHO	*Pro*	*Fat*		*CHO*	*Pro*	*Fat*
Chapati	4	80	12	—	4	80	12	—
Rice	4	80	7	—	4	80	7	—
Jowar	2	36	5	—	2	36	5	—
Milk	2	15	10	10	2	15	10	10
Dals/beans	2	30	10	—	1	15	5	—
Egg/fish/meat	—	—	—	—	1	0	6	6
Vegetable	3	9	6	—	3	9	6	—
Fruits	2	12	—	—	2	12	—	—
Fat	6	—	—	30	7	—	—	35
Total g		262	50	40		247	51	51
Total Calories -	1648	1088	200	360	1651	988	204	459
%age Calories from		66.0	12.1	21.9		59.8	12.4	27.8

Table 29.3: Sample Menu (based on Table 29.2)

Breakfast		**Snack**	
Pohe	2 S	Upma	2 S
Musumbi/guava	1 S	Tea/coffee	
Bread – butter	1 + 1 S		
		Supper	
Lunch		Bhakari (Jowar)	2 S
Chapati	2 S	Rice	2 S
Usal	1 S	Dal	1 S
Vegetable	1 S	Dahi	½ S
Dahi/lassi	½ S	Vegetable	1 S
		Salad	1 S

Note: In the above menu, one can reduce 1 fat exchange and add 2 tsp sugar/jaggery to improve acceptability.

The sugar can be used in tea/coffee and jaggery can be used in food preparation, especially in dal, usal and vegetables.

Control of Type I Diabetes

In chemical control, the blood glucose is kept normal and urine sugar free by taking proper diet and insulin. It is believed that it will prevent or postpone further complications of diabetes mellitus.

Insulin: Insulin is a protein. It has to be injected to ensure its being used as a regulator in the body. If taken orally, it would be digested like any food protein and will not be able to regulate the use of blood glucose. The amount of insulin needed depends on the patient's requirements; it can be reduced by exercise, while any infection or other stress may result in increased need. A number of types of insulins are available with different duration and speed of activity. The type that helps a patient to function effectively is chosen. Most diabetics, who need insulin, take one dose daily, while a few may need two doses per day.

Exercise: Exercise is an important part of any treatment plan. It should be selected to fit in with the person's capacity and requirements. It has many beneficial effects:

It helps to maintain weight, heart function, control of blood lipids and reduce adverse changes due to stress.

Persons with IDDM need to reduce their insulin dosage before and during exercise or take a carbohydrate containing snack to prevent hypoglycemia due to exercise.

Control of Type II Diabetes

Besides diet control, insulin and oral hypoglycemic agents may have to be taken by diabetic patients to metabolize excess glucose.

Oral Hypoglycemic Agents (OHA): When NIDDM is not controlled with diet and exercise, oral agents are sometimes used. These agents require the presence of endogenous insulin. Hence these are not suitable for use in IDDM.

OHA initially stimulate beta cells to increase insulin production (which may be temporary) and thus control glucose levels. These may increase the number of insulin receptor sites, thus improving glucose use.

Illness: Illness should be reported to the health care provider. Insulin or OHA should be continued if these are being used. Food should be taken as usual, with change to soft or liquid diet as needed. Sufficient amount of fluids should be taken.

Monitoring Control: (*a*) Check blood glucose to keep day-today control

(*b*) Check glycosylated hemoglobin to check long term index of control.

(*c*) Check urine glucose. Main value of this test is to confirm elevated blood glucose and monitor ketonuria. It is not a reliable test to detect hypoglycemia or the degree of hyperglycemia. Some substances give false or negative results; these are megadoses of ascorbic acid, salicylates and levadopa.

Acute Complications

Hypoglycemia– blood glucose less than 50 mg/dl.

When a diabetic participates in games or increased activity without taking food, hypoglycemia may occur.

When a diabetic takes an overdose of insulin or OHA, and does not eat at the scheduled time, there is a decreased supply of glucose, which results in fall of blood glucose level. When the blood glucose level falls below 50mg/dl, hypoglycemia occurs. Hypoglycemia may also occur, when a diabetic has diarrhoea or vomits, as this results in a decrease in blood sugar level.

Hypoglycemia is accompanied by a feeling of weakness, giddiness and fainting, if not attended to promptly.

If the person is conscious, he/she should be fed sugar, hard candy, fruit juice, sugar containing carbonated beverage or syrup, which give quick relief from symptoms. If the person is unconscious, intravenous glucose should be injected **immediately.**

A diabetic should carry sugar. hard candy or glucose tablets, for use when needed. **A diabetic should carry a medical identity card** indicating that she/he is a diabetic and should be given intravenous glucose if she/he is unconscious due to hypoglycemia. Such immediate treatment can avert extended hypoglycemia, which causes damage to the central nervous system and the brain.

Acidosis and Coma: Type I diabetics are in danger of suffering from acidosis.

It is caused by severe lack of insulin and stress. There is an increase in lipolysis (breakdown of fats for energy) and production of fatty acids. Liver oxidises fatty acids to meet energy needs. In the diabetic state, liver oxidises fatty acids and produces acetone, acetoacetate and beta-hydroxybutyrate. These tend to spill over into the urine causing **ketonuria.**

Prevention is very essential and involves ensuring that carbohydrate is distributed in the daily meal to fit in with type of insulin, its dosage and time of injection.

Thus by treating early symptoms promptly, **coma** can be prevented.

In older patients (NIDDM), the cause must be identified and treated quickly. It is very important to prevent dehydration.

Long-term Complications

Poorly controlled diabetes increases risks of long-term diabetic complications. These health problems relate mainly to tissue changes affecting blood vessels in vital organs.

Neuropathy: These changes in the nerves involve injury and disease in the peripheral nervous system, especially in the legs and feet. It results in sensory loss and causes numbness in feet. Inadequate blood supply leaves the foot susceptible to injury, infection, gangrene and ultimately amputation. Hence the need to pursue the diet, exercise and if need be insulin, very methodically and avoid or delay complications.

Retinopathy: The changes in the eyes include thickening of capillaries with small hemorrhages from broken arteries in the retina, with yellow waxy discharge or retinal detachment. This complication can eventually cause blindness. Retinopathy is not to be confused with blurry vision that occurs sometimes as one of the first signs of diabetes. Blurry vision is due to the increased glucose concentration in the eye fluids, which brings about brief changes in the light-refracting surface of the eye.

Atherosclerosis: Another complication is the development of fibrous plaques on the inside lining of major blood vessels, which thickens gradually, narrowing the interior part of the blood vessel and restricts blood flow. This complication occurs in diabetics about four times as often as in the general population. This risk factor accounts for the need to reduce dietary fats and cholesterol in diabetic diet.

Nephropathy: The thickening of capillaries in the glomerulus leads to **nephropathy**, later to renal failure, which is the leading cause of death among IDDM patients.

Study Questions

1. List symptoms of Diabetes mellitus.
2. What are the various types of diabetes mellitus?
3. Discuss the nutritional guidelines in planning diet for a diabetic person.
4. Write short notes on: Exchange lists of food, control of type I diabetes, hypoglycemia, neuropathy, retinopathy

CHAPTER 30

Nutrition in Cardiovascular Diseases

Introduction

Cardio means of heart and vascular means of blood vessels. Thus, cardiovascular diseases include ailments of heart (CHD) and of blood vessels (atherosclerosis).

The heart is the strongest and toughest muscle in the body. As the arteries carry blood from the heart to the lungs and other tissues, any damage to the artery results in a variety of heart diseases.

Cardiovascular diseases include **hypertension, ischemic heart disease**, leading to **angina pectoris** and lastly **myocardial infarction**. **Hypertension** is increased blood pressure (high BP). In **ischemic heart disease**, there is lack of blood to the heart muscle resulting in a heart attack. In **angina pectoris**, there is reduction of blood supply to the heart muscle due to narrowing of the artery wall. **Myocardial infarction** is caused by thrombosis, which is coagulation of blood in blood vessel or organ.

Cardiovascular diseases develop in three stages:

(*a*) In the first stage, arterial damage begins due to fat oxidation products, hypertension and/or smoking.

(*b*) As it progresses, there is deposition of fatty material in the arterial wall, increasing its thickness, making it narrow and rigid. The movement of oxygen and nutrients is made more difficult as the arterial passage is narrowed. An atherosclerotic plague is formed (Fig. 30.1). The heart must pump harder driving blood pressure up (high B.P. or hypertension).

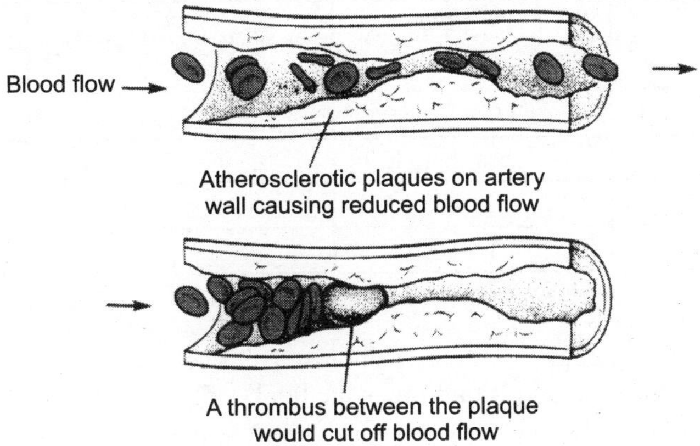

Fig. 30.1: Atherosclerotic plaque

(*c*) Lastly there is heart attack, which is also known **as coronary occlusion, coronary thrombosis or myocardial infarction**. It is virtually like a traffic jam, causing insufficient supply of blood to the tissues of the body beyond the point of blockage. If the blockage is in the artery connecting to the brain, it leads to stroke. As blood supply is crucial to the sustenance of life, it is crucial that the patient gets immediate medical aid to minimise the damage and save life.

Ailments of the heart are on the rise and even young persons succumb to these ailments. Hence, it is important to understand the contributing factors, to prevent these as far as possible and arrest their progress to minimize the damage.

Risk Factors

The major **risk factors** are:

(*i*) elevated serum cholesterol

(*ii*) emotional stress

(*iii*) hypertension

(*iv*) lack of activity leading to obesity and

(*v*) smoking

Heredity is an additional risk factor, for one inherits the food habits and often the life style of one's parents.

All researchers in this field uniformly agree that high blood lipids levels are a primary cause which contribute to most serious heart disorders. High sodium intake may be involved in hypertension.

Blood Lipids

In Chapter 5, you have noted that lipids are transported in the blood stream from one part to another to be utilized. Hence, blood lipids are a useful measure, first for detection and later for monitoring and evaluation of recovery after treatment. High levels of blood lipids (and its components, cholesterol and triglycerides) is an important **risk factor** in the development of coronary artery (heart) disease. (CAD/CHD) (Table 30.1)

Table 30.1: Serum Lipid Levels

Serum Level	*Desirable mg/dl*	*Borderline high mg/dl*	*High risk mg/dl*
Total Serum cholesterol	160	190 – 239	240 and above
LDL cholesterol	Less than 130	130 – 159	160 and above
HDL cholesterol	More than 35	less or equal to 35	
Serum triglycerides	30 – 190	250 – 500	500 and above

Cholesterol

Few heart attacks occur in people who have cholesterol levels in the 160 mg/dl range according to research studies conducted at Stanford and other medical centres in the world.

Increased serum cholesterol level above 200 mg/dl and low density lipoproteins (LDL) above 130 mg/dl are associated with increased risk of CHD. The level of high-density lipoprotein (HDL) in the blood is likely to be more important indicator than total serum cholesterol, as it protects the blood vessel against the formation of atheroma (fatty deposit).

Intake of high fat diet, especially saturated animal fats leads to obesity. The fat is first stored primarily in the adipose tissues and later minute amounts are deposited in the blood vessels. These fat deposits thicken the walls of blood vessels and this condition is known as **atherosclerosis.** Any plan to correct the situation must include modification in the fat component of the diet.

Basic Nutritional Plan to Monitor Serum Lipid Levels

The diet changes which have proved to be effective in preventing or reversing heart disease have the following nutritional goals:

- Reduce the total amount of fat, mainly the saturated fat in the diet.
- Use polyunsaturated fat in place of saturated fat in the diet.
- Decrease the intake of the amount of dietary cholesterol.
- Increase physical activity to alter cholesterol components in the blood.
- Attain ideal body weight and maintain it.

To accomplish these goals, the diet must have high carbohydrate (50–70% of total calories), adequate protein (12–20% of total calories) and reduced fat (20 to 30 % of total calories). The fat component must be such that it contains a third to half of polyunsaturated fat, a third monounsaturated fat sources and the remaining part may consist of saturated fat sources. The composition of food fats is given in Table 30.2. It can help to modify one's diet in the right direction.

In a 2000 calorie diet, the calories from fat would thus be 400 to 600, which amounts to about 45 to 65 grammes of fat in the diet, a third of it is taken in hidden form. Hidden fat as we have seen in chapter 5, occurs in foods such as milk, dahi, nuts, oilseeds, eggs and meat. Hidden fats content of diet varies, but is estimated to provide about a third or more of the total fat in the diet. Thus, the visible fat intake in the diet as butter, ghee and oil used in food preparation can be 30 to 40 grammes. In order to control the saturated fat intake, the amounts of animal foods such as ghee, butter, cheese, eggs and meats must be monitored to provide less than 15 grammes of the total fat intake.

Table 30.2: Saturated and Unsaturated Fatty Acid Composition of Food Fat

Foods	*Fatty Acids (%)*		
		Unsaturated	
	Saturated (%)	*Monounsaturated (% Oleic Acid)*	*Polyunsaturated (% Linoleic Acid)*
A. Vegetable Oils/Fats			
Groundnut	16–19	47–60	20-30
Mustard	5	32	18
Sesame	13–14	38–49	38–42
Olive	11–15	75	7–10
Corn	13–15	26–29	55
Soybean	14–15	25	50–60
Cottonseed	23–30	17–25	50–54
Sunflower	8–11	14–18	65–70
Safflower	6–10	13–25	67–74
Coconut	80–90	5–6	1–2
Vanaspati	25	73	2
B. Animal Fats			
Butter	45–65	27–32	1–4
Ghee	64	33	Nil
Whole milk cow's	64	29	4
Human milk	46	38	8
Cheddar cheese	65	28	3
Egg	10	13	2
Poultry	30–40	40–44	14–20
Fish (low fat)	2–5	2–3	4
Lamb, pork, beef	45–50	44	2–6
C. Nuts			
Groundnuts	9	25	14
Walnuts	4	10	40

Meal Planning and Food Exchange Lists

Food selection guide (Table 30.3) and food exchange lists for meal planning (Appendix B) can be a valuable tool in choosing foods to be used in the diet.

Cereals and Their Products: It is advisable to include whole cereal products such as chapati, *bhakri,* for most of the servings from this group.

Parboiled rice may be used in fermented preparations such as idli. The intake of refined cereal products such as bread, nan, bhature etc. must be reduced. The number of servings from this group varies from 7–12 and depends on the person's total energy needs, but must provide 55 to 70 per cent of the total calories.

Dals and Legumes: are important sources of protein, iron and B complex vitamins in the vegetarian Indian diet. It is advisable to use whole legumes which provide additional fibre. Cooked germinated pulses provide some vitamin C also. The number of servings may vary from two to four, depending on the age and the type of dietary (vegetarian or non-vegetarian).

Both fresh and germinated beans will help control cholesterol. The dry ones can be soaked and germinated to add variety. The fibre helps to excrete CHOL and thus reduce its blood concentration.

Milk and Its Products: Only toned milk or doubletoned milk, its curd, buttermilk and skim milk products can be used liberally. But limited amounts of whole milk, especially buffalo milk needs to be used **after removing the fat layer** after cooling. Similarly, ghee and butter, need to be used in very small amounts (only a teaspoon) as these are high in cholesterol and saturated fats.

Table 30.3: Food Selection Guide

Foods – Include As per Prescription	*Foods Include Liberally*	*Foods to Avoid*
Cereals – rice, wheat	Green leafy vegetables	A. Fatty sweets– mithais, laddus, chocolates, shreekhand, basundi, rabdi, cakes, pastries, cream biscuits, pies, doughnuts etc.
Jowar, bajra, nachni etc.	Salad vegetables- All gourds, Fruit vegetables, Fruits – melons, amla *	B. Fatty fried foods– Shev, chivada, farsan, wafers, chaklis, Fried papad, kurdais, khari biscuits etc. bhajias, wadas, samosas, cutlets, etc.
Dals and legumes		
Milk without cream	Thin buttermilk	C. Nuts (esp. dried ones) cashews, groundnuts, coconut, almonds, walnuts etc.
Lean meat	Coconut water	
		D. Salty sauces and oily dressings
Fish and egg white	Clear soups condiments-lime juice	E. Sodium rich foods– pickles, papad, sandage, baked products made with baking powder
Vegetable oils	Tamarind, cocum, vinegar etc.	
Sugar, jaggery		
Salt	Spices and spice mix to flavour food and garlic	F. Soft drinks and alcoholic drinks– beer, scotch etc.

* All gourds include ash, bitter-, snake-, ridge-, etc. Salad vegetables include cucumber, radish, tomato, onion etc. Fruit vegetables include drumstick, pumpkin, bhindi, dudhi, brinjal, tinda, etc.

Eggs, Fish, Poultry and Meat: Egg yolk is a concentrated source of cholesterol (275 mg/each egg yolk). Whole egg intake is suggested to be a maximum of two per week, including those used in preparations such as egg curry, cakes, custards, etc.

Meat intake is suggested to be limited to one to two servings of lean cuts with all visible fat removed. Fish (low fat ones) and chicken (with skin removed) may be used in these servings to control fat intake.

Vegetables and Fruits: Vegetables and fruits are good sources of minerals, vitamins and fibre. The number of servings suggested are five to six, one of which should be a seasonal one rich in beta-carotene (leafy vegetables such as amaranth, fenugreek, spinach, radish leaves etc.) and another vitamin C rich one. (amla, guava, orange, musumbi, papaya, tomato, drumstick leaves etc.). The remaining three to four servings may be selected from any of seasonal beans and fruit vegetables.

Fruits and vegetables are the best dietary source of antioxidants in the diet. The lycopene from tomatoes has been shown to be particularly effective at stopping LDLs from oxidizing.

Citrus fruits and apples contain soluble fibre in the form of pectin. Pectin can lower total and LDL cholesterol.

Vegetable Preparation: A variety of vegetable salads can be prepared. Dahi, lemon juice, herbs (coriander, mint, curry leaves) and spices (cumin seeds, mustard, fenugreek, asofoetida etc.) can be used to season these. Raw as well as cooked vegetables (pumpkin, gourds) are used to prepare salads and raitas. Vegetables can be seasoned with a little oil and spices (whole and powdered) to enhance the flavour and acceptability according to the family pattern.

Sugars, Sweets and Low-fat Desserts: These must be used in limited amounts not exceeding three teaspoons of sugar, honey or jam; half a cup of kheer made with toned milk, 2–3 mints or 1/3 cup gelatin dessert.

Oils and Fats: Butter, ghee and animal organ fats (such as liver) are rich sources of vitamin A. But as these contain cholesterol (about 300 mg/100 g) their intake must be restricted suitably to fit in the total dietary intake of 300 mg cholesterol per day (Table 30.4).

Table 30.4: Cholesterol Content of Foods (mgs/100g edible portion)

Food	*Cholesterol (mg)*
Milk, whole (6–8% fat)	11
Milk, fluid (4% fat)	1–2
Butter (86% fat)	280
Ghee (100% fat)	315
Cheese (whole milk – 24% fat)	135 – 160
Milk sweets	65
Skimmed milk powder (1% fat)	0.4
Eggs (hen's)	
Egg yolk frozen	133
Egg fresh, whole	468
Organ and Animal Fats	
Lamb (raw), pork, beef	70
Chicken (with skin)	80
Chicken (without skin)	60
Liver	300
Heart	150
Brain	2,000
Kidney	375
Lard and other animal fats	95

Use of Oils and Fats: Choose oils to maintain the proper balance of PUFA, MUFA and saturated fat. Corn, cottonseed, sunflower, safflower and soybean oils contain a high percentage of PUFA; sesame, groundnut and olive oil are rich in MUFA.

Meal Preparation Guidelines

A 1200 calories low fat vegetarian diet food exchanges are given in Table 30.5. The calories, protein, fat and cholesterol content of the diet is also included. Please note that when eggs and flesh foods are excluded, the cholesterol content of the diet is reduced to 45 mg by using toned milk and only **one** teaspoon of ghee or butter.

The menu plan based on the foods indicated in Table 30.5 is presented after the table. A number of variations of this menu can be made using the food selection guide given in Table 30.3 and food exchanges in Appendix B. The food exchanges can be increased gradually to maintain one's ideal body weight, when the desired weight loss has occurred.

Table 30.5: Low Fat Diet – Vegetarian (1200 Calories)

Food	*Exchanges*	*Calories*	*Protein*	*Fat*	*Cholesterol*
Cereals	7	595	18	—	—
Dal	2	170	11	—	—
Milk (toned)	2	200	10	9	30
Egg/Flesh foods	—	—	—	—	—
Vegetable A	2	—	2	—	—
Vegetable B	2	70	4–6	—	—
Fruits	2	40	—	—	—
Fat (half ghee)	2	90	—	10	16
Sugar	2	40	—	—	—
Total		1205	45 – 47	19	46

Total Calories: 1205, Protein: 45 g, Fat: 19 g
Calories from Protein = 15%
Calories from fat = 14%
Calories from carbohydrate = 71%
Cholesterol = 46 mg/day

Menu Plan

Morning – Tea 1C (+ 1 tsp sugar)

Breakfast Milk 1C
Bread 2 slices
Banana ½ big or 1 small

Lunch Chapati 1
Rice ½ C
Dal 1C
Palak Bhaji ½ C
Tomato Salad
Dahi ½ C

Tea + Snacks
Tea 1C (+ 1 tsp sugar)
Dhokla – 4 pieces (no oil)

Supper: Bhakari ½
Rice ½ C
Dal 1 C
French beans ½ C
Cucumber Salad
Dahi ½ C

Alterations in Knowledge and Habits: It is important to know food composition (from authentic sources), learn to develop healthy eating habits, make wise choices while eating out. For sedentary persons, increased physical activity will improve both physical fitness and food utilisation.

Some clinicians prefer that the patients adhere to the dietary and life style changes, which have been found to reduce the serum cholesterol in a number of studies. A low fat, 1600 calorie diet to maintain one's ideal body weight has been presented in Table 30.6. The possibility exists that the medications used to alter the blood lipids may cause long-term negative effects.

Table 30.6: A 1600 Calorie Low Fat Diet (Vegetarian)

Foods	*No. of Exchanges*	*Diet Pattern*			
		CHOs	*Proteins*	*Fats*	*CHOL*
Cereals	7	128	20	—	—
Pulses, dals	3	42	16	—	—
Milk, toned	2.5	19	12	12	38
Eggs/Meat	—	—	—	—	—
Vegetables	4	24	8	—	—
Fruits	2	22	2	—	—
Fat	5	—	—	25	24
Sugar	4	20	—	—	—
Total		255	58	37	62
Calories (from)		1020	+232	+ 333	= 1585
Total calories = 1585, Protein = 58 g, Fat =37 g, CHOL = 62 mg					

When medications have to be taken to improve the serum lipid profile and reduce hypertension, these may interfere with the nutrient use in the body. It is important to discuss these aspects with your doctor and take remedial steps suggested by him/her.

Heart and Blood Vessels Diseases

Therapy in ailments of heart and blood vessels involves nutritional care.

Hypertension is the most common problem in humans in India, though almost seventy-five per cent of the cases are mild. If unchecked, it can be a major risk factor for other serious heart conditions.

Normal blood pressure is less than 140 mm Hg **Systolic** and less than 85 mm Hg **diastolic.**

Hypertension has many causative factors though in 90 per cent of cases, the cause is unknown.

Atherosclerosis (narrowing of the arterial walls due to deposits of fatty material) causes resistance to blood flow, making the heart to pump harder, thus increasing the blood pressure. The increase in blood pressure injures the arteries further, thus worsening the atherosclerosis.

Therefore, it is essential to bring the blood pressure back to normal, to prevent the damage to the circulation system.

Diet Therapy: Hypertension may be often due to obesity, because the increased weight means increasing work of the heart to supply blood to the extra tissue formed. For many overweight hypertensive people, dietary changes which result in weight loss will lead to reduction in blood pressure. This may be adequate therapy in mild cases. But there are normal and underweight persons who suffer from hypertension.

The second possibility is excessive sodium intake, which draws more water into circulation, thus increasing blood volume, leading to increased blood pressure. There are about 20 per cent people who are sensitive to sodium and may be affected by excess sodium intake; other 80 per cent appear to be relatively free from the adverse effects of excessive sodium intake. Research studies have shown that increase in potassium intake can lower blood pressure. Increase in intake of alcohol in excess of 2 ozs. daily has a hypertensive effect, which increases with the amount consumed.

It is important to remember that **blood pressure control** is one of the most effective ways to decrease mortality in adults.

In patients, whose only problem is mild hypertension (diastolic pressure of 90–94 mm Hg), therapy without use of drugs is used to achieve control. This includes:

(*a*) **Moderate sodium restriction (1000–1500 mg/day):** No salt in cooking or at the table. No processed foods (pickles, papads, canned foods etc. containing salt). Four servings of regular bread can be taken.

(*b*) **Adequate potassium intake:** Plant foods are rich sources of potassium, especially fruits and vegetables. Potassium is present in higher concentration than sodium in fruits and vegetables by a factor of 5 to 50 fold. Hence, intake of three to four servings of fruits, which need no preparation (hence no addition of salt), can ensure adequate potassium intake.

(*c*) **Regular exercise** tailored to the individual is a must – walking 5 kilometres daily has been found to be an ideal way to keep fit. In all weather it needs no equipment.

(*d*) **Stress management:** is a very important aspect of therapy. It involves regular planning of one's activities allowing realistic scheduling of work, relaxation, physical activity, mealtimes, prayer/meditation and rest. This removes the stress from one's days, as there is time available for each aspect of the day. Thus, one does not rush from one activity to the other, gulp down food on the run or skip meals. People under stress are unable to function effectively. They are worried and tense all through the day, because so many tasks are unfinished due to no planning or poor planning. A planned, enjoyable routine of each day is the most important part of therapy to stress management.

(*e*) Abstaining from alcohol consumption is the most desirable part of the therapy. If one cannot follow it, alcohol intake must be restricted to **occasional** 2 oz limit.

Sodium Restricted Diets

Most people's daily intake of salt is 3–7 g (3,000–7,000 mg). Levels of sodium restriction commonly prescribed are:

(*a*) 500–700 mg is **severe restriction**. No sodium is used in cooking or at the table. Processed foods (pickles, papads, kurdais, wafers etc.) or canned vegetables containing salt are avoided. Low sodium bread, if available, should be used. Vegetables which have naturally high sodium content are omitted.

(*b*) 1000–1500 mg is **moderate restriction.** It is described above.

(*c*) 2000–3000 mg is **mild restriction.** Small measured amount of salt is used in cooking. A small plastic spoon (given with ice cream cups at stores) could be used to add salt in cooking, instead of a teaspoon to avoid excess sodium.

Sources of Sodium in the Diet

All living things, plants and animals require some sodium. Hence, all **foods** contain some sodium, even before they are processed or cooked in the home. Most plant foods are low in sodium. Animal foods – meat, fish and poultry are naturally high in sodium. Eggs are especially high in sodium (most of sodium is in the egg white)

Most vegetables which are low in sodium, are permitted in the diets restricted to less than 1000 mg; but not beets, spinach, chad and kale, which contain large amounts of sodium.

Fruits, unsalted butter, unsalted cereals and breads, oils, sugars can be used without restriction, as these contain very little or no sodium.

Vegetables and fruits, which are low in sodium, are listed in Table 30.7. This list may be useful in selection of foods to be included in sodium-restricted diets.

Table 30.7: Low Sodium Sources of Vegetables and Fruits

Sodium Content	*Vegetables*
Less than 5 mg/100 g EP	Bitter gourd (green), bottle gourd. brinjal, french beans, onion stalks, parwar, ridge gourd, onions
5 to 11 mg/100 g EP	Pumpkin, ladies finger (bhendi), peas, cucumber, colocasia, potato, sweet potato, tapioca (dried chips), yam, brussel sprouts
12–15 mg/100 g EP	Cabbage, green plantain.
	Fruits
Less than 6 mg/100 g EP	Amla, guava, orange, papaya, peaches, plums, chiku, pomegranates, tree tomato, phalsa.
7 to 13 mg/100 g EP	Pears, ripe tomato.

Salt: Salt is the main source of sodium in the diet. It is used in cooking, baking, at the table and in processing foods. Salt contains 40 per cent sodium, so a teaspoon of salt, which weighs 6 g, contains 2.4 g or 2400 mg of sodium. So, if a teaspoon of salt is added to a recipe which serves six persons, each person would get 400 mg in the serving.

Sodium compounds used in food preparations: Soda or sodium bicarbonate used in baking and food preparations (e.g., Papad) is a source of sodium in the diet. Hence the need to avoid such foods in a sodium restricted diet.

A number of drugs contain sodium e.g., Alkalizers, laxatives, sedatives and antacids.

The exchange list for meal planning (Appendix B) may be **modified** for **sodium restricted diet. High sodium foods/drugs to be avoided.**

- **Vegetables –** knol-khol, amaranth, field beans and tender tur.
- **Fruits –** muskmelon (kharbooja), lichis, dried fruits and cherries.
- **Salty snacks –** potato, banana or other chips/wafers, pop-corn, salted nuts, chiwda, shev, pharsan, bhajia, vada, chat, chana-dana, bhel etc.

- **Papads,** kurdayas, pickles, chutneys, sauces, khatta-mitha, etc.
- **Baked foods –** which contain baking powder, baking soda and/or salt such as bread, biscuits, cakes, pastries etc.
- **Salted** butter, cheese, khari lassi.
- **Salted** fish and meats.
- **Sodium** containing drugs laxatives, alkalizers, cough medicines, sedatives, antibiotics, etc.

Diet Plans: Food exchange list of 1000 mg sodium diet is given in Table 30.8 at two energy levels.

Table 30.8: Food List for a 1000 mg Sodium Diet

Food List	*1200 Calorie Exchanges*	*1600 Calorie Exchanges*	*Na (mg)*
Cereals	5	7	530
Dals 3		4	120
Eggs/Mutton	3	3	75
Vegetables	3	3	135
Fruits	3	3	110
Milk, toned	2	2	50
Fat	2	3	
Sugar	2	4	
			1020

These 1000 calorie diets might be permitted for patients after the third or fifth day after congestive heart failure or myocardial infarction. The 1600 calorie diet might be useful for the maintenance stage. When the patient returns home, the sodium level may be increased to 2000 mg.

Food Preparation for Sodium Restricted Diet

It takes about 3 months to get used to a sodium restricted diet. By that time the taste preference for salt decreases.

Use of spices, herbs, flavour extracts (cocum, tamarind, etc.) helps to improve acceptance of salt less recipe. These include lemon juice, pepper, green pepper, onion, garlic etc., which may be used in vegetables, stews and salads.

Angina Pectoris

Narrowing of arterial lumen and hence insufficient blood supply to the heart causes angina pectoris. It manifests by tight chest pain, often shooting pain in the shoulder, arm and hand. Physical exertion, excitement, the pressure of digesting a heavy meal or sudden exposure to cold wind may precipitate it. Weight loss, if the patient is obese, is helpful. Medication is used to relax heart muscle.

Myocardial Infarction

An **infarct** is necrosis (dead) local area, due to lack or poor blood supply resulting in the death of cells. When such an infarct forms in the heart, it is known as **myocardial infarction** (or heart attack). If it is in the brain it is called a **stroke.**

If the infarct (cluster of dead cells) is small, the rest of the tissue may heal, but the infarct leaves a scar. With therapeutic care, the rest of the organ can continue to function. But if more infarcts are formed, the ability of the organ is continuously reduced, which may imperil life.

Acute Stage: Care is highly individualized, suited to the condition of the patient. Electrocardiogram is used to monitor the condition of the patient. The work of the heart muscle can be minimised by letting the patient rest. Medications are given to help the heart muscle relax.

Diet: For 24 to 48 hours the patient is only given parenteral dextrose and no food is given by mouth, but sips of cool water are given. After that low fat liquid diet (500 to 800 calories and 1000-1500 ml fluid diet) is given in very small feeds for 2 to 3 days.

The patient progresses to a soft diet (about 1000-1200 calories), which may help establish circulation needed for digestion and absorption of food. The diet is given in five or six easily digestible meals. The fat content of the diet is less than 30 per cent of total calories, with less than.300mg cholesterol and less than 10 per cent calories from saturated fat.

The sodium is restricted to less than 1000 mg for a congestive heart failure patient, while it may be mild for less serious condition. Gas producing foods as per patient's perception are avoided. In edema cases fluid is restricted.

The patient is gradually helped to progress to maintenance diet, before leaving the hospital. The patient is helped to get used to a low salt diet, low cholesterol diet so that the recurrence of heart attack is prevented.

Congestive Heart Failure

In this condition, the heart is unable to maintain sufficient circulation to tissues. Reduced pumping ability leads to congestion of lungs and systemic circulation. Kidneys are unable to excrete sodium normally, resulting in accumulation of sodium in extracellular fluid and water retention. This results in at first of the extremities and later the abdomen and the chest retaining water and swelling.

The gastrointestinal tract and hence, digestion slows down due to reduced blood supply. There is loss of appetite, distention and at times vomiting.

Therapy: Patient must take bed rest. Oxygen may be needed.

Diet: The workload of heart must be reduced. The dietary progression is similar to that given above for myocardial infarction. In addition severe sodium restriction (500 – 1000 mg) and fluid restriction may be advisable.

Study Questions

1. List the cardiovascular diseases and the stages of their development.
2. Write notes on: major risk factors leading to cardiovascular diseases, desirable serum lipid levels, steps to monitor serum lipid levels, saturated and unsaturated fatty acids.
3. List how foods are chosen for inclusion in diet to control heart ailments.
4. Write short notes on: Hypertension, atherosclerosis, stress management, sodium-restricted diets, sources of sodium in the diet, myocardial infarction.

CHAPTER

31

Diet and Nutrition in Kidney Diseases

Introduction

Like the liver, kidneys play a vital role in maintaining the body's normal state (homeostasis). There are two kidneys in the human body. The **nephron** is the basic functional unit of the kidney. Each kidney has about a million nephrons. Each nephron has two main parts. Bowman's capsule (a cup-shaped top of the nephron) with a network of capillaries called the **glomeruli** (plural of the word glomerulus) in it, and the **renal tubule**. The tubule is a long winding tube, the first part of which surrounds the glomerulus. The fluid is driven by a pressure gradient from glomerulus into the tubule and the filtration begins. As the filtrate moves along, the materials needed are returned to the blood and waste material is carried to the bladder for storage and discharge at normal intervals.

Each nephron functions independently to produce urine. The glomerulus part of each nephron filters only a small drop of fluid a day. But the volume of plasma filtered by two million glomeruli amounts to a formidable 150-180 liters in 24 hours.

The **Glomerular Filtration Rate (GFR)** is the total amount of fluid filtered each minute by all the glomeuli of both kidneys. This is normally about 125 ml. per minute and is one index of kidney function. Most of the fluid (approx. 98.9 to 99.4 per cent) that passes through the winding tubule is reabsorbed; only **1 to 2 liters of urine** gets excreted each day. This means that over 99 per cent of the filtered water, all the glucose and vitamin C, almost all amino acids, sodium and other substances are returned to the blood. But if the intake of salt exceeds the body's needs the excess is excreted and extra water is needed to excrete it.

Functions of Kidneys

The kidneys help to regulate the internal harmony by performing the following functions:

1. **Filtration:** The kidneys are the filters through which all dissolved substances pass and selectively absorb those to be retained. Figure 31.1 depicts the urinary system. The end products of protein metabolism (urea, creatinine, uric acid and urates) are removed from blood by filtration to be discarded in urine. Excess of chloride, potassium, sodium and hydrogen ions are also filtered out from the blood. By being selective filters, kidneys try to maintain a constant blood composition and volume.
2. **Maintenance of Fluid, Electrolyte and Acid-base Balance.** Ions from the blood are secreted into the urine to maintain acid-base balance In this process they monitor the composition and volume of blood and other body fluids. Kidneys maintain fluid electrolyte and acid-base balance as they carry out selective filtration.
3. **Excretion:** The kidneys excrete dissolved unwanted substances filtered out of the blood as urine.
4. The kidneys help **regulate the blood pressure**.
5. **Kidneys produce erythropoietin (a hormone),** which stimulates maturation of red blood cells in the bone marrow.
6. **The conversion of vitamin D to its most active form calcitriol** occurs in the kidneys. Activated vitamin D regulates the absorption of calcium and phosphorus and thus helps regulate calcium and phosphorus levels in the blood.

When kidney function is disturbed due to disease or trauma, all the above functions are affected adversely.

Causes of Kidney Disease

Several ailments may cause kidney disorders. These include infection, degenerative changes, chronic diseases (e.g., diabetes mellitus, cardiovascular disorders such as atherosclerosis, hypertension), medications, toxic metal consumption, cysts, renal stones or trauma. Surgery, burns and poisons are some traumas, which may cause kidney damage.

Obesity increases the risk of renal disease. Habitual intake of high protein diet may increase the work of kidneys and cause damage. Reducing weight, decreasing protein intake to normal level can decrease the risk of kidney disease.

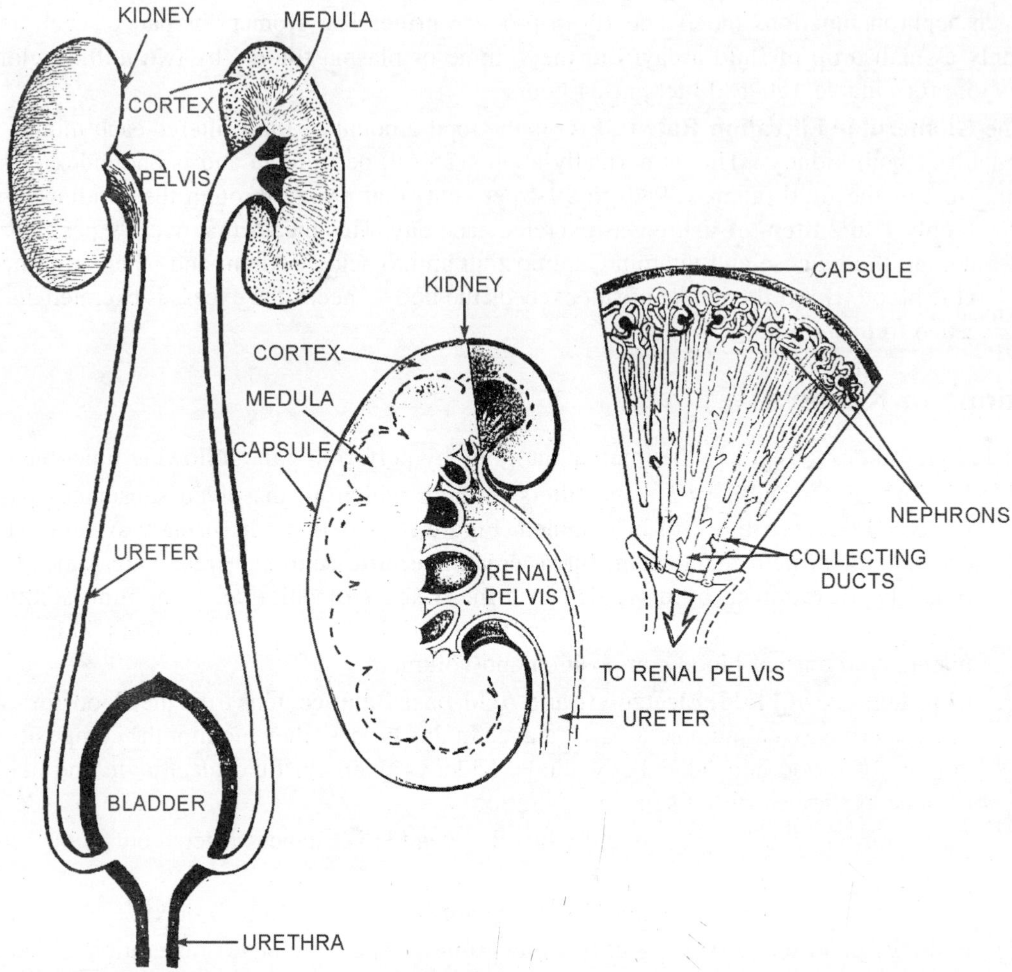

Figure 31.1 The urinary system and the nephron, the functional unit of the kidney

The most common cause of renal failure is diabetic nephropathy. Some antibiotics and pain medications may cause renal disease. The normal function of the nephrons, the working unit of kidneys, may be upset by the above ailments (Fig. 31.1).

Inflammation and Degeneration. The membranes and small blood vessels in the nephrons may get inflamed for a short time due to infection and thus lead to **acute glomerulonephritis**. In case entire nephron or nephron sections are affected, the normal function is hindered and **nephrotic syndrome** occurs. If not arrested at this stage, the lesions may affect more and more nephrons resulting in **chronic renal failure**. Any disturbance in kidney function impairs metabolism of proteins, electrolytes and water. Thus nutritional balance is impaired.

Other Diseases Damage Kidney Function. Any disorder in circulation, which results in degeneration of small renal arteries, disturbs normal nephron function. For example, poorly controlled hypertension is a disorder of circulation; uncontrolled type II diabetes can also damage small renal arteries resulting in **glomerulosclerosis**. In this condition, there is a loss of functioning nephrons. If not controlled, it may lead to **chronic renal failure**.

Chemical Damage. Environmental agents such as pesticides, solvents, etc. may cause kidney damage. Animal venom, certain plants and drugs may also damage kidney tissue.

Infection and Obstruction. Bacterial infection in urinary tract may cause mild discomfort, which can be alleviated by medication, if treated promptly. If not treated, it may cause more involved chronic disease. Kidney stones may block drainage and may cause further infection and tissue damage.

Diet therapy in renal disease is based on the nature of the disease and individual response.

Kidney Ailments

Any disease that affects the function of the glomerulus or tubule disturbs the body's ability to utilise food and can cause havoc.

Glomerulonephritis

Nephritis is a general term used to indicate inflammation of the kidneys. When capillaries in glomeruli are inflamed, it is called **glomerulonephritis**.

An acute form of glomerulonephritis often follows a streptococcal infection of the respiratory tract, tonsillitis, pneumonia or scarlet fever. It occurs mostly in children and young adults. If the infection is very mild, it may not be detected and treated, resulting in permanent damage to the system, which may be detected after many years. The symptoms include nausea, vomiting, fever, rise in blood pressure, albumin (**proteinuria**) and small amounts of blood in the urine (**hemanuria**) and edema. Usually recovery is complete.

Diet Therapy: When there is nausea and vomiting in the acute stage, sweetened fruit juices, sweetened tea, ginger-lemon sherbet, high carbohydrate, low electrolyte supplements are given. These help to reduce tissue breakdown. Fluid intake is monitored **in proportion to the urine output**.

As soon as the patient is able to eat, a diet to maintain weight containing sufficient calories is given. If urine volume is decreased (as in **oliguria**) fluid is limited. Protein is also restricted to 40g. The proteins included must be of high biological value. Sodium is limited to 1g/day. Table 31.1 presents diet and a menu plan for such a patient.

Chronic Glomerulonephritis

It can either be an untreated acute glomerulonephritis or an immunological cause of unknown origin. In the early stages, abnormal urine analysis results such as protein, red and white blood cells are observed in the urine. As the ailment advances, the patient may suffer from tiredness, edema, increase in blood pressure and blurred vision. As the kidneys cannot concentrate urine, there is frequent urination and need to urinate often in the night, thus disturbing sleep. If not checked by treatment, it can lead to chronic renal failure.

Diet Modification: The diet must be planned to suit the patient's kidney capacity.

Normal intake of protein is planned when kidneys are able to excrete wastes. If proteins are excreted in the urine, the protein losses must be covered by appropriate increase in the diet of proteins of high biological value.

When the blood urea nitrogen rises with the worsening of kidney function, the protein in the diet must be reduced to 30–40 g or less. At the same time, the energy intake through carbohydrate and fat must be enough to prevent tissue breakdown.

If there is edema, sodium intake needs to be restricted. Due to poor reabsorption of the nutrients, loss of iron can lead to anemia. Hence iron supplements are needed.

Table 31.1: Diet in Glomerulonephritis

Calories – 1800, Protein – 40 g, Na – 800 mg

Food Groups	*No. of Exchanges*	*Protein (g)*	*Calories (kcal)*	*Na (mg)*
Cereals	9	18	900	45
Legumes and Pulses	2	11	200	20
Milk, toned	2	10	200	48
Egg / chicken / fish	½	3	40	10 - 65
Vegetables A	2	—	—	20
Vegetables B	2	2	60	20
Fruit	2	—	100	20
Fat	2	—	180	—
Sugar	5	—	100	—
	Total	44	1780	183–238

Meal Plan

Meal	*Menu Items*	*Drink*
Breakfast	1 Egg, 2 toasts, orange/mosumbi	tea/coffee
Lunch	1c rice, 1 chapati, 1s french beans, 1s dal, ½ s dahi	
Tea	1s upma/pohe, 1 banana	tea
Supper	1c rice, 2 phulkas, 1c dal, 1s ridge gourd bhaji, ½c dahi	

Nephrotic Syndrome

This includes lipoid nephrosis, a rare condition, which affects children. It may also be due to progression of chronic glomerulonephritis or be related to toxins of streptococci.

There is a degeneration of kidney tissue, which permits protein loss through the filtrate. Large amounts of proteins (albumins) are thus lost through the urine from the body.

In the beginning, there is swelling of eyelids and legs due to fluid retention in the body. Loss of albumin in urine leads to low serum albumin values, at the same time, cholesterol level in the blood increases. In this rare disease, mortality is high.

Diet Modifications: Diet treatments must rectify edema, excessive protein loss and malnutrition (anemia, etc.)

- **Protein** allowance is increased to 2-3g/kg for children and 75-100g for adults, provided through high quality proteins (Table 31.2). High protein intake may sometimes hasten worsening of renal condition. Hence some authorities recommend 1.6 to 1.8g/kg of protein of high biological value. High protein supplements with low sodium content are useful.
- **Energy** allowance must be adequate to permit use of protein from the diet for tissue synthesis. About 50-60 calories/kg body weight need to be given.

- **Sodium** level needs to be kept at about 500 mg to prevent edema. Low sodium sources of vegetables and fruits are given in Table 31.3.
- Dietary fat and cholesterol may be limited to control hyperlipidemias.

The patients may not have good appetite and may need encouragement from attending relatives and dietitian to consume the diet presented completely. Appetizing and acceptable preparations will help the patient to enjoy the diet planned. A diet for nephrotic syndrome is given in Table 31.2 .

Table 31.2: Diet for a Patient with Nephrotic Syndrome

Wt. of the patient – 45 kg Calories 50 – 60/kg
Calories – 2400, Protein 85 g, Na – 500 mg/day

Food Groups	*No. of Exchanges*	*Proteins (g)*	*Calories (kcal)*	*Na (mg)*
Cereals	10	20	1000	50
Legumes and Pulses	2	11	200	20
Milk, toned	4	20	400	96
SMP	50g	19	180	260
Fish/chicken/duck	2	10	100	30 – 60
Vegetables A	2	—	—	20
Vegetables B	2	4	60	10
Fruits	2	—	100	10
Sugar	6	—	120	—
Oils, fats	2	—	180	—
	Total	84	2,340	496–516

Acute Kidney Failure

Acute kidney failure is sudden, often reversible in a patient who had limited function earlier. When kidneys are not able to carry out their normal function of maintaining the internal chemical environment of the body by filtering out the wastes and excreting them, it is known as renal failure. It often develops due to gradual destruction of renal tissue by the disease or may occur suddenly as in nephrosis or obstruction of the tract.

When the glomerular filtration rate rapidly drops to less than 20 ml/minute, there is a fast rise in the serum urea and creatinine. When the rate drops further to 10 ml/minute or less, an excess of urea and other nitrogenous wastes appear in the blood, which are symptoms of **uremia**. Simultaneously, there is inability to urinate, with urine output decreasing to less than 100 ml/day. At this stage, the patients may suffer from drowsiness, weakness, fatigue or may have headache, itching or blurred vision. Acute renal failure leads to death in one-fourth of the cases. The percentage increases to half, if the patient is over 75 years or there is associated trauma.

Dialysis has proved to be a boon for such patients. It is instituted until kidney function is regained.

Table 31.3: Low Sodium sources of Vegetables and Fruits

Sodium Content	*Vegetables*
1. Less than 5 mg/100 g EP	Bitter gourd (green), bottle gourd. brinjal, french beans, onion stalks, parwar, ridge gourd, onions
2. 5 to 11 mg/100 g EP	Pumpkin, ladies finger (bhendi), peas, cucumber, colocasia, potato, sweet potato, tapioca (dried chips), yam, brussel sprouts
3. 12 – 15 mg/100 g EP	Cabbage, green plantain.
	Fruits
4. Less than 6 mg/100 g EP	Amla, guava, orange, papaya, peaches, plums, chiku, pomegranates, tree tomato, phalsa.
5. 7 to 13 mg/100 g EP	Pears, ripe tomato.

Dietary Modifications: In the first 24-48 hours, food and liquid intake by mouth are restricted. Glucose is given intravenously as oral intake is limited due to nausea, vomiting and lack of appetite. Sometimes tube feeding or total parenteral nutrition (TPN) is used. Dialysis is essential when TPN is used.

A protein free diet may be given **before** a patient is put on dialysis. Another approach is to give glucose with essential amino acids orally, by tube feeding.

The fluid allowance is 500 ml to make up for insensible water losses plus the urine output. More fluid is provided if there is vomiting, diarrhea, fever, etc. to prevent dehydration.

Energy intake should be enough to prevent catabolism. 20-40g protein is given with gradual increase to normal levels with improvement in kidney function. The serum electrolytes and urine output are constantly monitored so that appropriate diet and fluid intake adjustments can be made.

Diet is modified as the patient regains normal kidney function, in the recovery phase of the ailment. A high-protein, high-calorie diet is needed by patients who have suffered tissue damage (Table 31.2). The recovery of kidney function may not be complete in some patients.

Chronic Renal Failure

Gradual loss of kidney function is the beginning, but if it silently continues, the glomerular filtration rate begins to reduce leading to chronic renal failure. Kidneys have a vast reserve capacity, which allows them to support life through much of this progressive deterioration. When the glomerular filtration rate (GFR) drops from normal 125 ml/minute to less than 30 ml/minute, dietary modification is initiated

When the GFR reduces to 3 ml/minute, dietary control is not sufficient and dialysis or kidney transplant is necessary to save the life of the patient.

Dietary Modifications: The diet planning takes into account the stage of the disease, its causes, blood levels of urea and electrolytes, nutritional status, other diseases occurring and if the patient is on dialysis. The patients awaiting dialysis have a more severely restricted diet compared to those who are on dialysis.

Energy: To prevent tissue breakdown and release of nitrogen and potassium into circulation, an intake of 1900-2000 cal/day is indicated. Main sources of energy are carbohydrates and fats. Their metabolic end products do not pose a problem for the kidneys, as these are excreted through lungs (CO_2), sweat glands (water) and bowel (semisolid residue).

Protein: Protein intake is reduced to reduce work of kidneys of excreting end products of protein metabolism (namely, urea, creatinine, uric acid, sulfate and organic acids) in the urine. Most of the protein (65 to 75 per cent) in the diet should be of high biologic value (Table 31.4).

Table 31.4: Diet for a Patient with Chronic Renal Failure

30–40 protein, 1900 calories, 500 mg Na per day

Food	*No. of Exchanges*	*Proteins (g)*	*Calories (kcal)*	*Na (mg)*
Cereals	8	16	800	40
Dals & Pulses	1	6	100	10
Milk, toned	1	5	100	24
Fish/chicken	½	5	40	10–37
Vegetables A	2	—	—	30
Vegetables B	3	3*	150	20
Fruits	2	—	100	15
Sugar	10	—	200	—
Oils, fats	4	—	360	—
	Total	35	1850	176

Meal Plan**

Meal	*Items*	*Drink*
Breakfast	1 parantha / chapati-bhaji. banana	Tea/coffee
Lunch	1 ½ chapati, thick dal, rice (½ c), ½ c buttermilk	
Tea	1 s upma, orange/musumbi	Tea
Supper	Rice (2s), Phulkas (2), cabbage, bhaji, egg curry	

* Choose low protein containing vegetables, eg. Gourds and fruit vegetables

** Use 0.325 g salt in food preparation. **Do not** serve salt at the table.

Minerals: Potassium and sodium intakes need to be restricted to avoid hyperkalemia, edema and hypertension respectively. Phosphorus is often restricted to 600-1200 mg/day to prevent metabolic acidosis.

Table 31.5: Possible Meal Plan for Protein Controlled Diet
(based on exchange system)

	Measure	*Protein*			
		20g	*40g*	*60g*	*80g*
Breakfast					
Cereal	1 Exchange	1	1	1	1
Low prot. Bread	1 Slice	2	2	2	2
Bread enriched	1 Slice	—	1	1	1
Fruit	1 Exchange	1	1	1	1
Egg	1 No.	1	1	1	
Milk	1 Cup	¼	¼	¼	1
Lunch					
Bread/starch	1 Exchange	—	1	2	2
Low prot. Bread	1 Slice	2	—	—	—
Egg	1	1	—	—	—
Vegetable, free	1 Exchange	—	1	1	1
Milk	1 Cup	—	¼	½	1
Low prot. Dessert	1 Serving	1	1	1	1
Fruit	1 Exchange	1	1	1	1
Dinner					
Bread/starch	1 Exchange	1	1	2	2
Low prot. Bread	1 Slice	1	1	1	1
Dal	1 Serving	—	1	1	1
Vegetable, free	1 Exchange	—	1	1	1
Vegetable- List 3	1 Exchange	—	1	2	2
Fruit	1 Exchange	—	1	2	2
Milk	1 Cup	¼	—	—	1
Low prot. Dessert	1 Serving	1	—	—	—

Supplements of calcium, iron and B vitamins need to be given, as restricted diets are low in these nutrients. Calcitrol may also be given as supplement as the kidney is not able to produce vitamin D hormone.

Fluid is restricted when urine output is low. The total fluid intake is equal to the volume of urine output plus about 500 ml for insensible losses. The fluid intake includes water present in foods and beverages also. Thus 100 ml of milk provides 87 ml, 100 g of fruits and vegetables provide 80-90ml of water.

Dialysis

Dialysis is used in acute and chronic renal failure for a short or long periods. It does not correct metabolic problems and there is need for modification of diet as also supplements. Most patients with end-stage renal disease lose whatever kidney function is left, after beginning dialysis.

In hemodialysis, the patient's blood circulates outside the body through a semipermeable membrane bathed in dialyzing fluid and removes nitrogenous wastes from it. Three times a week, the patient has to undergo dialysis for 4 hours each time. Some serum amino acids and water soluble vitamins are lost in the dialysate.

Between dialysis, dietary control helps to maintain acceptable levels of nitrogenous waste products, potassium, sodium and fluids in the blood. Supplementation of water soluble vitamins are lost in the dialysate.

Kidney Transplant

When both kidneys of a patient fail, kidney transplant provides a functioning kidney, which permits him/her to lead a normal life.

As in any other surgery, postoperatively, dietary progression is from a liquid to solid diet, which is planned to individual tolerance. To help the patient to recover, a high protein, low carbohydrate and sodium restricted diet follows, which counteracts the effects of drugs used in treatment. Reduced fat may also help control hyperlipidemias, while restriction of simple sugars prevents hyperglycemia.

Kidney Stones

Kidney stones are also known as **renal calculi, urolithiasis, or nephrolithias**. These may be found in the bladder, kidney, ureter or urethra. Deposition of varied sizes crystals in an organic matrix leads to the formation of these stones.

As stones of varied sizes form, they normally move towards the ureter. Small smooth stones pass into the ureter, but large ones can block the ureter opening which impedes normal flow and causes intense pain. The pain may be accompanied by nausea, vomiting, even chills and fever. Only 10 per cent stones are large and cause such reactions.

Dietary correlation to kidney stone formation is not easy to prove. They occur in conjunction with other diseases, which infect or weaken the urinary tract. Excessive excretion of calcium (e.g. in osteoporosis) and concentration of urine may promote stone formation.

Low intake of water, leading to concentration of urine may lead to the formation and deposition of crystals in the renal tract. Calcium salts (with carbonate, phosphate, ammonium), magnesium oxalate, sulfate etc. account for 90 per cent of the stones; uric acid and rarely cystine or xanthine account for the rest.

Diet Therapy: Therapy is planned on the basis of the predominant component of the stone.

A very liberal fluid intake of 2500 to 3000ml per day is recommended to avoid formation of concentrated urine from which salts get precipitated out as stones. This recommendation is universal and does not depend on the type of stone.

Calcium Stones: If stones are not preceded by other disease (are idiopathic) dietary calcium intake is reduced to 600mg/day or less. Fiber in the diet is increased to bind excess calcium. If water supplies are high in calcium, it may be necessary to use special filter to eliminate it, before using it for drinking and cooking.

Oxalate Stones: A diet low in oxalate is indicated. Ascorbic acid content of the diet should be normal. Dietary fat should be reduced to 50g/day or less if the patient suffers from steatorrhea.

Uric acid Stones: Altered purine metabolism and sometimes gout may lead to the formation of these stones. A diet reduced in purines is prescribed sometimes.

Most of the small stones pass through the ureter. Those which are too large and obstruct function and cause pain need to be removed surgically. A modern procedure (**laproscopy**) in which the stone is broken into bits and flushed out, has done away with the need for painful surgery.

Dietary Modifications

It is important to note that dietary modifications cannot dissolve existing stones but it can be helpful in preventing development of new stones.

Some of the steps one can take to **prevent formation of kidney stones** are:

(*i*) **Drink lots of water**. Kidneys filter harmful substances out of the blood and flush them out of the body via the ureters. In the presence of fluid, the waste dissolves and flows out from the body. But when the body is dehydrated, the waste products solidify in crystalline form and can react with each other to form a stone of calcium oxalate or uric acid.

Fluids are the most important input in the prevention of kidney stones. The aim is to drink enough water to produce two liters of urine per day. Those living in hot climate, will need additional two to four glasses of water per day.

You can check the colour of the urine, which is an indicator of its concentration. If it is dark yellow, the crystals are not dissolving, and you should increase your fluid (mainly water) intake.

(*ii*) **Increase your potassium intake**. In scientific studies, it was observed that those, who ate a lot of fruits and vegetables rich in potassium reduced their risk of developing kidney stone by 50 per cent. Bananas, citrus fruits, potatoes are good sources of potassium.

(*iii*) **Reduce intake of meat**. The risk of kidney stones is reduced if intake of meat is reduced to a serving of three ounces per day.

Study Questions

1. List the functions of kidney.
2. Discuss the causes of kidney disease.
3. What is glomerulonephritis? What changes in diet are made to meet it?
4. List low sodium sources of vegetables and fruits.
5. What are kidney stones? What steps can one take to reduce their incidence?

CHAPTER

32

Nutrition in Cancer

The Nature of Cancer

Cancer is the cause of about 3 to 6 per cent of all deaths in India and its incidence is on the rise.[(1)]. In 2004, annual mortality due to cancer was reported to be 0.7 million. The incidence of the type of cancer varies with sex and age. In Indian females, breast, cervix-uterine, oesophagel and gastrointestinal cancers account for 30 per cent of all cancer deaths. In males, 31 per cent of all cancer deaths occur due to oropharyngeal, lung, oesophegal and stomach cancers. Leukemias and pediatric malignancies (lymphomas and osteo-sarcomas) occur in children.

Cancer is characterized by abnormal cell growth. It can occur in any organ. In cancer, the genes lose control of cell growth in some way and reproduction of cells is unstructured and excessive. The abnormal growth leads to a developing mass called a **tumor** or **neoplasm**. Hence cancer is also called **neoplasia**. Cancerous tumors are malignant, affecting the structure and hence the functions of organs. More than 100 types of malignant forms of cancer are known. Cancer cells are said to **metastasize** when they break away from their original site, move through the blood and spread at a new site. Cancer does not always cause death, but the mortality rate of cancer patients is high. If it is detected at an early stage of development, prompt treatment can cure or eradicate it. The study of cancer is called **oncology** and a physician, who is a specialist in cancer is called an **oncologist**.

The Causes of Cancer

The exact cause of cancer is not known, but several factors are thought to contribute to its development. These include: heredity, viruses, environmental **carcinogens** and perhaps emotional stress.

(1) Ambiye, R.Y. et al. Diet, Nutrition and Cancer AFST(I) Newsletter, Bombay Chapter, p.26, Jan. 2005.

Some families seem to have a **genetic** predisposition for cancer though it is not inherited. In such cases, it is advisable to carefully avoid environmental carcinogens and be regular in medical checkups.

Environmental carcinogens include some substances breathed in (tobacco smoke and asbestos), radiation (from x-rays, sun or nuclear wastes), certain chemicals ingested in food and water and some chemicals, which are in regular contact with the skin. Only a prolonged exposure to carcinogens leads to cancer, not an occasional exposure.

Relationships of Food and Cancer

There appear to be associations between food and cancer, both good and bad, though these have not been proved. About fifty per cent of cancers may be related to diet. Cancers of the colon, rectum, prostrate and breast are the ones which have been shown to be associated with diet.

Healthy immune system is maintained by adequate intake of protein foods. Any damage to immune system, such as malnutrition, may be a contributing factor in the development of cancer.

On the positive side, diets high in fibre are thought to help to protect against **colorectal cancer**. Intake of sufficient amounts of vitamin C-rich foods may protect against cancers of stomach and esophagus. Intake of sufficient amounts of carotene and vitamin A rich foods may protect against cancers of lung, bladder and larynx. Phytochemicals (substances that occur naturally in plant foods) are thought to be anticarcinogenic agents. Flavonoids, phenols and indoles, which are abundantly found in fruits and vegetables are examples of phytochemicals. Hence it is advisable to eat six or more servings of fruits and vegetables. Legumes such as lentils, mung and other dried beans and dals contain proteins, minerals and fibre. High intakes of these and soya foods are associated with decreased risk of breast and colon cancer.

However, excessive intake of protein and fats may be involved in colon cancer development.

Omega-3-fatty acids protect the cell from cancer development, whereas monounsaturated fats (MUFA) are neutral. Linoleic acid, an essential fatty acid, has been shown to be a causative factor of cancer. Once cancerous cells are formed it promotes their proliferation. High intake of polyunsaturated fats (PUFA) in the diet have been shown to increase the development of breast, colon, pancreas and prostate cancer in animals. More research is needed to establish the role of fat and its degradation products in the development of cancer.

Nitrites in cured and smoked foods (bacon and ham), which can be changed to nitrosamines (carcinogens) during cooking, are examples of substances in foods, which are thought to be carcinogenic. Regular intake of these foods is associated with cancers of breast, uterus, prostate and colon. People, who smoke and drink excessive amounts of alcohol, appear to be at greater risk of cancers of the mouth, pharynx, esophagus than those who do not smoke and drink alcohol.

When food is fried in the same oil continuously, the oil polymerises and these polymers have been shown to be carcinogenic.

Calcium intake up to 1200 mg/day seems to have a protective influence. So does drinking more than five glasses of water per day.

The most important principle is **moderation**. An occasional serving of bacon or buttered popcorn or wine is not likely to cause cancer, but the regular excessive use of carcinogenic foods may contribute to cancer. Vitamins that are thought to prevent cancer should be ingested in foods that **naturally** contain them.

Excessive intake of vitamin supplements **can be harmful**. For example, abnormally large amounts of vitamin A can cause pain, hair loss, headaches and liver and skin problems.

In the news

***Carrots and tomatoes may reduce ovarian cancer risk**: Women who eat plenty of carrots, tomatoes, and other foods high in carotene and lycopene may reduce their risk of ovarian cancer. This was most apparent in post-menopausal women. Since carotene (which the body converts to vitamin A) and lycopene are antioxidants, women should get their carotenoids from foods and **not from supplements**. They should take at least five servings of carrots and one cup of tomato sauce per week.*

(Source : Reuters Oct. 2001, Intl. J of Cancer 2001, 94:128-134)

The Effects of Cancer

Unexplained weight loss is one of the first indications of cancer, because the tumor cells use the nutrients the host has taken in for their own growth and development. As a result the host is famished, feels weak and may lose appetite, which compounds the weight loss.

The weight loss includes the loss of muscle tissue and **hypoalbuminemia** and **anemia** may develop. In cancer patients, nutrient deficiency may affect the sense of taste and smell. These may become abnormal. As a result, foods taste less sweet and more bitter than they would taste to healthy persons.

Decreased digestive secretions may reduce appetite of cancer patients and they may feel full when they eat a small amount of food. **Hyperglycemia** can develop due to abnormal insulin production, which may delay stomach's emptying and dull the appetite. Some cancers can cause **hypercalcemia**. If this is chronic, it can lead to formation of renal stones and damage kidney function. The location of a tumor determines the effects of cancer on the host. For example, there is blockage in the gastrointestinal tract causing malabsorption, when the tumor is in the esophagus or intestine. If the cancer is not treated, the continued loss of appetite (anorexia) and weight loss will create a state of severe malnutrition and body wasting (cachexia) and untimely death.

The Treatment of Cancer

Three methods can be used to treat cancer. – **chemotherapy, radiation, surgical removal** or a **combination of these methods.**

Chemotherapy reduces the ability to regenerate the absorptive cells of the small intestine and can cause hemorrhagic colitis. Both chemotherapy and radiation may cause nausea, vomiting and diarrhea, which result in fluid and electrolyte imbalances. Both may also depress appetite. However, the patient can get back to normal well-balanced diet after the therapy is over and these problems may disappear.

Radiation can affect a number of body functions adversely. It can change senses of taste and smell; it can cause a decrease in salivary secretions and can reduce the absorptive tissue in the small intestine. It can cause constipation or diarrhea. Decrease in salivary secretions can cause dry mouth (xerostomia), difficulty in swallowing (dysphagia), tooth decay and even loss of teeth sometimes.

Cancer surgery affects the function of the part of the body affected. The ability to chew and swallow is affected in mouth surgery, the absorption is affected in gastric or intestinal surgery, resulting in nutritional deficiencies.

However, these treatments have side-effects, which have adverse effects on the nutritional status of the patient.

Nutritional Care of Cancer Patient

A cancer patient needs a high-calorie, high-protein diet, as there is an increase in metabolic rate due to cancer, need to rebuild damaged tissues and to replace nutrients lost to the cancer. Patients on high-calorie, high-protein diet tolerate the side effects of therapy and higher doses of drugs better than those who cannot eat normally. Patients, who can maintain their weight or minimize its loss have a greater chance of responding to treatment and thus their recovery.

Though their nutritional needs are high, anorexia is a major problem for cancer patients. It is very difficult to overcome because patients develop strong dislike to foods, which are side effects of chemotherapy. Therefore chemotherapy needs to be scheduled two to three hours before or after meals. Parenteral or enteral nutrition may be necessary in the early stages to meet the needs of the patient.

The appetite and absorption is improved after chemotherapy. So the nutritional status of the patient improves in the period between chemotherapy treatments.

Diet plans for cancer patients require special attention. The plans need to be made in consultation with the patient, taking care to include favourite foods, prepared in familiar ways and served attractively.

Those with a chewing problem, may find soft diet suitable. Those with diarrhea may respond to a low-residue diet.

Cancer causes a hypermetabolic state, which increase energy demands. Though energy needs vary from one patient to another, 45-50 kcal/kg body weight may be recommended. Carbohydrates and fats must provide this energy and spare protein for tissue building and immune system. Protein needs vary from 1.0 to 1.2 g/kg for those with good nutrition and 1.3 to 2.0 g/kg for malnourished patients.

Sufficient fluids need to be ingested to help the kidneys eliminate the metabolic wastes and the toxins from drugs.

Patients may tolerate several small meals than three large ones. If possible, supplement meals with high-calorie, high-protein liquid foods as snacks.

To sum up, abnormal cell growth is a character of cancer. It can occur in any body tissue. Energy needs are high due to the hypermetabolic state and the demands of tumor. At the same time, the patient suffers from anorexia. It causes severe wasting, anemia and several metabolic problems. Chemotherapy, radiation and surgery are used to treat cancer singly or in combination as needed. Due to the illness and anorexia, it is difficult to improve the nutritional status of the patient. Parenteral or enteral nutrition may be necessary in the early stages to start the process of recovery.

Study Questions

1. What is cancer? What are the factors which contribute to its development?
2. Discuss relationships of food and cancer.
3. Discuss treatment of cancer including nutritional care of the cancer patient.

CHAPTER

Nutrition in Immune System Dysfunction, AIDS and Allergy

33

Introduction

The ability of the body to resist infection is known as immunity. Natural immunity is the sum total of the defenses of the body, which enables the body to resist infection under normal conditions. This phenomenon explains why most of us resist the agents of disease that we are exposed to every day. The various types of immunity are depicted in Fig. 33.1. One can observe from the table that all types of immunity are closely related.

Cells and tissues involved in immunity comprise about 2% of the body's weight. Cells, which participate in immune responses are collected together in lymphoid organs - thymus, spleen, lymph nodes and Peyer's patches. In this environment they can perform their functions effectively, and they also disseminate immunity by migrating throughout the body.

Non-Specific Immunity – Primary Defences

Physical Barriers prevent the entry and action of microbial invaders in the body. The first response to microbial invaders is non-specific and does not need to recognise the invader (antigen).

Physical barriers are the primary defences of the body against infection. Intact **skin and mucous membranes** prevent entry and action of microbial invaders, As we know mucous membranes line the respiratory, alimentary and genitourinary tracts. Additional non-specific resistances include visceral movements, the complement system.

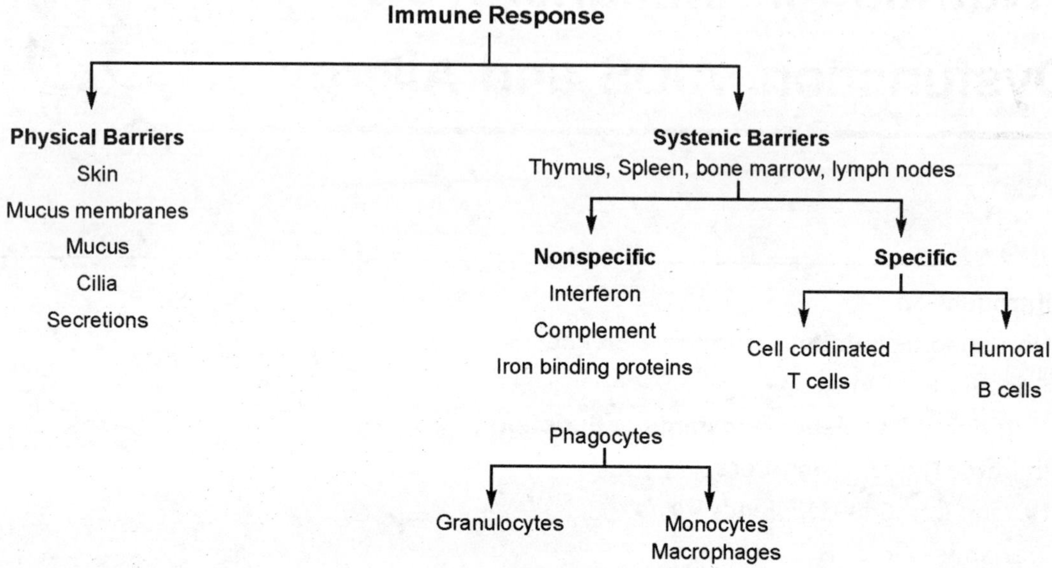

Figure 33.1 Types of immunity

Cilia are hair-like structures on the lining of cells of the nose and windpipe (trachea), which help to cough up the microbes, that may have entered there. **Mucus** produced in the nose and sinuses traps dust and helps destroy bacteria. **Secretions** such as sweat, mucus, tears and intestinal secretions mechanically flush away foreign substances.

Nonspecific resistances also include the complement system, interferon (protein formed when cells are exposed to virus), iron-binding proteins (e.g., lactoferrin and transferrin) and phagocytes (granulocytes, monocytes and macrophages).

Complement System is a group of proteins, which interact with each other in a step-wise progression to bring about antigen-antibody reactions. If the complement system becomes defective, the susceptibility to bacterial infections is increased.

Phagocytes ingest and destroy microorganists. Phagocytes include granulocytes and macrophages all of which circulate. Macrophages eat up (kill) bacteria and viruses. Macrophages ready the invading agent (antigen) so that the T and B lymphocytes can recognize it and act on it. Phagocytes and complement release digestive enzymes which contain lysosomes. Lysosomes destroy antigen.

Specific Immunity

Cell-mediated and **humoral** are two types of specific immunity. Cell-mediated occurs inside or on the surface of the cell. Humoral immunity occurs in blood and fluid outside the cell.

Cell-mediated Immunity: Lyphocytes called **T-cells** are the main agents of cell-mediated immunity. T cells get activated on contact with antigen.

Our resistance to fungal and viral infections and regulation of humoral immunity is due to cell-mediated immunity. Hence greater understanding of T-cells can help prevent and treat diseases.

Organ transplants, which are foreign tissues may be rejected due to the body's T-cells recognizing these as such. Hence immunorepressive drugs are given to a patient receiving organ transplant to suppress action of their T-cells.

Humoral Immunity involves lymphocytes called B cells. There are a variety of B-cells. B-cells specific to the invading cell produce plasma cells, which in turn produce a variety of immunoglobulins. (Ig-antibodies). These antibodies bind the antigen and form a complex. The complex cells are destroyed by interaction with complement proteins. The destroyed cells are ingested by macrophages.

Most viral and some bacterial infections occur, when there is a deficiency of B-cells.

Nutritional Deficiency and Immune Function

The organs which are centres of immune function, namely thymus, spleen, lymph nodes, atrophy in protein-energy malnutrition. As a result T-cells numbers and phagocytosis is reduced. In the absence of protective mechanisms in malnourished persons, infectious diseases are usually more virulent. For example, measles is frequently a life-threatening disease in a malnourished child, though it is a mild disease in a healthy child.

Those persons, who are at risk due to lack of natural immunity include :

Infants, the elderly,

food faddists as also hospitalised patients,

alcoholics and drug users.

Infants are protected by antibodies received in the womb from their mother, though immunity is low at birth. Breast milk also provides IgA (immunoglobulin A). Low birth weight infants may have suboptimal immune function and thus are prone to get infections easily.

Elderly. There is progressive decline in immune function with age. There is decrease in lean body mass nutrient levels in blood fall and poor nutrition is a problem at times. Thus the malnutrition coupled with decreased immunity leads to a greater incidence of infections, degenerative diseases and cancer.

Food Faddists. Food faddists may take deficient diets, self-treat themselves with unnecessary supplements, creating imbalance in nutrients (too much of some and too little of other nutrients). Such regimen may affect immune function adversely and make them susceptible to infectious diseases.

Effect of Specific Nutrients on Immunity. Cell-mediated and humoral immunities are decreased by any nutrient deficiency or imbalance, which reduces production or maturation of T-cells or B-cells, depresses DNA synthesis, cell division or replication.

Energy. In animal experiments , it is observed that animals fed diets adequate in all nutrients, but with moderate restriction in energy, live longer, have fewer tumors and exhibit slower decrease in immune function with age. Humans are likely to exhibit a similar trend. The incidence of respiratory infections is higher in obese than normal weight people.

Protein Synthesis is an essential prerequisite of normal immune function. Cell-mediated immune function is depressed in kwashiorkor (a protein deficiency disease).

The quality and quantity of protein are both important in immune response. Increased incidence of infections is observed, when the diet does not meet the essential amino acid needs of the individual.

Immune System Disorders

Autoimmune Diseases: When the body's immune defenses attack the body itself, the antibodies produced attack its cells and organs. These antibodies are responsible for autoimmune diseases, which include insulin dependent diabetes mellitus, rheumatoid arthritis etc.

Secondly the absence or insufficiency of a component/s of immune system levels leads to these disorders. Some infants have these defects from birth. Some patients may develop as part of disease in an advanced stage of **cancer** and/or as side effects of the treatments.

The third type is caused by a virus (the human immuno-deficiency Virus – **HIV**), which destroys body's specific cell-mediated defense system. (a helper T-cell and the T-4 cell). Hence it is called acquired immuno-deficiency syndrome (**AIDS**). As it affects vital body systems (thymus, spleen, lymph nodes, etc.) it leads to a variety of infections.

Ordinary harmless organisms cause these infections due to the body's loss of defense mechanism. It is important to take precautions to prevent food-borne infections as persons with AIDS are at high risk.

Human Immuno-deficiency Virus

As you may recall, a virus is a microscopic parasite that attacks and infects various tissues of our body. It gets its nourishment from our tissues and multiplies countless times causing a variety of ailments.

There are many viruses that infect humans. Some cause only mild illness, for example, those which are responsible for causing cold. There are other viruses, which are deadly; the **Human Immunodeficiency Virus (HIV)** is one of the deadly ones.

Our blood contains T cells which are white cells, which protect our body from infections. HIV invades the T cells, impairing the normal function of the T cells, which is to protect the body from other microorganisms present in the body. Persons, who have a healthy immune system, are thus protected from invaders by the T cells.

HIV positive persons are those who are infected by the HIV virus. If not treated effectively in the early stages, HIV infection ultimately progresses to an Acquired Immune Deficiency Syndrome (AIDS), which is incurable and fatal.

Transmission of HIV Infection

So far there is no cure for HIV infection, but it can be prevented. It can affect anyone of any age and sex, who is exposed to it. It is not transmitted through casual contact such as shaking hands. It is transmitted through body fluids such as:

- sexual contact
- by transfusion of contaminated blood
- by the use of contaminated needles during ear piercing, tattooing, acupuncture, or injection of illegal drugs.
- By infected mothers to their fetuses in pregnancy or to their infants during breast feeding.

Advancement from HIV to AIDS: This occurs in three stages. Soon after exposure to HIV, the body produces antibodies in an attempt to destroy the virus. Some persons may have symptoms like mild 'flu, others may have no symptoms for a few months to even ten years. At this stage, the person will know that he/she is HIV-positive only **if tested**.

In the first dormant stage, the virus, which is incubating, multiplies in various parts e.g. tonsils, adenoid glands and spleen and destroys the T cells. If a person suspects that he/she is exposed to HIV, early detection helps to start treatment, which can prolong life, as the treatment may delay the action of the virus. Good nutrition at this stage helps to increase body's ability to delay action of the virus.

In the second stage, infected persons, who are undetected and therefore not treated, suffer from damage to their immune system. Infections occur, which may result in a variety of symptoms such as fatigue, headache, oral infections, cough, sore throat, fevers, shortness of breath, diarrhea, weight loss, skin rashes, night sweat, etc.

In the third stage, HIV infection leads to AIDS (Acquired Immune Deficiency Syndrome). It is evident from a very low T-cell count, which results in the body's inability to fight infections. At this stage, other parasites invade (e,g, T.B.) and in the absence of immunity, the body succumbs.

Nutrition in HIV Infection

A healthful, nutritious diet ensures a healthy immune system, which may delay the progression of HIV infection to AIDS.

When a person is diagnosed as HIV positive, it is important to assess the nutritional status of the person. At this early stage, any unhealthful dietary habits can be corrected with a dietitian's guidance and the importance of meeting future nutritional needs emphasised to help the action of the body to resist the action of the virus.

As the condition progresses, patients may begin to suffer some of the problems listed above. The metabolic rate, nutrient and energy needs increase due to infections, while the appetite and ability to absorb nutrients may decrease. Medicines given may cause nausea and reduce the appetite. Taste may change, swallowing may be painful due to oral infection. These difficulties may result in malnutrition, such as protein-energy malnutrition and hence loss of weight.

To improve the appetite of the patient, there are several things the dietitian can do, such as:

Offer soft food,
Serve frequent small meals,
Offer food the patient tolerates,
Add sugar and flavourings to improve acceptability of liquid.supplements,
Avoid extremely hot or cold foods, spicy or acidic foods,
Give medicines after meals,
Talk to the patient to help him/her unburden worries about family, friends and finances.

Allergy

Allergy is hypersensitivity to certain substances or conditions. The allergic person may have distressing symptoms from what she/he breathes, eats or touches. To the allergic person a summer day with its pollen grains means hay fever or asthma. A person allergic to a particular food may have stomach pains, eczema or skin rashes and/or migraine headaches, if she/he eats it. A person allergic to a particular dye may develop an intense itching, rash on even a slight contact with the dyed cloth.

About 10 to 20 per cent of the population suffer from allergy. The allergic person produces antibodies, which combine with foreign material such as pollen or food protein leading to an antigen-antibody reaction with release of mediators such as histamine and prostaglandins. These mediators injure the body cells and cause illnesses. Such illnesses are called **allergies**.

Respiratory System: The linings of the nose, the windpipe and the bronchial tubes are affected by a variety of substances such as pollens of ragweed and grass, mold spores, house dust, dust from feathers, animal hair, mites from pillows, bed linen etc.. These result in allergies of the respiratory system.

Asthma: The lining of the nose continues into the bronchial tubes. Asthma in most cases is an extension of nasal allergy into bronchial tubes. About 40 per cent patients who have nasal allergy develop asthma . As the substances that cause swelling and cause increased secretions affect bronchial tubes, the passage becomes narrower, gets plugged with thick mucus. These cause difficulty in breathing and induce coughing attacks, the main symptoms of asthma (meaning 'breathless').

Skin: Two types of allergies affect skin – eczema and hives. Some materials, which affect almost everyone are poison ivy and poison oak or sumac. These materials can produce severe blistering rashes due to allergy in any person following sufficient exposure.

Many other substances also affect skin and produce less severe rashes, which may cause itching and redness in the affected areas. These include dyes (used to dye hair or clothes), chemicals in creams, shampoos and cosmetics, furniture polishes, detergents, mercury and nickel compounds and many others.

Allergic eczema may be caused by substances taken internally. In mild attacks, the face, neck, back of elbows/knees are involved; in severe cases, rash may cover the entire skin.

Hives (urticaria) are temporary swellings starting below the skin surface. The most common causes of hives are foods and drugs.

The Digestive Tract: Foods are the most common cause of allergic symptoms in the gullet, stomach or intestines; while some drugs may also cause allergy. The symptoms may appear within few seconds to several hours after the intake of food. The symptoms of gastrointestinal allergy vary from mild discomfort (bloating and constipation or diarrhea) to severe abdominal pains. The gastrointestinal symptoms may begin in the area first exposed like the mouth, gums, lips, tongue and pharynx, which may itch, swell and burn.

Food Allergy Diagnosis

Many steps are involved in assessment and diagnosis of a food allergy.

Assessment: In the diet history, symptoms and their timing, suspected foods and the amounts eaten to produce a reaction as also family history of allergies is recorded. The cause may be a common food or foods or a non-food. Anthropometric measurements are recorded to evaluate growth and development in the child. Nutritional assessment can help to detect persons at risk of malnutrition.

Diary of Food Intake and Symptoms is kept for 2 weeks. It helps to identify food causing allergy and also gives an idea of nutritional adequacy of the diet.

Treatment

To treat any allergy requires finding causes as indicated above. A very careful diet study is necessary with tests in which suspected foods are eliminated **or** purposely tried to observe their effect. Intelligent observation is essential, in which the patient's patience and physician's skill play important roles. The only effective treatment is to avoid the substances causing the allergy.

For infants, who are not breast-fed and are allergic to cow's milk, casein hydrolysate formulas are used.

Persons, who have allergy to foods, should be educated about **cross-reactivity**, that is allergy to the foods from the same group or botanical family. Thus a person who is allergic to groundnuts may also be allergic to other beans such as soybeans.

Patient education: Patient's meal pattern must fit in with their family pattern. Nutritional adequacy must be achieved. If one is allergic to citrus fruits, other sources of ascorbic acid must be included in the diet.

Patients need to be educated to read food labels and avoid those containing foods, which they are allergic to.

While eating out it is best to select foods, which are free from the offending food. While minute amounts may produce adverse reactions, the person, should wear a medical alert locket indicating the allergen(s) and carry an **epinephrine kit** to be used if the offending food is eaten by mistake or unknowingly. The injection of epinephrine can give great relief from an allergic reaction.

Study Questions

1. What is non-specific immunity?
2. Write short notes on: Cell-mediated immunity, humoral immunity, auto-immune diseases, HIV, transmission of HIV.
3. Discuss role of nutrition in HIV investigation.
4. What is allergy? Which systems are affected by allergy? How is it treated?

CHAPTER 34

Nutrition Support in Metabolic Disorders

Introduction

In 1990 over 4900 metabolic disorders were catalogued. About 250 of these have a defined biochemical basis. These disorders result from variation in the structure of enzymes or protein molecules. The amino acid sequences of enzymes, which are proteins, and their quantity are decided by genes. About 30% of our population is heterozygous for common alleles, as suggested by the extent of normal variation in genes. Relatively rare traits, which result in disease, are produced by mutations of genes. The frequency of occurrence of mutant genes varies in populations. For example, maple syrup urine disease (MSUD) occurs in about one in 250,000 newborns worldwide, but in an inbred Mennonite population, it occurs one in 176.

Genetic disorders can affect the metabolism of proteins, carbohydrates, lipids, pyrimidines, minerals and vitamins, depending on the metabolic pathway that is affected.

To prevent irreversible changes, such as brain damage, in infants, population-wide nonselective screening of newborns has been instituted for PKU, MSUD, galactosemia, homocystinuria and tyrosinemia in UK and USA. In these disorders, speed in diagnosis and treatment is of the utmost importance.

Metabolic Disorders Benefited by Nutrition Support

In metabolic disorders accumulation, excess production or lack of normal substrates and metabolic products, leads to toxic symptoms. In many of these, appropriate changes in the dietary supply helps to alleviate the problem.

Identifying the affected persons before irreversible changes have occurred is a very important step in optimum management of these disorders. Analysis of the amniotic fluid cells in the sixteenth to eighteenth weeks of gestation can help to detect a number of genetic disorders. Such search for genetic disease is done when there is a family history of inherited disease. Such tests help to prevent inborn error such as congenital cataracts in galactosemia by removing lactose from mother's diet. Other metabolic disorders can be detected by analysis of blood, urine, etc. of susceptible infants.

It must be noted that persons suffering from metabolic disorders benefit from nutrition support, when it is given promptly after detection. In this chapter, only a few disorders will be discussed to illustrate that early nutrition support can prevent irreversible, severe pathogenic problem.

Eight approaches to therapy of metabolic disorders are discussed here. Selection of the method depends on how the disease occurs. Several methods may be used in sequence or at the same time, depending on the case.

1. *Correct the basic imbalance in metabolic reactions.*

   For example, in **phenylketonuria (PKU)**, which occurs due to phenylalanine hydroxylase deficiency, intake of phenylalanine is limited and tyrosine is supplemented.
2. *The excretion of accumulated metabolic products, which are overproduced, is enhanced.*

   In **gout**, the blood uric acid levels are lowered by blocking renal reabsorption with use of drugs. Then the tissue deposits of uric acid are mobilised for use.
3. *Alternate metabolic pathways are provided to reduce accumulation of toxic precursors in blocked reaction.* For example, in urea cycle defects, the accumulated ammonia is decreased by using nitrogen to form phenylacetyl glutamine from glutamine by giving curative amounts of phenylacetic acid.
4. *To reduce overproduction of reaction products by use of inhibitors.* Thus in gout, overproduction of uric acid is inhibited by use of allopurinol.
5. *Products of blocked pathways are provided.* Administration of pancreatic enzymes, when the normal secretion is blocked, helps to correct the digestive defect in cystic fibrosis.
6. *Altered enzyme proteins are stabilised.* Appropriate intake of the co-factor vitamin B_6 in homocystinuria or thaimine in MSUD increases intracellular coenzymes of these vitamins and hence the specific activity of the related enzymes.
7. *Deficient cofactors are replaced.* Appropriate intake of specific vitamin precursor cures a number of vitamin dependent disorders, which occur due to blocks in production of their coenzyme.
8. *Genetic counseling to limit the frequency of inherited diseases.* Genetic counseling can prevent marriages between high-risk individuals and thus reduce the birth of affected progeny.

The main component of treating inherited disorders is nutrition management. In addition to dietary restrictions, some amount of chemically tailored foods need to be used to correct imbalances in metabolic relationships.

Metabolic Disorders Involving Amino Acids

Amino acids are the building blocks of proteins. They have many functions in the body. Metabolic disorders related to amino acids can occur due to defects in the way they are metabolised or their entry into the cells. As these disorders lead to symptoms early in life, newborns are screened for them routinely in some countries.

Phenyl ketonuria (PKU) was discovered in 1933. Prevention of mental retardation caused by it, is a classic example of diet therapy.

Of the amino acid disorders, **phenyl ketonuria (PKU)** will be discussed, as it is one of the few causes of mental handicap for which reasonably effective treatment is available.

In classic PKU, the activity of the enzyme phenylalanine hydroxylase is less than 1 per cent of normal. This enzyme is present in the liver and converts excess phenylalanine to tyrosine, another amino acid which is eliminated from the body. In 1 to 3 per cent cases with defective hydroxylation, there is deficiency of the cofactor tetrahydrobiopterin, and in this rare condition, the brain damage is not prevented by dietary treatment.

Phenylalanine is an essential amino acid, which needs to be provided through food, as it cannot be synthesized in the human body.

Phenylketonuria (PKU) is a group of inherited disorders of phenylalanine metabolism. It is caused by impaired phenylalanine activity. The symptoms occur at 3 to 6 months of age. These include developmental delay, microcephaly, abnormal electroencephalogram, eczema, musty odour and hyperactivity.

In some countries (UK, USA) neonates are screened between 6th to 14th day after birth for PKU. If diagnosed for PKU, treatment must be started immediately, to minimise the deleterious effects of the disease.

Treatment involves intake of controlled low-phenylalanine diet and regular monitoring of the blood phenylalanine concentrations. Phenylalanine is an essential amino acid. If the amount in the diet is insufficient, brain damage will occur. Hence the essential requirement must be ingested each day, a part of the daily requirement being given with each meal. The synthetic protein substitute for PKU must contain all the other essential amino acids needed. In addition, tyrosine becomes essential due to the metabolic block. The recommended intake of all other nutrients is similar to that of other infants.

The practical management of the PKU diet is very important. The levels of phenylalanine in the blood should be monitored on specimens taken 3.5 to 4 hours after a feed or main meal, using a micromethod (Guthrie), so that a capillary sample can be used. The suggested frequency of checking is weekly during the first few months for infants, every two weeks after weaning to toddler age; every 3 – 4 weeks in preschool age and 4 weekly thereafter up to teens; after that, it may be every 2 – 3 months or less. Young children are likely sometimes to pilfer food or suffer from infections. At such times the blood levels of phenylalanine needs to be checked and monitored.

During infection, when a child is likely to eat poorly, a high-energy drink must be fed to avoid breakdown of tissues, which may elevate phenylalanine level.

Human milk has lower phenylalanine content than cow's milk. Hence time-controlled breast-feeding can be judiciously combined with use of protein substitute for a newly diagnosed infant.

The sweetener, aspartame (nutrasweet/other brand name) contains phenylalanine and should not be fed to phenylketonuric patients of any age. Manufactured foods containing these sweeteners also need to be avoided from the PKU diet.

A lady suffering from PKU, who wishes to have a child, must be advised to stick to low – phenylalanine diet, much before conception and continue it through pregnancy. The blood levels must be strictly controlled. Strict monitoring of the diet is essential to ensure adequate supply of energy, phenylalanine and tyrosine and other nutrients to ensure appropriate growth of the fetus.

When a mother with phenylketonuria, takes normal diet during pregnancy, her child has a high probability of suffering from severe congenital abnormalities such as mental retardation, microcephaly and heart defects.

Maple Syrup Urine Disease (MSUD) is a group of inherited disorders of the metabolism of the branched-chain amino acids leucine, isoleucine and valine. Impairment of the branched-chain alpha-keto acid dehydragenase occurs due to several different mutations.

At birth infants with MSUD appear normal and well. But after intake of a protein-containing feed, in severe cases seizures, aponea (suspension of breathing), occurs. If not treated death occurs within ten days of birth.

Hence it is urgent to screen susceptible newborns for MSUD, diagnose it and start appropriate feeding promptly within the first week of life. This may consist of orogastric feeding of branched-chain aminoacid-free protein and energy source, which should be started as soon as possible after diagnosis is made. The aim is to initiate anobolism in the infant and prevent accumulation of neurotoxic branched-chain aminoacids.

For patients with 15% or more enzyme activity, protein intake of upto 1.5 g/kg/day may be sufficient.

The long-term diet therapy for MSUD involves maintenance of plasma concentrations of the branched-chain amino acids within specified limits, to permit maximum intellectual development and provide all other nutrients for optimal growth.

The nutrition support is achieved by use of special medical foods and natural foods.

Galactosemia

Lactose is the principal carbohydrate and energy source for infants and young children. Galactose is found only as a component of lactose in natural foods and has a central metabolic role in human nutrition.

Galactose is formed by hydrolysis of lactose by lactase in the intestine.

Galactose must be converted in the liver to glucose before it is used; this occurs through three enzymatic steps. (Fig. 34.1).

Galactosemia may occur due to deficient function of any of three enzymes (galactokinase, galactose-1-phosphate uridyl transferase or UDP galacto-4-epimerase)

Deficiency of galactokinase results in only cataracts.

Galactosemia due to deficiency of galactose-1-P-transferase leads to accumulation of galactose-1-P with progressive damage to the central nervous system, liver and renal tubule, if galactose restriction is not started in the first few days of life. In most of the untreated infants, who survive, retarded mental and physical growth occurs.

Diagnosis of galctosemia is made by measuring galactose-1-P transferase activity in erythrocytes. Recently a rapid ancillary method has been developed for prenatal diagnosis of galactosemia. In this method, the amniotic fluid of a fetus is analysed for elevated level of galactitol by GC/MS, which indicates impaired transferase activity.

Nutrition support aims to prevent or improve symptoms and at the same time provide adequate energy and other nutrients to ensure normal growth and development of the infant. Treatment consists of the removal of all sources of lactose and galactose from the diet. It should be started from the first week of life.

Human milk contains 6 to 8 per cent lactose, cow's milk 4 to 5 per cent lactose and infant formulas 7 per cent lactose. These milks must be replaced by a formula low in galactose. Soya protein isolate formulas have been found to be suitable, as it contains only 1.4 mg galactose per 100ml. in oligosaccharide forms which are not hydrolysed in the human intestine.

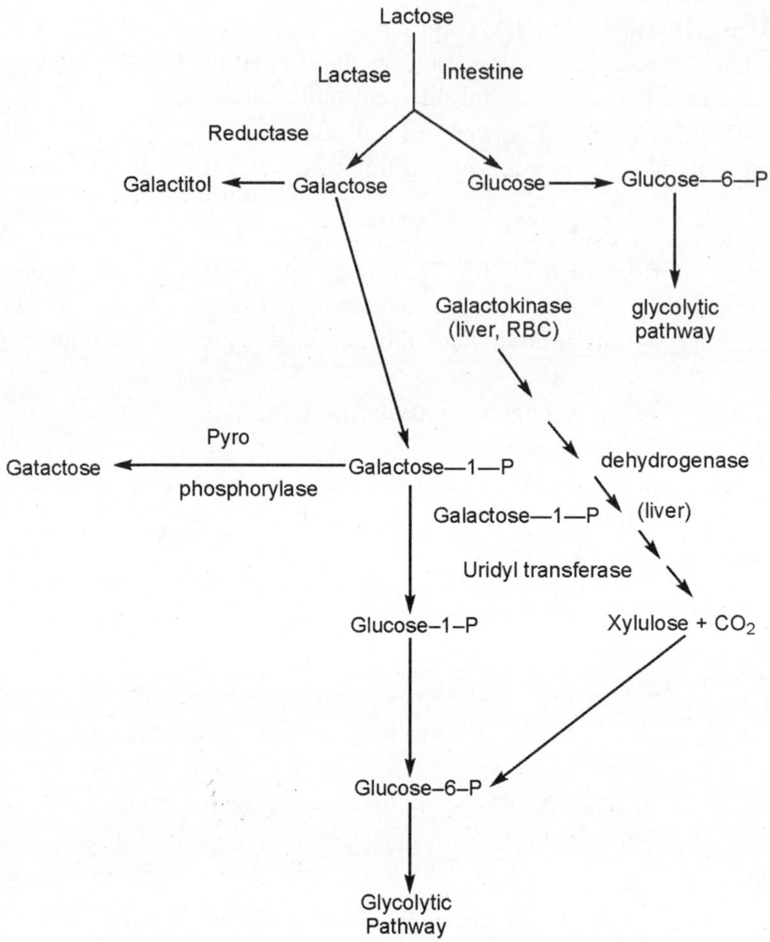

Figure 34.1 Metabolic blocks in galactose metabolism that lead to galactosemia. Genetic disorders of catalyssed reactions are indicated by hatched bars

As the child grows, solid foods are added to the diet, after proper scrutiny to avoid lactose containing foods. Even fermented dairy products and aged cheeses must be excluded from the diet, as the conversion of lactose to lactic acid is not complete in these.

Foods allowed - in galactose restricted diets are – cooked rice, chapaties, millet breads made without milk addition, home-made cakes, puddings, pasta, all dals, legumes, nuts and seeds.

Fats – Oils, nuts, shortenings.

Sugar Beverages – carbonated drinks, fruit juices other than apple, grape, pear and papaya.

Meat, fish, poultry – all primary products, not prepared ones, which contain milk or milk products.

Soups – clear soups, dal soups, vegetable soups made with vegetables allowed.

Vegetables – asparagus, beets, cabbage, cauliflower, celery, corn, cucumbers, brinjal, lettuce, ladies' finger, potatoes, spinach and yams.

Miscellaneous foods – Popcorn, pure sugar candy, jelly or marmalade, sugar, corn syrup, pickles, pure spices and seasoning, molasses, honey.

Foods excluded - All milk and milk products, all cheeses, commercial cakes, biscuits, custard, puddings, ice cream, Omelets and souffles containing milk,

Butter, cream, cream cheese, salad dressings containing lactose, non-dairy cream sweeteners containing sodium/calcium caseinate, diet through life All canned or frozen fruits containing lactose,

Apples, bananas, dates, figs, grapes, kiwi fruit, papaya, pears, persimmon, water melon, All legumes, fermented soyabean products; hazelnuts, safflower seed kernel,

Vegetables – bell peppers, broccoli, carrots, onions, peas, pumpkin, sweet potatoes, tomatoes,

Miscellaneous – chewing gum, milk chocolates, some cocoas, toffee, peppermint, caramels, certain drugs and vitamins and mineral preparations,

Spice blends with added lactose, artificial sweeteners containing lactose.

Galactosemic patients need to follow galactose-restricted diet to avoid damaging effects of accumulated galactitol in lens, liver and kidneys.

Endocrine Disorders

Hypothyroidism: Hypo, that is decreased secretion of thyroid hormones (thyroxine) by the thyroid gland, leads to lowering of metabolic rate. Mild form of this disorder is common and affects women more often than men. Overweight is common due to lower metabolic rate. Screening of newborns helps to detect it and start treatment early.

Severe hypothyroidism in adults is known as myxoederma. In this condition, the metabolic rate is very much reduced. It results in weight gain, flabby muscles, lethargy, constipation and high blood lipids. Severe lowering of metabolic rate in fetal life is known as cretinism and is discussed in Chapter 13.

Treatment: A synthetic hormone is given to make up for the missing thyroid hormone. Dietary fiber is increased to prevent constipation. A calorie restricted diet helps to maintain normal weight in overweight patients.

Hyperthyroidism: The metabolic rate is increased by 50 per cent due to excessive secretion of the thyroid gland. As a result of increased metabolic rate, the appetite is increased resulting in hyperactivity, nervousness, rapid heartbeat and loss of weight. The thyroid gland is enlarged; the eyes are prominent and there is double vision. Liver glycogen is rapidly lost due to increased metabolism and there is tissue wasting. Increased excretion of calcium and phosphorus may cause osteoporosis

Treatment: A high calorie (4000 – 5000 kcal) and high protein (100 – 125 g) diet is required to reverse the weight loss and tissue wastage until normal nutritional status is attained.

Intake of snacks between meals helps to increase calorie intake and satisfy hunger. Multivitamin mineral supplements are often given. Foods containing caffeine are avoided due to their stimulating effect.

To reduce the metabolic rate to normal, antithyroid drugs are used in most cases. Tranquilisers are given to control cardiac and hyperactivity effects.

Study Questions

1. What are the approaches to treat metabolic disorders?
2. What is PKU? How can it be treated?
3. Write short notes on: maple syrup urine disease, galactosemia, hypothyroidism.

CHAPTER

35

Nutrition in Stress, Burns and Surgery

Definition

Stress can be mental, emotional or physical. Stress disturbs the normal steady state (homeostasis) of the body. The extent of alteration in nutritional needs depends on the kind and extent of stress imposed on the body.

Emotional and **mental stress** is caused by anxiety, worries and tension due to a variety of situations real and sometimes imaginary. The ability of individuals to handle stress varies.

Emotional stress is one of the factors, which is found to cause some serious conditions such as peptic ulcer, hypertension, cardiovascular disease and even cancer. Some of the common emotional stress situations include sudden death of a near relative (child, mate, parent), losing a job, divorce, financial problems, loss of limb in accident and even inability to cope with change such as job, location, new family member etc.

Physical stress **includes burns or thermal injury and surgery.**

Nutritional Requirements During Stress

These are affected by three main factors:

(*a*) the kind of stress – its severity, extent and period.

(*b*) nutritional status of the patient

(*c*) age of the patient.

Food intake is often reduced due to stress; the body reserves are of great importance. Thus a person in optimal nutrition state before stress can face the stress situation better as he/she can call on the body reserves.

Burns

Burns are one of the leading cause of accidental death in India. Burns or thermal injury impose an unparalleled stress on the human body. The percentage of body surface area involved, the extent of cellular damage and the area of the body affected would determine the severity of the burns.

Burns are usually classified as follows:

First Degree: If only the epidermis is affected, it is a first degree burn. It is important to provide oral fluids to replace losses due to oozing and give medication for pain relief.

Second Degree: Second degree burns are very painful as both epidermis and dermis are injured, resulting in exposure of nerve endings. It is important to maintain aseptic and hygienic condition of the affected part to avoid infection. The dietary treatment consists of ample fluids and provision of adequate nutrients in the diet to ensure quick healing.

Third Degree: In third degree burns, both epidermis and dermis are destroyed, nerve fibers are also destroyed, resulting in lack of sensation and pain. When the layer of dead skin begins to separate, pain is felt. If the burns involve more than ten per cent of the body surface, nutrition support is essential to expedite recovery. This includes generous intake of fluids and adequate nutrient intake through a well planned diet.

Fourth Degree: In fourth degree burns, the subcutaneous tissue, muscle and bone are damaged. There is need for constant, well planned nutrition support to help recovery.

Burns interfere with normal functions of the skin; these include protection against infection, control of body temperature, fluid balance, sense of touch and the beauty of looks.

Diet: In the first few days after burn injury, it is very difficult to provide sufficient energy and proteins because of the hypermetabolic state of the body. When the stress response becomes moderate, it is easier to meet the needs for these nutrients.

The ascorbic acid intake is increased up to 1 g per day and a zinc supplement is often given to help wound healing process. Passive exercise helps to reduce protein loss. Use of layered dressings help to maintain body temperature and thus reduce protein losses. However, the nutrients and electrolytes lost through exudate or fluid leaking out of capillaries and urine needs to be replaced.

Mode of Feeding: Initially parenteral nutrition is required, if peristalsis is absent due to shock. When gastrointestinal function has returned, there is a transition made to oral feeding or tube feeding, on the basis of the nature and site of burns. Special formulas are used for hypermetabolic states; protein supplements or modular feedings can be utilized.

Nutritional Assessment: As nutritional care plays a major part in recovery from burns, nutritional assessment from time to time is essential to monitor the patient's progress. The techniques used will be decided by the state of the patient.

Complications: One of the complications which occur are stress ulcers. Prevention of stress ulcers involves several steps, which include – fluid replacement to prevent hypovolemia, oxygen therapy to prevent hypoxia of gastric mucosa, nutrition support to nourish gastric mucosa and use of antacids to maintain gastric pH above 5.

Nutritional Care of Patient with Burns

Days 1-3 (Immediate shock period)

Loss of enveloping skin surface and exposure of extracellular fluids leads to immediate loss of interstitial water and electrolytes, mainly sodium and large protein depletion.

Fluid therapy:

(*i*) Colloid (protein) through blood and plasma transfusion

(*ii*) Electrolytes, sodium and chlorine by use of saline solutions – lactated Ringer's solution

(*iii*) Water {dextrose solution) to cover additional insensible losses

Recovery period (days 3 to 5): Intravenous therapy is discontinued and oral solutions such as Holdene's is used

Holdene's solution (oral fluid and electrolyte replacement)

3 – 4 g (1/2 tsp) salt

1.5 – 2 g (1 ½ tsp) baking soda (sodium bicarbonate)

1,000 ml water

+ lemon juice for flavour and chill

A careful check of fluid intake and output is essential with constant check of dehydration over hydration.

Secondary Feeding Period (6–15 days): Optimal nutritional therapy necessary to

(*a*) make up for tissue destruction in which protein and electrolytes are lost

(*b*) due to continued nitrogen losses due to tissue catabolism

(*c*) due to increased metabolic demands of infection (extra calories + B vit.), fever and tissue regeneration (protein + vit.C)

(*d*) to have optimal tissue health necessary for subsequent grafting to be successful.

Principles of Diet Therapy

A high protein, high calorie and high vitamins diet is needed to ensure rebuilding of tissues damaged/destroyed and catabolised. The protein requirement varies from 150 – 400 g/day. Simultaneously the calorie need varies from 3,500 – 5,000cal/day. Intake of high carbohydrate foods is suggested. The need for vitamins is very high to ensure recovery. The recommended vitamin C intake is 1 – 2 g. per day. There is a need for increased intake of thiamine, riboflavin and niacin to metabolize the extra carbohydrates and protein in the diet.

Intake record – A careful record of protein and calories in the amount of food consumed is a necessary tool for planning care.

A diet plan to be followed in recovery period is given below.

Diet Plan

Breakfast	*Lunch and Dinner*
Egg	Chapati 2
Bread + Butter	Dal
Bananas	Rice
Milk	Dahi
In between	Vegetables
Buttermilk, custard,	
Dahi + roasted methi powder	
Milk + milk powder + flavour	

Accidental Injury

A number of accidental injuries lead to physical stress. These include vehicular accidents, stab wounds or other accidental injury. These result in pain, shock with possibility of loss of blood, fluids and/or electrolytes. If there are fractures, in addition, the healing is more complicated.

There is a loss of protein rich fluids from open wounds, which needs to be replaced. Healing of fractures may involve bed rest, which increases loss of calcium due to lack of movement.

Nutritional Care: The losses in injury have to be replaced and needs of healing have to be met.

In the first 24-48 hours after injury, the blood volume and electrolyte balance needs to be maintained.

Next, the diet must help to resist infection, ensure healing, restore muscular strength and avoid weight loss.

Nutrients Needed: (*a*) Sufficient protein and calories to meet the above-mentioned needs

(*b*) In case of fracture, additional calcium and vit. D need to be provided

(*c*) Intakes of Vit. B complex be increased in proportion to increase in calories and protein

(*d*) Vits. A and C to ensure wound healing and prevent infection

Intake of drinks providing high protein and calories between meals ensure adequate nutrient intake and utilization. The mode of feeding - oral, tube feeding or parenteral route – depends upon the severity and location of the injury. (Refer to Chapter 25 for details of diets).

Surgery

It is good to remember that to aid recovery from surgery, nutritional support is necessary.

Some illnesses need surgery as a corrective measure, for example, appendicitis, removal of infected part, etc. Prior to surgery, the patient may have lost appetite due to illness or may have had restricted food intake. If there has been vomiting or diarrhea or loss of blood, these may result in losses of sodium, potassium chloride, iron in addition to fluid loss.

Prior to the operation, the patient is expected to fast. After operation, the patient may be given only clear-liquid diet. Thus the nutritional leak is further aggravated.

Nutritional Considerations

The most critical factor is protein status of the patient. It is known that the stress of surgery will increase protein losses for several days after surgery. So the patient is likely to be in negative nitrogen balance.

Nutrients needed are:

(*a*) Proteins for wound healing, to ensure resistance to infection and to protect liver from toxicity of anesthesia.

(*b*) Energy to maintain or restore desirable weight, spare proteins.

(*c*) Ascorbic acid supplements to ensure wound healing.

(*d*) Iron supplements or transfusions to cover blood loss.

(*e*) Zinc supplements to promote wound healing and cell-mediated immunity.

If nutritional status prior to surgery is improved, the surgical risk is reduced. If the patient is underweight, weight gain may be beneficial. Likewise, weight loss may improve the status of obese patients. However, rapid loss is not recommended as it may result in tissue breakdown.

Hence post-operative nutritional care assumes great importance. A 30 to 50 per cent increase in calorie and protein intake above maintenance level is needed to help gain weight if the patient is underweight.

Postoperative Diet: After a minor surgery, liquids may be tolerated within few hours and return to normal diet is rapid. In other cases, when peristalsis resumes, patients are progressively given ice chips, sips of water, a clear liquid, full liquid, soft and then normal diet. The diet is similar to that given in Tables 25.3 and 25.4. The rate of progression is dependent on the patient's condition and tolerance of food. If the patient is unable to take food orally or is not able to eat sufficient food, it is necessary to resort to tube feeding or parenteral feeding.

If a patient is dehydrated,, it is important to ensure rehydration, before planning surgery.

If the surgery is minor, a deficient intake for a few days may not pose a serious problem. But if the person is nutritionally depleted and has to undergo a major surgery, the matter may be serious. Therefore screening persons on admission to identify those at nutritional risk is very important.

Specific Surgery

Though the basic dietary needs of all surgery patients are similar in each case, attention to some specific aspects helps to ensure comfort of the patient.

Teeth: the diet is restricted to liquids (cool), followed by soft foods for multiple tooth extractions

Tonsillectomy: After the operation, cold bland food, low-fibre foods are given followed by soft foods, not too hot or cold and then to regular normal diet.

Gastrectomy: Removal of part or all of the stomach and vagotomy (cutting of the vagus nerve to relieve pain). In gastric cancer and sometimes for intractable peptic ulcer, part or all of the stomach(gastrectomy) and the vagus nerve (vagotomy) are removed surgically. Digestion of proteins and fats, absorption of iron, vit. B_{12} is adversely affected. In absence of vagus nerve, food flow through gastrointestinal tract is increased and diarrhea and steatorrhea are likely to occur. These problems result in the patient losing weight.

Hence diet modifications are a must to cope with these problems.

Dietary Modifications: 60-90 ml clear liquids are given each hour, after gastrectomy for first two days. A full-liquid or very low residue diet is allowed by third day. Vit. B_{12} is given by injection. Since tolerance is low, foods are introduced one by one, meals are very small and frequent. The order of introduction of foods is as follows:

(1) Cereals, milk, cream soups, fruit, purees, eggs, custards.

(2) Cottage cheese, pureed vegetables, tender chicken (in non-vegetarian diet)

Foods included should be rich in proteins, moderate in fat and low in sugars. Fluids are given between meals.

Dumping Syndrome

This is one of the problems faced by some patients after gastrectomy. This is mainly due to inappropriate composition of diet, with sugars being used as a CHO source. These patients suffer from nausea, weakness, sweating and faintness soon after eating. They often suffer from diarrhea, vomiting and lose weight. Due to absence of stomach, foods enter into the intestines directly. The water from blood circulation is tied up by the large amount of carbohydrates present and blood volume is reduced. This results in the symptoms given above.

The diet for this condition is given in Table 34.1. Intake of bulking agents before meals helps to slow intestinal motility.

Table 35-1: High Protein, Moderate Fat, Low CHO Diet

Diet Pattern
Include 100-120g complex CHO daily
Avoid simple sugars, syrups, sweet desserts etc.
Include liberal protein and moderate fat.
Take 6 small meals regularly every day. Take liquids 30-60 minutes after meals. Avoid very hot or very cold food
Eat slowly, chew food well and rest before and after meals
Include vitamins and mineral supplements
Plan the diet to suit individuals e.g. some patients cannot tolerate milk.
Foods allowed each day
Egg-1, soft or hard cooked, scrambled or poached.
Low fat milk: 300 ml, if tolerated - take ½ - 1 hr after meals
Dals : Mung, masur, cooked - 50 g.
Fish, Poultry, Meat: all kinds, baked, boiled (not fried), stewed – 8 oz.
Chapati – 1 chapati per meal or 1 slice enriched bread per meal
Bread substitutes: rice, boiled or mashed potato or sweet potato, spaghetti, macaroni noodles
Cereal: one serving
Vegetables: all kinds one serving per meal
Fruits: fresh, one serving per meal
Fruit juices between meals
Fats: butter, cream, oil
Nuts: if tolerated

In conclusion, surgery, burns, fevers and infections are traumas which lead to increased pace of metabolism in the body. Thus there is a need for increased supply of nutrients in the diet. At the same time, the injury causes a loss of nutrients from the body.

Therefore, the diet must be modified to provide extra fluid, proteins, energy, vitamins and minerals as required in these conditions. When surgery is preplanned or elective, the nutritional status must be improved before surgery. When food cannot be taken orally, enteral or parenteral nutrition should be used.

Study Questions

1. What is stress? How are nutritional needs affected by stress?
2. Discuss the various degrees of burns and the nutritional care of the patient with burns.
3. What is accidental injury and how are the nutritional needs of the patient met?
4. Discuss the nutritional needs of a patient who has undergone surgery.
5. What is a dumping syndrome?

CHAPTER

36

Nutrition: Addictive Behaviours in Anorexia Nervosa, Bulimia and Alcoholism

Definitions

Addictive behaviours are compulsive ways of living (eating, drinking, etc.). Anorexia nervosa and Bulimia are addictive behaviours related to food intake, while alcoholism is the result of addiction to alcohol and alcoholic drinks. There are no simple causes or solutions to eating and drinking disorders. Each case has to be studied and the patient helped to normalcy with patience and perseverance.

Though eating disorders have been known since the Middle Ages, the incidence of eating disorders is on the rise in the developed countries. One of the contributing factors is the breakdown of social structure resulting in isolation of individuals. Luckily there is hardly any report of these in India, but one needs to watch and prevent these, as the treatment and rehabilitation of persons suffering from eating disorders is very slow and expensive.

The incidence of alcoholism is on the increase in all strata of population in India. It needs to be stemmed as it affects the well being of the whole family adversely

All these disorders result in the deterioration of the nutritional status of the person; therefore nutritional rehabilitation of the patient is a very important part of therapy.

Eating Disorders

Anorexia nervosa implies loss of appetite. It can aptly be described as denying one's appetite. In USA one per cent girls in the age range of 12 to 18 years suffer from it. Its occurrence in males and adults is not common. Girls whose profession demands maintaining ultra slim figures (such as models, dancers, athletes) have long standing histories of eating disorders. **Bulimia means** "ox-hunger" or being as hungry as an ox. The persons suffering from bulimia go on a eating binge often and feel guilty. So they try to get rid of the food by forced vomiting, fasting, taking diuretics or using laxatives. They keep their binge –purge behaviour a secret and hence it is difficult to identify the disorder until the stress of these episodes results in some visible impact on the system. Even male athletes(runners, wrestlers, swimmers, etc.) and pilots also resort to binge-purge practices.

Causes: Addictive behaviours have multiple causes – emotional, psychological, social and biological, which result in disordered eating. Stress may have a strong role and lack of appropriate coping mechanism is another common factor.

Symptoms of Anorexia Nervosa: The anorectic patient is often 20 to 40 per cent below desirable weight for the age and stature and appears to be skin and bones. Other symptoms are lowered body temperature, slower basal metabolism, decreased heart rate (hence easy fatigue, fainting, sleepiness), iron-deficiency anemia, rough dry scaly and cold skin from a poor nutrient intake, low white blood cell count (increasing risk of infection and death), loss of hair, constipation (and laxative abuse), loss of menstrual periods and deterioration of teeth due to frequent vomiting, An anorectic person is psychologically and physically ill and needs help.

Treatment of Anorexia Nervosa: The patient is often a victim of isolation and fear. Hence the health team must include a psychologist in addition to a physician, dietitian and other health personnel. They should all work together to restore a sense of balance, purpose and future with the cooperation of the patient. The first step is to help the patient to gain weight, as a psychiatrist cannot counsel a starving person.

Nutrition Therapy: The first step is to increase the person's food intake. This will help to stop weight loss and may help weight gain. The next is to restore regular food habits. The third is to ensure that the patient keeps in weekly contact with the dietitian. In all this it is critical to allow the person to feel in control of her life in the early stage of treatment. There should be no surprises, as these may be detrimental to progress. Anorectics are very clever and resistant. They try to disguise weight loss or fake weight gain by wearing many layers of clothes, putting coins in the pocket and drinking a lot of water before weighing. One needs to gain their trust to be able to help them.

The nutritional rehabilitation is slow. The nutritional care consists of going through the stages of liquid to soft to full diet. (refer to Chapter 24)

The mode of feeding will depend on the condition of the patient. It is important to educate the patient and help her/his family. Some points to note in the treatment of anorectics are:

1. Patients need to be given intravenous feedings to restore fluid and electrolyte balance, when the patient is in a critical state and is likely to get dehydrated.
2. When patient's nutritional state is precarious, give peripheral parenteral nutrition to support oral intake.
3. Get patients to be partners in the efforts to restore satisfactory nutritional status; attain normal weight and develop normal eating patterns.
4. Anorectics are intelligent patients. Educate them about their normal growth pattern and the intake to meet the needs for their growth. This will enable them to set goals to attain their normal growth gradually.
5. Lastly **avoid** food being the centre point of their day. They need to take interest in recreational activities – music, games, reading, enjoying family company, making friends etc. to get back to enjoying normal life of which food is an important part.

Bulimia Nervosa

An increasing number of youngsters, especially females (models, actresses, dancers, athletes and others) go through stages of eating large amounts of foods (high fat sweets) and then get rid of it by vomiting. This disorder is called **bulimia nervosa**. Bulemics may eat 3,000 to 5,000 calories in one extended binge and then vomit to get rid of it. With repeated episodes, they may have chloride and potassium deficiencies, which may lead to heart damage and other complications.

Bulemics suffer from low self-esteem and depression. It is necessary to help a bulemic develop self-esteem through understanding self worth, develop a positive attitude, learn to take pleasure in simple activities (listening to music, reading, writing, drawing, sewing, knitting, gardening, playing games, etc.) and avoid depressing inactivity. Most bulemics have irregular food habits and they may be underweight and undernourished.

Diet for Bulemics

Bulemics need to understand about effects of starvation on the body, their nutrient needs and how to meet these through planned diet modification. Bulemics need to recognise that their primary aim is the stabilization of their body weight without having to go through binging and purging, which disturbs and hurts the body's well being. Some points to note in their treatment are:

1. Help patients to understand and plan a diet which meets their normal nutritional needs. The actual calorie expenditure needs are determined by measuring oxygen consumption.
2. Plan the diet using basic food guide. (Chapter 24, Table 24.1). The foods thus selected meet the mineral and vitamins needs (refer to Table 24.1). Hence supplements are not necessary.
3. The patient can be helped to select a varied diet, after taking her likes and dislikes into account.
4. Teach how to measure or weigh foods to give confidence that there will be no over- eating.
5. Personalized meal plans (3 meals + snacks) with wide variety of foods helps acceptance.
6. Avoid excessive bulk in the initial stages to have a third of stomach empty.
7. Gradually increase intake by 200 calories until the norm is reached.
8. Avoid fasting, skipping meals and eating inadequate amounts at a meal as it leads to binges. Keep food record.

These measures help to develop confidence in themselves and make them self-reliant in managing their diet.

Alcoholism

People offer beverages to companions in social gatherings. Some people choose alcohol over other beverages such as juice, coffee, tea, soft drinks or milk. For some of these people, alcohol use becomes a life-shattering addiction, alcoholism, which leads to severe malnutrition, physical illness and erosion or loss of self-esteem.

Persistent intake of amounts of alcohol that exceed the daily permitted levels indicates a dependence that needs to be recognized as addiction and dealt with. Malnutrition, as well as impaired digestion and absorption, is now considered a result of chronic alcohol consumption.

Alcoholism is a major chronic disease. It is also a major social problem which afflicts a large section of society, irrespective of economic status. It accounts for more than half of fatal car accidents. As the drinker gets abusive, violent and/or incapable, the effects of alcoholism on the family are devastating. The help of an outside agency such as **Alcoholics Anonymous** is needed to help rehabilitation. However, for such help to have any success, the addict needs to admit that she/he has a problem and really wants to give up drinking. Until she/he reaches that point and starts to co-operate in rehabilitation, the life of the family can be of unbearable misery.

Effect of Alcohol Intake

Alcoholic beverages contain ethanol, which liberates 7.1 kcal/g.. If it replaces half the intake of food in a balanced diet, it results in malnutrition and malfunction. Chronic alcohol consumption may alter digestion and absorption of food. Ethanol disrupts the gastric mucosal barrier and causes acute gastritis. Massive bleeding and hence iron deficiency may accompany acute gastritis. Alcohol may increase acid secretion. Even in the absence of any legions, alcohol abuse reduces intestinal enzymes. Intake of excessive alcohol (1g/ kg) results in lesions in the duodenum and functional changes in the small intestines. This may give rise to diarrhea, malabsorption of folate, thiamine, B_{12}, fat and xylose, changes in pancreatic secretion and bile salt metabolism.

The most significant complication in alcoholics is liver disease (fatty liver. hepatitis and cirrhosis) which aggravates the malnourished state. The second organ affected is heart leading to heart disease. Beriberi may result due to thiamine deficiency. Deficiencies of pyridoxine and folate may result in abnormalities in blood synthesis. The nervous disorders result in decreased fine movements. Besides thiamine, deficiency of other B vitamins may also lead to these disorders.

The success of nutritional therapy depends on two points. The first is removal of the cause – abstinence from alcohol. The second is nutritional care of the patient to reverse the organ damage to ensure healing and regain normal function.

Alcoholic fatty liver is the earliest stage of liver injury. This is a completely reversible stage. Abstinence from alcohol and specific therapy for nutritional deficiencies helps recovery. However, the alcoholic should not be led to believe that mere correction or prevention of nutritional inadequacies will fully protect against liver damage.To this end, abstinence from alcohol and specific therapy for nutritional deficiencies helps recovery.

Diet, which provides normal protein low fat and extra vitamins, remains the mainstay of the treatment. Several times the daily requirements of water soluble vitamins are given. Sufficient calorie intake is necessary to prevent the breakdown of proteins in the body. One indicator of calorie sufficiency is weight gain, if the patient is underweight, and weight maintenance, if the patient has not lost weight due to excess alcohol intake,

Complications: When the patient has neuropsychiatric symptoms, she/he may need hospitalisation to ensure abstinence and special nutritional care.

In case of ascites and edema, dietary intake and salt restriction will need to be monitored according to the severity of the condition. In extreme cases, sodium may be restricted to 250 mg per day. As the severity decreases, sodium intake may be increased to 500 mg or more per day.

Neurologic disorders in the alcoholic include peripheral neuropathy, in which thiamine B_{12}, pyridoxine, nicotinic acid, pantothenic acid and riboflavin deficiencies are associated. It is treated with abstinence and B-vitamin therapy. Though optimal dosage is not established, one recommendation is 10 times the normal requirement for 1 week and 5 times the daily needs after that.

Iron deficiency in the alcoholic needs to be treated cautiously. In patients with liver disease, excess iron may lead to liver damage. The patient may respond simply to abstinence and vitamin supplementation.

In case of beri-beri heart disease, thiamine repletion of 5 to 10 mg per day is likely to be sufficient, along with adequate diet and alcohol abstinence.

The **interactions of alcohol and nutrition** are presented in Table 36.1. Thus multiple nutrient deficiencies result from reduced food intake and interference with nutrient use in the body.

Table 36.1 Effects of Alcohol Intake on Nutrition

1. Alcohol is empty calories, it displaces food, hence nutrients.
2. Alcohol reduces food intake resulting in inadequate nutrient intake.
3. Alcohol disrupts every tissue's metabolism of nutrients.
   - (*i*) Stomach cells over-secrete both acid and histamine (which causes inflammation); extra acid may cause ulcers in stomach and esophagus linings.
   - (*ii*) Intestinal cells fail to absorb thiamin, folate, Vit. B_6 and other vitamins.
   - (*iii*) Liver cells lose efficiency in activating Vit. D and change their synthesis and elimination of bile.
   - (*iv*) Retinal cells process alcohol instead of Vit. A alcohol (retinoal) thus damaging vision
   - (*v*) Kidneys excrete essential ,minerals (magnesium, calcium, potassium and zinc) thus creating deficiency of these minerals.
4. Alcohol metabolites interfere with Vit. B_6 metabolism and thus reduce RB cells production.
5. Excessive alcohol expels folate from of all its sites of action and storage. Thus liver storage of folate is leaked to blood to kidneys. Blood is excreted from the kidneys. Intestines fail to retrieve folate leading to folate deficiency. This inhibits synthesis of new intestinal and blood cells.

Nutrition Therapy: Patients treated for alcohol addiction need simultaneous optimal nutrition therapy to reverse nutritional deficiencies that occur. These include night blindness (Vit. A)), beriberi, (thiamine), pellagra (niacin), scurvy (Vit. C) and protein-energy-malnutrition. Therefore there is a need for adequate intake to ensure recovery of the patient.

Study Questions

1. What are addictive behaviours?
2. Discuss the symptoms and the points to note in the treatment of an anoretic.
3. What are the important points to note while treating bulimics?
4. List the effects of alcohol on the human system.

CHAPTER

37

Nutrient Drug Interaction

Introduction

Diet and drugs are both necessary to treat and cure diseases. With increase in the medications available to patients and widespread use of drug therapy to control of chronic disease, it is necessary to identify risks of nutritional side effects. In addition, we need to know that the predicted and intended therapeutic effects of drugs are not altered by diet. Some drugs may have adverse effect on the utilisation of some nutrients. So it is necessary to understand their relationship and maximise their utility by judicious planning.

Interaction between diet and drugs is significant in

(*a*) Those who need long term drug therapy.
(*b*) Those who are malnourished.
(*c*) Those suffering from chronic diseases.
(*d*) Those who have undergone surgery.
(*e*) Those who are obese
(*f*) High-risk segments of population

Interactions of frequently used drugs with nutrients are given in Table 37.1.

High Risk Segments of Population

These include developing fetus, infants (especially premature ones), pregnant women, chronically ill persons and elderly persons.

In late pregnancy increased concentrations of the transport protein for most drugs results in drug concentration in the fetus.

Young children (including infants) have high requirements of nutrients per kg body weight; hence drugs that decrease absorption or increase excretion of a nutrient affects them adversely.

Many elderly persons suffer from chronic diseases and have to take several drugs for prolonged periods. Their food intake is often inadequate. They may take wrong drugs at times. Thus this segment of elderly need special assistance to avoid adverse nutrient drug interaction.

Some commonly used drugs include analgesics (pain killers), cough, cold, sinus and allergy drugs, digestive aids, antacids, sleep aids (sedatives), appetite suppressants, diuretics, antibiotics etc. Many of these drugs are available without prescription. In addition, health enthusiasts take vitamin and mineral pills in the belief, if a little is good, a higher amount may be better for health. These create a scenario for an undesirable nutrient-drug interaction.

Nutrient Absorption

Most nutrients and drugs are absorbed in the small intestine. Hence it is the major site for nutrient-drug intervention.

The absorption of nutrients may be adversely affected by drugs, if the transit time is altered. Laxatives tend to reduce nutrient absorption by reducing the transit time. If the pH of stomach contents is increased due to drugs (e.g. antacids), the absorption of iron, calcium, zinc and folates is reduced.

Fat and fat-soluble vitamins are poorly absorbed, when drugs are taken to reduce cholesterol by the patient; neomycin (an antibiotic) has the same effect.

High doses of antacids (aluminium or magnesium hydroxide) can cause phosphate depletion, leading to muscle weakness, loss of appetite (anorexia) and even congestive heart failure. Diuretics (thiazide and furosemide) can cause sodium, potassium and magnesium depletion leading to loss of appetite and muscle weakness.

Drug Absorption

A drug is a chemical, which interacts with the metabolic process in the body to bring about a desirable effect. Drug action can occur **only** after it is dissolved, carried to the target site and absorbed. About 75 per cent of oral drugs will generally be absorbed in 1 to 3 hours.

The metabolism of many drugs and a variety of foreign compounds is carried out by the mixed-function-oxidase system (MFOS). Almost all nutrients are components of the MFO system. These include proteins, lipids, B-complex vitamins (nicotinic acid, riboflavin and pantothenic acid), fat soluble vitamins (A and E) and minerals (iron, copper, calcium, zinc and magnesium).

When food enters the stomach, the gastric pH is lowered by dilution and stomach emptying is delayed. These factors may reduce the absorption rate and hence the effectiveness of the drugs. In view of this, it is advisable to take pain relievers (analgesics), fever reducing drugs (antipyretics), antiinfectives for acute infections and antihistamines on an empty stomach for rapid recovery. Aspirin and antibiotics are also better absorbed in a fasting state.

Almost a billion dollars is spent each year in the United States of America on antacids, making these products among the most popular over-the-counter (OTC) drugs. These tablets and liquids are gulped down for the relief of heartburn, sour stomach and indigestion. Antacids may also be prescribed to treat stomach ulcers.

Table 37.1: Interactions of Frequently Used Drugs with Nutrients[2]

Drug	*Possible Effects*	*Time of Intake*
Antipyretic Aspirin Acetaminophen	Nausea and vomiting Gastric pain or bleeding G.I. irritation	Take on empty stomach for quick relief; with food to reduce gastric disturbance.
Antibiotic		
Amoxicillin	Diarrhea, nausea, vomiting	
Ampicillin or Penicillin	-do- Glossitis, stomatitis	Take on empty stomach
Erythromycin	Stomach ache, diaarhea, nausea and vomiting	Take on empty stomach
Tetracycline	Loss of hunger, diarrhea, glossitis, nausea, vomiting. Difficulty in swallowing	Take with water on empty stomach Do not take dairy foods or iron containing foods within 3 hours
Bronchodilator		
Theophylline	Loss of hunger, stomach upset nausea and vomiting	Take with food
Antihypertensive		
Atenolol	diarrhea, nausea.	
Propranolol	stomach ache, constipation, diarrhea, nausea and vomiting; decreased CHO tolerance	Take with food
Cardiotonic		
Digoxin	Loss of hunger, diarrhea, nausea and vomiting; increased urinary losses of minerals	Take on empty stomach, avoid increased sodium, avoid bran, take adequate K.
Diuretics		
Chlorthalidone	Loss of hunger, constipation, diarrhea, stomach pain, decreased CHO tolerance, electrolyte imbalance	Take with food, reduce Na intake, take adequate protein.
Antiinflammatory		
Ibuprofen Naproxen	Abdominal upset and pain, edema flatulence, G.I.bleeding, heartburn, nausea and vomiting	Take with food; avoid alcohol
Steroidal Antinflammatory		
Prednisone	Indigestion, fluid and electrolyte imbalance, fluid and Na retention, -ve N balance, peptic ulcer	Take with food, reduce Na intake, increase K, protein vit. D intake, reduce CHO intake, avoid alcohol

2. Adapted from Lecos, C.W. FDA Consumer, **21**: 22–27, 1987–1988

Although many consumers take antacids almost casually, these drugs are not as harmless as they may seem. Antacids can affect the way other drugs behave in the body. They can speed the absorption of some prescription drugs, possibly causing an overdose, or slow it for others thus reducing their effectiveness.

Some nutrients and food components can decrease food absorption and hence its effectiveness. These include amino acids from high protein diet, dairy products and iron from iron supplements.

Therefore it is advisable to time intake of food and drugs at appropriate intervals to get the best results, since one needs both for proper recovery.

Effect of Drugs on Food Intake

Food intake is affected by drugs taken by the patient. The effects can include decrease or increase in appetite and taste, nausea and vomiting. For example, antacids, caffeine, cough medicines, antihistamines can decrease appetite.

Drugs taken to reduce weight are intended to reduce appetite. But their effectiveness is reduced rapidly. Hence their utility in weight reduction regimen is limited.

Antibiotics and many chemotherapy agents (for cancer) may cause diarrhea or vomiting and thus reduce food intake.

Some drugs may be a source of nutrients which may not be appropriate for some patients. For example, cough medications may contain sugar; antibiotics and antacids may contain sodium.

Nutrient Metabolism

Some drugs used as anticonvulsants may cause calcium loss and folate deficiency. Calcium loss may lead to osteomalacia on prolonged use of anticonvulsants. Hence the need for nutrient supplements with these drugs. In contrast, the effectiveness of some drugs such as levadopa and coumarin is reduced due to vitamin supplements (pyridoxine and vitamin K) respectively.

Some drugs block enzymatic action involved in DNA synthesis and thus lead to the death of a cell. This is the principle used in the chemotherapy of cancer.

Two common antivitamins, used as drugs, are the folate antagonists, methotrexate (MRX) (used in the treatment of leukemia and rheumatoid arthritis) and pyrimethamine (used in the treatment of malaria and ocular toxoplasmosis) are folate antagonists. These drugs displace folic acid from the related enzyme and the unbound folic acid is excreted. In the absence of folic acid, DNA synthesis is inhibited, cell synthesis stops and the cell dies.

Isoniazid, which is used in the long-term treatment of TB, forms a complex with the B-vitamin, pyridoxine, which may lead to its deficiency in some patients. Anticoagulants used in treatment are intentional vitamin K antagonists. If there is damage to intestinal mucosa, it can decrease the rate of drug absorption. The acidity of the gastrointestinal tract also affects drug disposition. A more acidic environment reduces the availability of penicillin and isoniazid but increases the absorption of tetracyclines. Food decreases, delays or enhances the absorption of some antibiotics.

Alcohol

Alcohol is not prescribed as a drug. But it is a chemical, which affects nutrition in many ways. It yields 7 calories/gramme, but not much of other nutrient. It is a habit-forming drink; hence its use is best avoided.

Alcohol can cause nausea and thus decrease appetite. Alcohol abuse commonly results in deficiencies of thiamin, folate, vitamin B_6, vit. A and zinc.

Caffeine

Caffeine, an addictive chemical, is present in tea, coffee, soft drinks and chocolates, which are consumed by all age groups. It is reported that an average healthy person can take moderate amounts of caffeine without any harmful effects.

An intake of 1000mg/day or more of caffeine can cause diarrhea, headache, heartburn and sleeplessness.

Even in smaller amounts, caffeine can act as a diuretic. It can also increase a basal metabolic rate and heart rate.

More than 1000 over-the-counter drugs, which need no prescription, contain caffeine. These drugs include those used to increase alertness and avoid sleepiness, headache and cold remedies and even weight-control drugs.

It is important to note that caffeine does not reverse the effects of alcohol, as it is commonly believed and hence does not help in 'sobering up' after excessive intake of alcohol.

MAOI Inhibitors

The most harmful drug-nutrient interaction is the one between the enzyme Monoamine Oxidase Inhibitors and blood-pressure elevating (pressor) amines, especially tyramine.

MAOI (Monoamine Oxidase inhibitors) are used as drugs. These include antidepressants, antimicrobials, antineoplastics and antihypertesnsive drugs.

Normally, the enzyme MAO (Monoamine Oxidase) inactivates the pressor agents and thus prevents the release of excess of norepinephrine, a hormone. The MAOIs block this reaction and the levels of norepinephrine rise unchecked. This can lead to reactions such as headaches, hypertension, palpitations etc. Major strokes have been reported in extreme cases. The severity of reaction is affected by the dosage of the drug and the level of dietary tyramine.

The tyramine content of foods is increased by aging (as in fermentation or spoilage). Hence it is best to take fresh foods in diet, when a person is on MAOI therapy. It is also advisable to avoid foods stored for long periods and those likely to have bacterial contamination. Alteration to restrict tyramine in the diet must be made some days before starting MAOI therapy and be continued for 3 – 4 weeks after the therapy.

Precautions to be taken

The unrestricted buying and ingestion of drugs bought over the counter is a cause of concern in developing countries like India where there is little supervision of the sale of drugs, especially for those needing a medical doctor's prescription. Nutrient absorption can be reduced in such situations and in extreme cases may lead to incompatability reactions endangering life. This is more so with elderly persons as they are prone to taking drugs for various ailments.

In conclusion to quote Sizer and Whitney (1997)[(1)] " When you need to take a medicine, do so wisely. Ask your physician, pharmacist or health care provider for specific instructions about the doses, times and how to take them – for example, with meals or an empty stomach. If you notice new symptoms or if a drug does not seem to be working well, consult your physician.

1. Sizer and Whitney, *Nutrition Concepts and Controversies* p-511, 7th ed., West/Wadsworth, an International Thomson Publishing Co. 1997.

The only instruction people need about illicit drugs is to avoid them altogether for countless reasons. As for smoking and chewing tobacco, the same advice applies: don't take these habits up, or if you already have, take steps to quit. For drugs with lesser consequences to health, such as caffeine, use moderation.

Try to live life in a way that requites less chemical assistance. If sleepy, try a 15-minute nap or meditation instead of a 15-minute coffee break. The coffee will stimulate your nerves for an hour, but the alternatives will refresh your attitude for the rest of the day.

If you suffer from constipation, try getting enough exercise, fiber and water for a few days. Chances are that a laxative will be unnecessary.

The strategy being suggested here is to take control of your body, allowing your reliable, self-healing nature to make fine adjustments that you need not force with chemicals. Bodies have few requests, adequate nutrition, rest, exercise and hygiene. Give yours what it asks for, and let it function naturally, day-to-day, without interference from drugs."

Table 37.2: Caffeine Content of Some Foods and Beverages

Beverage/Food	*Amount (oz.)*	*Caffeine (mg)*
Coffee		
Brewed	5	40 – 180
Instant	5	30 – 120
Tea		
Brewed	5	20 – 110
Iced	6	34 – 38
Soft Drinks		
Coca-cola (regular and diet)	6	22
Pepsi-cola	6	19
Other		
Cocoa beverage	5	2 – 20
Chocolate milk	4	1 – 4
Milk chocolate	1	1 – 15

Study Questions

1. When is interaction between diet and drugs significant?
2. List the high-risk segments of population with reference to nutrient-drug interaction.
3. How do drugs affect nutrient absorption?
4. List the ill-effects of drugs on nutrient metabolism.
5. Discuss the action of MAOI inhibitors in the body.

Appendices

Appendix 1 – Mathematical Tools

Mathematical Tools Nutrition

You need a few mathematical concepts to study nutrition. These include addition, subtraction, multiplication and division. Besides these, you need to calculate simple ratios (percentages) and convert English units of measurement to metric units(which are decimal), for example, conversion of kcalories to kjoules, as in energy measurements. It is important to know this, as many scientific journals will accept energy units in kjoules only.

Percentages

When the total represents 100 parts, the term percent (%) refers to a part of this total. For example, if you get 90% on your nutrition test, it means you have correctly answered 90 out of the 100 questions asked and have answered 10 remaining questions incorrectly.You can master this concept by calculating the problems given below:

Question	**Answer**
What is 10% of 30?	$0.10 \times 30 = 3.0$
What is 35% of 10?	$0.35 \times 10 = 3.5$
What percent of 15 is 6?	$6/15 = 0.4$ or 40%

Thus you eat 20% of your RDA for vitamin C at breakfast, you would have had 12 milligrams of vitamin C in your breakfast (0.20×60 milligrams = 12 milligrams).

If you had 200 grammes carbohydrates, 25 grammes fat and 45 grammes protein in your diet yesterday, the percentage of total calories from each component would be :

Total calories = $(200 \times 4) + (25 \times 9) + (45 \times 4) = 1205$

Carbohydrates (% of total calories) = $(200 \times 4)/1205 = 66.3$ %

Fat (% of total calories) = $(25 \times 9)/1205 = 18.7$ %

Protein (% of total calories) = $(45 \times 4)/1205 = 15.0$ %

Thus a concept of percentages is important in study of nutrition, for it gives you an idea of the contribution of various nutrients to the over all diet. This is a concept, which is used frequently in nutrition.

The metric system

You are familiar with the metric system, in which the basic units are meter for length, gramme for weight and liter for volume. In the English system, the basic units are foot for length, pound for weight and cup for volume.

The metric weights, measures and their abbreviations are given below :

1 meter (m)	–	100 centimeters = 1,000 millimeters
1 kilogramme (kg)	–	1,000 grammes
1 gramme/gram (g)	–	1,000 milligrammes (mg)
1 liter	–	1,000 milliliters
20 drops	–	1 milliliter (ml)
1 teaspoon (tsp)	–	5 milliliters
1 tablespoon (T or tbsp)	–	3 teaspoons or 15 milliliters
1 cup (c)	–	16 tablespoons or 240 milliliters

Household measures

1 ladle	–	40 milliliters
1 tea cup	–	145 to 150 milliliters
1 katori (large)	–	175 milliliters

1 kilocalorie is the heat needed to raise the temperature of 1 kilogramme water from 14.5 to 15.5degree Centigrade.

1000 calories = 1 kilocalorie, which is the unit used in nutrition. Normally it is written as a calorie in nutrition textbooks.

English weights and measures and their metric equivalents

1 yard	–	3 feet	–	0.9144 m
1 foot (ft)	–	12 inches	–	30.48 cm.
1 inch	–	2.54 centimeters		
1 pound (lb)	–	16 ounces or 454.6 grammes		
1 ounce (oz)	–	28..3 grammes		
1 quart	–	4 cups		
1 cup	–	8 ounces		

Energy units are kilocalorie or normally called calorie is a metric unit.

The English energy unit are joule and kilojoule.

4.184 kilojoules (kj)	–	1 kilocalorie
1000 joules	–	1 kilojoule (kj)
1000 kilojoules	–	1 megajoule (mj)

With this knowledge you can calculate any metric quantity into English units and vice a versa.

Equivalents

20 drops	– 1 milliliter (1 ml)
1 teaspoon (tsp)	– 5 milliliters (ml)
1 tablespoon (T or tbsp)	– 3 teaspoons or 15 milliliters
1 cup (c)	– 16 tablespoons or 237 milliliters
1 Ladle	– 40 milliliter
1 tea cup	– 145-150 milliliter
1 katori (large)	– 175 milliliters

Abbreviations

tsp	–	teaspoon
T. or tbsp	–	tablespoon
c	–	cup
g	–	gramme/gram
ml	–	milliliter

Appendix 2 – Food Values

Food Exchange Lists

Two lists are included

1. Food Exchange List from the **Diet Manual of AIIMS,** New Delhi-110016.
2. Food Exchange System suggested by **SNDT University**, Mumbai-400049.

1. What is an Exchange List? (AIIMS)

It is a group of foods of the same caloric value and similar protein, fat and carbohydrate content that can be substituted for one another in a meal plan. Foods have been divided into six groups of exchanges. Any one of the exchange groups cannot by itself supply all the needed nutrients for a well-balanced diet. It requires all six of them put together as a team to supply the normal nutritional needs for good health. The **six** major exchanges are:

1. Milk exchange
2. Vegetable exchange
3. Fruit exchange
4. Cereals and pulses exchange
5. Meat exchange
6. Fat exchange

Milk Exchange

1. Glass (250) milk exchange or substitute contains –

Food	**Quantity**	
Toned Milk	1 glass 250 ml	CHO 10–12 gm
Skimmed Milk	1–1/2 glass	Protein 8 gm
Butter Milk	4 glasses	Fat 8 gm
Curds	250 gm (1 cup)	Calories 140–150
Fresh Paneer	50 gm	
Icecream	100 gm (1 small cup)	

Vegetable Exchange

Food Root Vegetables	Quantity	Group A
Arbi	40 gm	CHO 3 gm
Potato	40 gm	Proteins 2 gm
Zimikand	40 gm	Calories 20 gm
Kachalu	40 gm	
Sweet potato	40 gm	
Tapioca	25 gm	
Leafy Vegetables		**Group B**
Spinach	100 gm	CHO 6 gm
Bathua	100 gm	Proteins 2 gm
Cabbage	100 gm	Calories 32 gm
Sarson	100 gm	
Methi	100 gm	
Seasonal Vegetables		**Group C**
Lauki	100 gm	CHO 6–8 gm
Tinda	100 gm	Protein 2 gm
Brinjal	100 gm	Fats nil
Cauliflower	100 gm	Calories 32–40 gm
Knolkohl	100 gm	

Fruit Exchange

Foods	Approx. measures		
Apple	100 gm	1 medium	CHO 10 gm
Orange	100 gm	1 medium	Protein 1 gm
Banana	100 gm	1 small or big	Fats nil
Guava	100 gm	1 small	Calories 40 Kcal
Mausambi	100 gm	1 small	
Mangoes	100 gm	1 small dusheri or 1 big slice.	
Big grapes	100 gm	20 no.	
Cherries	100 gm	20 no.	
Musk melon	250 gm	1/4 of medium size	
Papaya	100 gm	1 slice	
Peaches	100 gm	2 medium	
Pears	150 gm	4 small	
Plums	100 gm	4 small	
Water melon	200 gm	1 cup	

Cereal Exchange

Foods	Approx. measures	
Bread	1-1/2 slice (1 lb bread)	CHO 17-18 gm
Bajra	small chapati	protein 2 gm
Barley	1/2 cup cooked	Fats Nil
Maize	1 small roti	Calories 80–85
Cornflakes	1/2 cup cooked	
Oat meal	1/2 cup cooked	
Rice	1/2 cup cooked	
Wheat flour	1-1/2 medium chapati	
Rice (puffed)	1 cup	
Sanvai	1/2 cup cooked	
Dalia (wheat)	1/2 cup cooked	
Macroni	1/2 cup cooked	
Biscuits	5–10 salt and 3–5 sweet	
Soyabean flour	2 table-spoon	

Legumes and Pulses

Foods	Approx. measures	
Bengal gram	1/2 cup cooked	CHO 15 gm
Bengal gram (roasted)	1/2 cup cooked	Proteins 5 gm
Besan	2 table spoon	Calories 80 Kcal
Black/Green/White gram/ Rajmah/Lobia/Soyabean	1/2 cup cooked	Fats : nil

Meat Exchange

Foods	Approx. measures	
Mutton	4 pieces or ribs	CHO 1–2 gm
Chicken	1 leg or breast	Fats 2–4 gm
Fish	2 pieces	Proteins 5 gm
Egg Hen	2 medium	Calories 65 Kcal
Paneer	40 gm	
Ham	25 gm (1 slice)	

Fat Exchange

Foods	Approx. measures	
Butter	15 gm	CHO nil
Ghee	11 gm	Fats 11 gm
Oil	11 gm	Proteins nil
Vanaspati	11 gm	Calories 100
Almonds	15 gm	
Cashew nuts	30 gm	
Peanuts	20 gm	

2. Food Exchange System Suggested by S.N.D.T. University, Mumbai

Cereals:	Each exchange provides 100 kcal 6–12 exchange can be taken 1 katori cooked rice 1 big or 1-1/2 small bread slice 1 katori rawa upama 1 chapati or 2 phulkas 4-5 puris 1 katori rice flakes
Pulses and Legume:	Each exchange gives 100 kcal 2–3 exchanges can be taken 1 katori *dal* (cooked) 1 katori legume/usal 1 katori varan
Nuts and Oilseeds:	Each exchange gives 100 kcal 1 handful of groundnuts/cashewnuts/til/almonds/pista 1/4 katori fresh coconut grated
Vegetables:	Each exchange supplies 25–30 kcal 2 exchanges or more can be taken
Vegetable A	1 katori vegetable (preferably dark green leafy vegetables)
Vegetable B	1 katori any other vegetable, e.g., ladies finger, brinjal, etc.
Vegetable C	1/2 katori root vegetable, e.g., carrot, beetroot

Fruits:	Each exchange supplies 50 kcal 1-2 exchange can be taken 1 fresh medium fruit (guava, apple, orange) 1/2 banana/small mango/1 sapota 1/2 glass fruit juice (unsweetened)
Milk & Milk Products:	Each exchange supplies 100 kcal 2 or more exchanges can be taken 1 glass of full milk or standard milk (unsweetened) 2 katoris of curds 1 cube of cheese/paneer
Meat:	Each exchange gives 100 kcal One exchange can be taken 1 serving of poultry or fish 1 serving of meat/beef muscle 1 serving of mutton/egg Vegetarians may substitute meat by extra exchange of legumes/pulses/milk
Fat:	Each exchange gives 100 kcal 2–3 exchanges can be taken 2 tsp ghee/vanaspati oil 3 tsp butter
Sugar:	Each exchange gives 100 kcal one exchange can be taken 5 tsp of sugar/jaggery 2 tsp of honey

Appendix 3

Indian Names of Foodstuffs

S.No. 1	*Name of Food* 2	*Hindi* 3	*Marathi* 4	*Gujarati* 5	*Tamil* 6
15	Rice, parboiled	Usna Chawal	Ukdala tandool	Ukadello chokha	Puzhungal arisi
19	Rice, flakes	Chewra	Pohe	Pawa	Aval
20	Rice, puffed	Murmura	Churmura	Murmura	Pori
25	Vermicelli	Siwain	Shevaya	Semiya	Semiya
32	Dal, bengalgram	Chane-ki-dal	Harbhara dal	Chana dal	Kadalai paruppu
34	Dal, black gram	Urad dal	Udid dal	Adad dal	Ulutham paruppu
46	Dal, red gram	Arhar dal	Tur dal	Tuver dal	Tuvaram paruppu
35	Cowpeas	Lobia	Chavli		Karamani
43	Peas	Mattar	Vatana	Vatana	Pattani
45	Rajmah (French beans dry)	Rajmah	Shravan ghevda	Phansi	
42	Moth beans	Moth	Matki		Narippayir
282	Groundnut	Moongi phali	Bhui mug	Bhoising	Nilakkadalai
280	Garden cress seeds	Halim	Ahliva	Saalio	Alivirai
648	Poppy seeds	Post dana	Khaskhas		Khasakhasa
51	Amaranth	Chaulai Sag	Math		Thandu keerai
71	Colocasia leaves	Arvi-ka-sag	Alu-pan		Seppan ilaigal
74	Coriander leaves	Hara dhania	Kothimbir	Kothmer	Kothamalli
77	Drumstick leaves	Saijan patta	Shevaga pan	Saragavo	Murungai keerai
229	Giant chillies	Sagiya Mirchi	Bhopali mirchi		Koda milagai
218	Cluster beans	Guar-ki-phali	Govar	Govar	Kothavara
346	Grape fruit	Chakotra		Chakotra	
400	Pummelo	Chakotra	Papnas	Papnus	Bombilimus
332	Cape goose berry	Rasbari	Tipari	Popta	
351	Jack fruit	Kathal	Phanas	Phanas	

(Contd...)

1	2	3	4	5	6
775	Watermelon	Tarbul	Kalingad	Tarbuj	Darbusini Mathalam
398	Pomegranate	Anar	Dalimb	Dalamb	Pazham
402	Raisins	Khishmise	Manuka	Khishmish	Drakshai
301	Corainder seeds	Dhania	Dhane	Dhania	Kothamalli vidai
302	Cumin seeds	Jira	Jire	Jiru	Jeerakam
592	Arrow root flour	Tavkeel	Toukil		Kuva mavu

Appendix 4

Stability of Nutrients

Nutrients	*Neutral pH*	*Acid pH*	*Alkaline pH*	*Air or O_2*	*Light*	*Heat*	*Cooking Losses (per cent)*
Vit. C	U	S	U	U	U	U	0–100
Thiamin	U	S	U	U	S	U	0–80
Riboflavin	S	S	U	S	U	U	0–75
Vit. A	S	U	S		U	U	0–40
Carotene (Provit. A)	S	U	S	U	U	U	0–30
Vit. D	S		U	U	U	U	0–40
Mineral salts	S	S	S	S	S	S	0–03
Lysine	S	S	S	S	S	U	0–40
Threonine	S	U	U	S	S	U	0–20
Tryptophan	S	U	S	S	U	S	0–15
All other EAA[1]	S	S	S	S	S	S	0–10

S—Stable; U—Unstable

1. EAA—Essential Amino Acid, Isoleucine, Leucine, Methionine, Phenylalanine and Valine.

Appendix 5 – Recommended Dietary Allowances for Indians—1989

Group	*Particulars*	*Body Wt/kg*	*Net energy kcal*	*Protein g/d*	*Fat g/d*	*Calcium mg/d*	*Iron mg/d*	*Vit.A Retinol*	*µg/d B-carotene*	*Thiamin mg/d*	*Riboflavin mg/d*	*Nicotinic acid mg/d*	*Pyridoxin mg/d*	*Ascorbic acid mg/d*	*Folic acid µg/d*	*Vit B_{12} µg/d*
Man	Sedentary Work		2350							1.2	1.4	16				
	Moderate Work	60	2700	60	15	400	28	600	2400	1.4	1.6	18	2.4	40	100	1
	Heavy Work		3200							1.6	1.9	21				
Woman	Sedentary Work		1800							0.9	1.1	12				
	Moderate Work		2100	50	15	400	30	600	2400	1.1	1.3	14	2.0	40	100	1
	Heavy Work		2450							1.2	1.5	16				
	Pregnant Woman	50	+300	+15	25	1000	38	600	2400	+0.2	+0.2	+2	2.5	40	400	1
	Lactation															
	0–6 months		+550	+25	35	1000	30	950	3800	+0.3	+0.3	+4	2.5	80	150	1.5
	6–12 months		+400	+18						+0.2	+0.2	+3				
Infants	0–6 months	5.4	118/kg	2.05/kg		500				59 µg/kg	71 µg/kg	780 µg/kg	0.3	25	25	0.2
	6–12 months	8.6	108/kg	1.65/kg				300	1200	54 µg/kg	65 µg/kg	71 µg/kg	0.4			
Children	1–3 years	12.1	1125	23			12	400	1600	0.6	0.7	7.0	plant			
	4–6 years	18.2	1600	31	20	400	18	400	1600	0.8	1.0	11	0.9			
	7–9 years	25.2	1925	41	15		25	600	2400	1.0	1.2	13	1.6			
Boys	10–12 years	33.5	2150	53	15	600	28	600		1.1	1.3	14				
Girls	10–12 years	35.0	1950	55	15		20		2400	1.0	1.2	13		40	100	0.2–1.0
Boys	13–15 years	46.8	2400	71	15	600	43	600		1.2	1.4	16				
Girls	13–15 years	47.8	2050	67	15		28		2400	1.0	1.2	14	2.0			
Boys	16–18 years	56.1	2600	79	15	500	50	600		1.3	1.6	17				
Girls	16–18 years	49.7	2050	65	15		30		2400	1.0	1.2	14				

In mixed cereal diet with absorption of 3% in man, 5% in woman, 8% in pregnant.

Narasingha Rao B.S., Y.G. Deosthale and K.C. Pant, *Nutrient Composition of Indian Foods,* p. 94, National Institute of Nutrition, Hyderabad-500007, India, 1989.

Appendix 6 – Table of Food Composition[1] (Nutrients per 100 g edible portion)

S.No.[2]	Food	Moisture	Energy	CHO	Protein	Fat	Minerals	Fibre	Calcium	Iron	Thiamin	Riboflavin	Niacin	Vit.C	Vit.A
			Cal.	g	g	g	g	g	mg	mg	mg	mg	mg	mg	mcg
1	2	3	4	5	6	7	8	9	10	11	12	13	14	15	16
	Cereals and Their Products														
	Rice														
17	Raw, milled	13.7	345	78.2	6.8	0.5	0.6	0.2	10	3.1	0.06	0.06	1.9	0	0
15	Parboiled, milled	13.3	346	79.0	6.4	0.4	0.7	0.2	9	4.0	0.21	0.05	3.8	0	0
19	Flakes	12.2	346	77.3	6.6	1.2	2.0	0.7	20	20.0	0.21	0.05	4.0	0	0
20	Puffed	14.5	325	73.6	7.5	0.1	3.8	0.3	20	6.6	0.21	0.01	4.1	0	0
	Wheat														
27	Whole		346		11.8	105			41	4.9	0.45	0.17	5.5	—	64
28	Flour, Whole	12.2	341	69.4	12.1	1.7	2.7	1.9	48	11.5	0.49	0.29	4.3	0	29
29	Flour, Refined	13.3	348	73.9	11.0	0.9	0.6	0.3	23	2.5	0.12	0.07	2.4	0	25
23	Suji (Rawa)	13.1	348	74.8	10.4	0.8	—	0.2	16	1.6	0.12	0.03	1.6	0	—
25	Vermicelli	11.7	352	78.3	8.7	0.4	0.7	0.2	22	2.0	0.19	0.05	1.8	0	0
606	Bread, white	39.0	245	51.9	7.8	0.7	—	0.2	11	1.1	0.07	—	0.7	—	—
	Millets														
1	Bajra	12.4	361	67.5	11.6	5.0	2.3	1.2	42	5.0	0.33	0.25	2.3	0	132
8	Jowar (Cholam)	11.9	349	72.6	10.4	1.9	1.6	1.6	25	5.8	0.37	0.13	3.1	0	47
9	Maize, dry	14.9	342	66.2	11.1	3.6	1.5	2.7	10	2.0	0.42	0.10	1.8	0	90
13	Ragi (Nachni)	13.1	328	72.0	7.3	1.3	2.7	3.6	344	6.4	0.42	0.19	1.4	0	42
	Other millets	11.9	334	66.0	10.7	3.3	2.3	6.7	22	6.7	0.35	0.12	2.6	0	34
6	Maize, tender (Makka)		125	24.6	4.7	0.9	0.8	1.9	9	1.1	0.11	0.17	0.6	6	32
	Pulses														
	Dals														
32	Bengal gram	9.9	372	59.8	20.8	5.6	2.7	1.2	56	9.1	0.48	0.18	2.4	1	129
34	Black gram	10.9	347	59.6	24.0	1.4	3.2	0.9	154	9.1	0.42	0.37	2.0	0	38
38	Green gram	10.1	348	59.9	24.5	1.2	3.5	0.8	75	8.5	0.72	0.15	2.4	0	49
46	Red gram	13.4	335	57.6	22.3	1.7	3.5	1.5	73	5.8	0.45	0.19	2.9	0	132

(Contd...)

1	2	3	4	5	6	7	8	9	10	11	12	13	14	15	16
	Whole														
31	Bengal gram	9.8	360	60.9	17.1	5.3	3.0	3.9	202	10.2	0.30	0.15	2.9	3	189
35	Cowpeas (Chawli) small	13.4	323	54.5	24.1	1.0	3.2	3.8	77	5.9	0.51	0.20	1.3	0	12
37	Green gram	10.4	334	56.7	24.0	1.3	3.5	4.1	124	7.3	0.47	0.39	2.1	0	94
41	Lentil (masur)	12.4	343	59.0	25.1	0.7	2.1	0.7	69	4.8	0.45	0.20	2.6	0	270
43	Peas, dry	16.0	315	56.5	19.7	1.1	2.2	4.5	75	5.1	0.47	0.19	3.4	0	39
45	Rajmah	12.0	346	60.6	22.9	1.3	3.2		260	5.8	—	—	—	—	—
42	Moth bean	10.8	330	56.5	23.6	1.1	3.5	4.5	202	9.5	0.45	0.09	1.5	2	9
47	Soyabean	8.1	432	20.9	43.2	19.5	4.6	3.7	240	11.5	0.73	0.39	3.2	—	426
	Other beans		334	23.4	23.4	0.6			173	5.5	0.47	0.18	1.6	—	—
	NUTS AND OILSEEDS														
282	Groundnut	3.0	567	26.1	25.3	40.1	2.4	3.1	90	2.8	0.90	0.13	19.9	0	37
283	Groundnut, Roasted	1.7	570	26.7	26.2	39.8	2.5	3.1	77	3.1	0.39	0.13	22.1	0	0
287	Til (Seasame, ginelly)	5.3	563	25.0	18.3	43.0	5.2	2.9	1450	10.5	1.01	0.34	4.4	0	60
280	Gardencress seeds	3.2	454	33.0	25.3	24	6.4	7.6	377	100.0	0.59	0.61	14.3	0	27
648	Poppy seeds (khaskhas)	4.3	408	36.8	21.7	19	9.9	8.0						—	—
662	Watermelon seeds	4.3	628	4.5	34.1	53	6.4	7.6	100	7.4	0.13	0.20	1.3	—	—
	Treenuts														
279	Coconut, fresh	36.3	444	13.0	4.5	42	1.0	3.6	10	1.7	0.05	0.10	0.8	1	0
278	Coconut, dry	4.3	662	18.4	6.8	62	1.6	6.6	40	2.7	0.08	0.01	3.0	7	0
276	Cashew	5.9	596	22.3	21.2	47	2.4	1.3	50	5.0	0.63	0.19	1.2	0	—
275	Almond	5.2	655	10.5	20.8	59	2.9	1.7	230	4.5	0.24	0.57	4.4	0	0
	MILK AND MILK PRODUCTS[3]														
568	Milk, cow's	87.5	67	4.4	3.2	4.1	0.8	—	120	0.02	0.05	0.19	0.1	2	52
567	Milk, buffalo's	81.0	117	5.0	4.3	8.8	0.8	—	210	0.2	0.04	0.10	0.1	1	48
569	Milk, goat's	86.8	72	4.6	3.3	4.5	0.8	—	170	0.3	0.05	0.01	0.3	1	55
572	Curds	89.1	60	3.0	3.1	4.0	0.8	—	149	0.2	0.05	0.16	0.1	1	31
573	Butter milk	97.5	30	0.5	0.8	1.1	0.1	—	30	0.8	—	—	—	—	0
577	Cheese	40.3	348	6.3	24.1	25.1	4.2	—	790	2.1	—	—	—	—	82
576	Channa	54.1	292	7.9	13.4	23.0	1.6	—	480	—	—	—	—	—	—
579	Khoya	30.6	421	20.5	14.6	31.2	3.1	—	650	5.8	—	—	—	—	—

1	2	3	4	5	6	7	8	9	10	11	12	13	14	15	16
583	Whole milk powder	3.5	496	38.0	25.8	26.7	6.0	—	950	0.6	0.31	1.36	0.8	4	420
582	Skimmed milk powder	4.1	357	51.0	38.0	0.1	6.8	—	1370	1.4	0.45	1.64	1.0	5	0
	EGG AND MEAT														
547	Egg, hen	73.7	173	—	13.3	13.3	1.0	—	60	2.1	0.10	0.40	0.1	0	960
556	Mutton	71.5	194	—	18.5	13.3	1.3	—	150	2.5	0.18	0.14	6.8	—	0
552	Goat meat	74.2	118	—	21.4	3.6	1.1	—	12	—	—	—	—	—	—
551	Chicken	72.2	109	—	26.0	0.6	1.3	—	25	—	—	0.14	—	—	—
541	Beef, Muscle	74.3	114	—	22.6	2.6	1.0	—	10	0.8	0.15	0.04	6.4	2	0
559	Pork, Muscle	77.4	114	—	18.7	4.4	1.0	—	30	2.2	0.54	0.09	2.8	2	0
555	Liver, sheep	70.4	150	—	19.3	7.5	1.5	1.3	10	6.3	0.36	1.70	17.6	20	6,690
	Fish														
502	Pomfrets	78.4	87	1.3	17.0	1.3	1.3	1.5	200	0.9	—	0.15	2.6	—	—
460	Hilsa	53.7	273	2.9	21.8	19.4	2.9	2.2	180	2.1	—	—	2.8	24	—
483	Mangalore	78.1	98	—	22.1	1.1	0.5	—	40	1.6	0.10	—	2.5	—	—
503	Prawn, fresh	77.4	89	0.8	19.1	1.0	1.7	—	323	5.3	0.01	0.10	4.8	—	0
	Fish, fresh, low fat		76–126		14.7–25.2	0.6–4.7			71–1070	0.8–6.8	—	—	0.6	—	—
	Fish, fresh, high fat		130–170		11.2–19.4	5.8–12.1			180–1605	0.5–4.4	—	—	2.2	—	—
	Fish, dry		255–413		55–76	2.7–17.0			315–38.45	3–50	—	—	—	—	—
519	Shell fish, dry	6.0	349	—	68.1	8.5	17.4	—	4380	—	—	—	—	—	—
447	Crab muscle	83.5	59	3.3	8.9	1.1	3.2	—	1370	21.2	—	—	3.1	—	780
448	Crab, small	65.3	169	9.1	11.2	9.8	4.6	—	1606	—	—	—	—	—	—
	LEAFY VEGETABLES														
	Miscellaneous														
	Dark green		22		2.4	0.3			166	2.9	0.09	0.19	0.8	70	3560–14,000
	Light green		18		1.5	0.1			55	1.1	0.16	0.08	0.4	5–61	126–3000
51	Amaranth, tender	85.7	45	6.1	4.0	0.5	2.7	1.0	397	25.5	0.03	0.30	1.2	99	5,520
52	Ambatchuka	95.2	15	1.4	1.6	0.8	0.9	0.6	63	8.7	0.03	0.06	0.2	12	3,660
55	Bathua leaves	89.6	30	2.9	3.7	0.4	2.6	0.8	150	4.2	0.01	0.14	0.6	35	1,740
61	Cabbage	91.9	27	4.6	1.8	0.1	0.6	1.0	39	0.8	0.06	0.09	0.4	124	1,200
71	Colocasia (green) leaves	78.8	56	8.1	3.9	1.5	2.5	1.8	227	10.0	0.22	0.26	1.1	12	10,270

1	2	3	4	5	6	7	8	9	10	11	12	13	14	15	16
74	Coriander leaves	86.3	44	6.3	3.3	0.6	2.3	1.2	184	18.5	0.05	0.06	0.8	135	6,918
77	Drumstick leaves	75.9	92	12.5	6.7	1.7	2.3	0.9	440	7.0	0.06	0.05	0.8	220	6,780
78	Methi leaves	86.1	49	6.0	4.4	0.9	1.5	1.1	395	16.5	0.04	0.31	0.8	52	2,340
101	Lettuce	93.4	21	2.5	2.1	0.3	1.2	0.5	50	2.4	0.09	0.13	0.5	10	990
130	Radish leaves	90.8	28	2.4	3.8	0.4	1.6	1.0	265	3.6	0.18	0.47	0.8	81	5,300
144	Palak (spinach)	92.1	26	2.9	2.0	0.7	1.7	0.6	73	10.9	0.03	0.26	0.5	28	5,580
	BULBS AND TUBERS														
163	Beetroot	87.7	43	8.8	1.7	0.1	0.8	0.9	18	1.0	0.04	0.09	0.4	10	0
167	Carrot	86.0	48	10.6	0.9	0.2	1.1	1.2	80	2.2	0.04	0.02	0.6	3	1,890
189	Radish, white	94.4	17	3.4	0.7	0.1	0.6	0.8	35	0.4	0.06	0.02	0.5	15	0
182	Onion	86.6	50	11.1	1.2	0.1	0.4	0.6	47	0.7	0.08	0.01	0.4	2	0
	STARCHY TUBERS, ROOTS														
185	Potato	74.7	97	22.6	1.6	0.1	0.6	0.4	10	0.7	0.10	0.01	1.2	17	*
170	Colocasia	73.1	97	21.1	3.0	0.1	1.7	1.0	40	1.7	0.09	0.03	0.4	0	—
192	Tapioca (Cassava)	59.4	157	38.1	0.7	0.2	1.0	0.6	50	0.9	0.05	0.10	0.3	25	—
197	Yam, elephant (Suran)	78.7	79	18.4	1.2	0.1	0.8	0.8	50	0.6	0.06	0.07	0.7	0	260
	OTHER VEGETABLES														
212	Brinjal	92.7	24	4.0	1.4	0.3	0.3	1.3	18	0.9	0.04	0.11	0.9	12	74
214	Cauliflower	90.8	30	4.0	2.6	0.4	1.0	1.2	33	1.5	0.04	0.10	1.0	56	30
223	Drumstick	86.9	26	3.7	2.5	0.1	2.0	4.8	30	5.3	0.05	0.07	0.2	120	110
229	Giant chillis (capsicum)	92.4	24	4.3	1.3	0.3	0.7	1.0	10	1.2	0.55	0.05	0.1	137	420
238	Knol-Knol	92.7	21	3.8	1.1	0.2	0.7	1.5	20	0.4	0.05	0.09	0.5	85	20
208	Bitter gourd (Karela)	92.4	25	4.2	1.6	0.2	0.8	0.8	20	1.8	0.07	0.09	0.5	88	125
	Other gourds		14		0.4	0.1			23	0.6	0.04	0.02	0.3	3	60
	Stems		18		0.6	0.2			60	0.9	0.02	0.07	0.2	8	—
227	Beans, french	91.4	26	4.5	1.7	0.1	0.5	1.8	50	1.7	0.08	0.06	0.3	24	130
218	Beans, cluster	81.0	60	10.8	3.2	0.4	1.4	3.2	130	4.5	0.09	0.03	0.6	49	200
250	Peas	72.1	93	15.9	7.2	0.1	0.8	4.0	20	1.5	0.25	0.01	0.8	9	80
258	Redgram tender	65.1	116	16.9	9.8	1.0	1.0	6.2	57	1.1	0.32	0.33	3.0	25	470
	Other beans		48–158		3.5–8.3	0.1–0.7			40–210	1.4–2.6	0.07–0.34	0.06—0.19	0.7–0.9	12–27	9565

1	2	3	4	5	6	7	8	9	10	11	12	13	14	15	16
	VITAMIN C-RICH FRUITS														
317	Amla	81.8	58	13.7	0.5	0.1	0.5	3.4	50	1.2	0.03	0.01	0.2	600	9
334	Cashew Fruit	86.3	51	12.3	0.2	0.1	0.2	0.9	10	0.2	0.02	0.05	0.4	180	23
347	Guava, country	81.7	51	11.2	0.9	0.3	0.7	5.2	10	1.4	0.03	0.03	0.4	212	0
357	Chinch, Vilayti	79.2	78	16.0	2.7	0.4	0.7	1.0	14	1.0	0.22	0.06	1.6	108	0
	CITRUS FRUITS														
346	Grape Fruit	92.0	32	7.0	0.7	0.1	0.2	—	20	0.2	0.12	0.02	0.3	31	—
361	Lemon	85.0	57	11.1	1.0	0.9	0.3	1.7	70	2.3	0.02	0.01	0.1	39	0
362	Lemon, sweet	90.5	35	7.3	0.7	0.3	0.5	0.7	30	0.7	—	0.04	0	45	0
365	Lime	84.6	59	10.9	1.5	1.0	0.7	1.3	90	0.3	0.02	0.03	0.1	63	15
366	Lime, sweet, malta	90.3	36	7.8	0.7	0.2	0.4	0.6	30	1.0	—	—	0	54	0
367	Mausambi	88.4	43	9.3	0.8	0.3	0.7	0.5	40	0.7	—	—	0	50	0
380	Orange	87.6	65	10.9	0.7	0.2	0.3	0.3	26	0.3	—	—	—	30	1,104
381	Orange juice	97.7	48	1.9	0.2	0.1	0.1	—	5	0.7	0.06	0.02	0.4	64	15
400	Pummelo papanas	88.0	44	10.2	0.6	0.1	0.5	0.6	30	0.3	0.03	0.03	0.2	20	120
	OTHER VIT. C-RICH FRUITS														
332	Cape gooseberry	82.9	53	11.1	1.8	0.2	0.8	3.2	10	2.0	0.05	0.02	0.3	49	1,425
352	Jamb, safed	93.5	19	3.7	0.1	0.4	0.1	2.2	17	0.1	0.01	0.02	0.2	30	—
363	Lichi	84.1	61	13.6	1.1	0.2	0.5	0.5	10	0.7	0.02	0.06	0.4	31	0
374	Melon, musk (kharbooja)	95.2	17	3.5	0.3	0.2	0.4	0.4	32	1.4	0.11	0.08	0.3	26	170
375	Papaya, ripe	90.8	32	7.2	0.6	0.1	0.5	0.8	17	0.5	0.04	0.25	0.2	57	665
394	Pineapple	87.8	46	10.8	0.4	0.1	0.4	0.5	20	1.2	0.20	0.12	0.1	39	*
407	Seetaphal	70.5	104	23.5	1.6	0.4	0.9	3.1	17	1.5	0.33	0.44	1.3	37	0
410	Strawberry	87.8	44	9.8	0.7	0.2	0.4	1.1	30	1.8	0.03	0.02	0.2	52	15
413	Tomato, ripe	94.0	20	3.6	0.9	0.2	0.5	0.8	48	0.4	0.12	0.06	0.4	27	350
	OTHER FRUITS														
318	Apple	84.6	59	13.4	0.2	0.5	0.3	1.0	10	1.0	—	—	0	1	0
319	Apriot, fresh	85.3	53	11.6	1.0	0.3	0.7	1.1	20	2.2	0.04	0.13	0.6	6	2,160
322	Bael fruit	61.5	137	31.8	1.8	0.3	1.7	2.9	85	0.6	0.13	1.19	1.1	3	55
325	Banana, ripe	70.1	116	27.2	1.2	0.3	0.8	0.4	17	0.9	0.05	0.08	0.5	7	78

1	2	3	4	5	6	7	8	9	10	11	12	13	14	15	16
335	Cherries, red	83.4	64	13.8	1.1	0.5	0.8	0.4	24	1.3	0.08	0.08	0.3	7	0
341	Figs (Anjeer)	88.1	37	7.6	1.3	0.2	0.6	2.2	80	1.0	0.06	0.05	0.6	5	162
	Grapes (average)	81.0	65	15.0	0.5	0.3	0.4	0.8	20	0.5	0.04	0.03	0.2	1	*
351	Jackfruit	76.2	88	19.8	1.9	0.1	0.9	1.1	20	0.5	0.03	0.13	0.4	7	175
	Plantain ripe		135		1.2	0.3			8	1.3	0.08	0.04	0.6	20	780
370	Mango, ripe	81.0	74	16.9	0.6	0.4	0.4	0.7	14	1.3	0.08	0.09	0.9	16	2,740
375	Melon, water	95.8	16	3.3	0.2	0.2	0.3	0.2	11	7.9	0.02	0.04	0.1	1	0
	Peaches, pears, plums	86.0	50	11.1	0.8	0.3	0.5	0.9	10	0.6	0.04	0.03	0.3	4	—
387	Passion fruit	76.3	54	12.4	0.9	0.1	0.7	9.6	10	2.0	0.07	0.14	1.6	25	54
388	Passion fruit juice	89.0	37	7.7	1.2	0.2	0.7	1.2	10	0.7	0.01	0.02	0	13	1,970
398	Pomegranate	78.0	65	14.5	1.6	0.1	0.7	5.1	10	0.3	0.06	0.10	0.3	16	0
406	Sapota (Chiku)	73.7	98	21.4	0.7	1.1	0.5	2.6	28	2.0	0.02	0.03	0.2	6	95
418	Kavath (wood apple)	64.2	134	18.1	7.1	3.7	1.9	5.0	130	0.6	0.04	0.17	0.8	3	61
	FRUITS, DRIED														
320	Apricots	19.4	306	73.4	1.6	0.7	2.8	2.1	110	4.6	0.22	—	2.3	2	60
337	Currants, black	18.4	316	75.2	2.7	0.5	2.2	1.0	130	8.5	0.03	0.14	0.4	1	20
338	Dates (khajur)	15.3	317	75.8	2.5	0.4	2.1	3.9	120	7.3	0.01	0.02	0.9	3	25
402	Raisins	20.2	308	74.6	1.8	0.5	2.0	1.1	87	7.7	0.07	0.19	0.7	1	*
	CONDIMENTS														
301	Coriander seeds	11.2	288	21.6	14.1	16.1	4.4	32.6	630	18.0	0.22	0.35	1.1	0	940
302	Cumin seeds	11.9	356	36.6	18.7	15.0	5.8	12.0	1080	31.0	0.55	0.36	2.6	3	520
303	Fenugreck seeds (methi)	13.7	335	44.1	26.2	5.8	3.0	7.2	160	14.1	0.34	0.29	1.1	0	95
311	Onva (ajwain)	7.4	360	24.6	17.1	21.8	7.9	21.2	1525	27.7	0.21	0.28	2.1	0	70
298	Chillies, green	85.7	29	3.0	2.9	0.6	1.0	6.8	30	1.2	0.19	0.39	0.9	111	175
297	Chillies, dry	10.0	246	31.6	15.9	6.2	6.1	30.2	160	2.3	0.93	0.43	9.5	50	345
	FATS AND OILS														
584	Butter	19.0	730	—	—	81.0	2.5	—	—	—	—	—	—	—	960
585	Ghee (cow)	—	900	—	—	100.0	—	—	—	—	—	—	—	—	960
586	Ghee (buffalo)	—	900	—	—	100.0	—	—	—	—	—	—	—	—	270

1	2	3	4	5	6	7	8	9	10	11	12	13	14	15	16
587	Vanaspati (fortified)	—	900	—	—	100.0	—	—	—	—	—	—	—	—	750
588	Vegetable oil	—	900	—	—	100.0	—	—	—	—	—	—	—	—	0
	Vegetable oil (refined, fortified)	—	90		—	100.0	—	—	—	—	—	—	—	—	750
	MISCELLANEOUS														
592	Arrow root flour	16.5	334	83.1	0.2	0.1	0.1	—	10	1.0	—	—	—	—	—
596	Betel leaves	85.4	44	6.1	3.1	0.8	2.3	2.3	230	7.0	0.07	0.03	0.7	5	5,760
603	Biscuits, salted	4.5	534	54.6	4.5	6.6	1.9	—	—	—	—	—	—	—	—
604	Biscuits, sweet	5.4	450	71.9	5.4	6.4	1.1	—	—	—	—	—	—	—	—
607	Sugar-cane	0.4	398	99.4	0.4	0.1	0.1	0	1	—	—	—	—	—	—
613	Coconut, tender	90.8	41	6.3	0.9	1.4	0.6	—	10	0.9	—	—	—	2	—
615	Coconut water	93.8	24	4.4	1.4	0.1	0.3	0	24	0.1	0.01	0	0.1	2	0
621	Fish liver oil	—	900	—	—	100	—	—	—	—	—	—	—	20,000[4]-1,00,0000	
623	Honey	20.6	320	79.5	0.3	0	0.2	—	5	0.9	0	0.04	0.2	4	0
624	Jackfruit seeds	64.5	133	25.8	6.6	0.4	1.2	1.5	50	1.5	0.25	0.11	0.3	11	10
625	Jaggery, cane	3.9	383	95.0	0.4	0.1	0.6	—	80	11.4	0.02	0.04	0.5	0	165
642	Mushroom	88.5	43	4.3	4.6	0.8	1.4	0.4	6	1.5	0.14	0.16	2.4	12	0
645	Papad	20.3	288	52.4	18.8	0.3	8.2	—	80	17.2	0	—	—	—	0
654	Sago	12.2	351	87.1	0.2	0.2	0.3	—	10	1.3	0.01	—	0.2	—	—
657	Sugarcane juice	90.2	39	9.1	0.1	0.2	0.4	—	10	1.1	—	0.04	—	—	—
663	Yeast, dried Brewer's	13.6	320	39.1	39.5	0.6	7.0	0.2	440	43.7	6.00	4.0	40.0	0	65
664	Yeast, dried, food	7.8	344	46.3	35.7	1.8	8.4	—	160	21.5	3.20	—	27.0	0	—

1. Selected from *Nutritive Value of Indian Foods,* by Gopalan, C. *et al.,* Indian Council of Medical Research Publication, 1971, pp. 60–114.
2. The numbers refer to serial numbers in ICMR publication mentioned above.
3. Milk and Milk products: Vitamin A value is given I.U.s.
4. Preformed Vitamin A in Cod liver oil–20,000 to 70,000 mcg; about 70,000 mcg; in shark liver oil; and 1,000,000 mcg per 100g in halibut liver oil.

Note: Abbreviations and Symbols: Cal.–Kilo calories: mg–milligram; *–negligible; mcg–microgram; Vit.–Vitamin–Value not reported.

Appendix 7 — Weight for Height for Age, 1–18 years, Girls[1,2]

Height cm	Weight kg Mean Weight	Age Years 1	2	3	4	5	6	7	8	9	10	11	12	13	14	15	16	17	18
60	5.3	5.3																	
65	6.5	6.3	6.7																
70	7.4	7.3	7.4																
75	8.4	8.2	8.5	8.7															
80	9.7	9.4	9.5	9.8	10.1														
85	10.8		10.4	10.8	10.8	11.0													
90	11.8		11.6	11.7	11.8	11.9	12.0												
95	12.8			12.7	12.8	12.9	13.0	13.0											
100	14.4				14.0	14.0	14.2	14.5	14.8										
105	15.4				15.3	15.3	15.4	15.4	15.4	15.5									
110	17.0					16.8	16.8	16.9	16.9	16.9	17.2								
115	18.6					18.4	18.4	18.5	18.5	18.6	18.5	18.8							
120	20.6						20.2	20.3	20.4	20.4	20.5	20.7	21.0						
125	22.6							22.2	22.2	22.3	22.6	22.6	22.9	23.0					
130	24.7								24.2	24.4	24.5	24.8	24.9	25.3					
135	28.5									27.1	27.4	27.8	28.0	28.5	29.0	31.0			
140	33.1										29.3	29.8	30.5	31.8	33.1	34.9	36.0	36.7	37.4
145	36.3										32.6	33.0	33.4	34.9	36.3	37.8	38.8	39.2	39.8
150	40.1												37.3	38.3	39.3	40.1	41.3	42.5	45.5
155	42.9													40.5	42.1	42.9	44.0	44.7	45.5
160	46.1																45.3	46.2	46.1

1. *Growth and Physical Development of Indian Infants and Children,* ICMR Technical Report Series No. 18, adapted from Table 13, pp. 70–73, 1972.

2. The fiftieth percentile is given.

Appendix 8 — Weight for Height for Age, 1–18 years, boys[1,2]

Height	Weight kg	Age Years																	
cm	*Mean Weight*	*1*	*2*	*3*	*4*	*5*	*6*	*7*	*8*	*9*	*10*	*11*	*12*	*13*	*14*	*15*	*16*	*17*	*18*
65	7.0	7.0																	
70	7.6	7.5	7.6																
75	8.7	8.5	8.7	8.8															
80	9.9	9.8	9.9	9.9	10.0														
85	10.8		10.7	10.8	11.0	11.0													
90	12.0		11.9	12.0	12.1	12.1													
95	13.1			13.0	13.1	13.2	13.2												
100	14.3			14.2	14.3	14.3	14.4	14.6											
105	15.5				15.4	15.5	15.5	15.5	15.6										
110	17.0					16.9	17.0	17.0	17.0	17.1									
115	18.5						18.4	18.5	18.5	18.7	18.5	18.9							
120	20.2						20.4	20.1	20.1	20.2	20.5	20.6	21.0						
125	22.5							22.2	22.3	22.3	22.5	22.7	22.5	22.7					
130	24.6								24.3	24.3	24.4	24.6	24.7	25.1	24.8				
135	27.1									26.6	26.6	27.0	27.1	27.2	27.5	27.7			
140	29.5										28.8	29.3	29.5	29.8	29.9	30.2	29.9		
145	33.2											32.0	32.3	32.6	33.2	33.3	33.3	34.9	
150	36.3												35.5	36.1	36.2	36.3	38.0	39.2	41.4
155	40.8												38.7	39.2	39.8	40.8	41.3	42.1	43.3
160	44.7													43.7	43.2	43.5	44.7	45.3	46.7
165	47.3														46.2	47.1	47.3	48.4	49.0
170	51.0															49.8	50.9	51.6	51.8

1. *Growth and Physical Development of Indian Infants and Children,* ICMR Technical Report Series No. 18, adapted from Table 13, pp. 70–73, 1972.
2. The fiftieth percentile is given.

Appendix 9

Low Calorie Vegetables and Fruits (20 Kcal)

Name of the vegetables	*Kcal/100 gm*
GLV	
Amaranth (stem)	19
Ambat chukka	15
Celery stalk	18
Spinach stalk	20
Roots and tubers	
Radish table	16
Radish white	17
Other vegetables	
Ash gourd	10
Bottle gourd	12
Cluster beans	16
Colocasia stem	18
Cucumber	13
Ghosala	18
Kovai	18
Parwal	20
Ridge guard	17
Snake guard	18
Vegetable marrow	17
Fruits	
Bilimbi	19
Jamb safed	19
Musk melon	17
Water melon	16
Orange juice	9
Tomato ripe	20

Source: Nutritive Value of Indian Foods

Appendix 10

Vegetables and Fruits with High Calorie Value (≥ 100 Kcal)

Food Stuff	*Kcal/100 g*
Leafy vegetables	
Chekkur manis	103
Colocasia leaves (dried)	277
Curry leaves	108
Fetid cassia (dried) (Chakunda)	292
Rape leaves (dried)	297
Tamarind leaves	115
Roots & Tubers	
Arrow root flour	334
Parsnip	101
Sweet potato	120
Tapioca	157
Yam ordinary	111
Yam wild	110
Other vegetables	
Beans, scarlet runner	158
Jack fruit, seeds	133
Karonda (dry)	364
Lotus stem (dry)	234
Sundakai (dry)	269
Water chestnut (fresh)	115
Water chestnut (dry)	330
Fruits	
Apricot (dry)	306
Avacado pear	215
Banana	116
Bael fruit	116
Currants, red	316
Dates (dried)	317
Dates fresh	144
Mahua (ripe)	111
Raisins	308
Seetaphal	104
Wood apple	134

Source: Nutritive Value of Indian Foods

Appendix 11

Approximate Calorific Value of Some Cooked Preparations

Preparation	*Quantity for one serving*	*Calories (Kcal)*
1. *Cereal*		
Rice	1 cup	170
Phulka	1 No.	80
Paratha	1 No.	150
Puri	1 No.	80
Bread	2 slices	170
Poha	1 cup	270
Upma	1 cup	270
Idli	2 Nos.	150
Dosa	1 No.	125
Kichidi	1 cup	200
Wheat porridge	1 cup	220
Semolina porridge	1 cup	220
Cereal flakes with milk (corn/wheat/rice)	1 cup	220
2. *Pulse*		
Plain dhal	½ cup	100
Sambar	1 cup	110
3. *Vegetable*		
With gravy	1 cup	170
Dry	1 cup	150
4. *Non-Vegetarian*		
Boiled egg	1 No.	90
Ommelette	1 No.	160
Fried egg	1 No.	160
Mutton curry	¾ cup	260
Chicken curry	¾ cup	240

Preparation	*Quantity for one serving*	*Calories (Kcal)*
Fish fried	2 big pieces	190
Fish cutlet	2 Nos.	190
Prawn curry	¾ cup	220
Keema kofta curry	¾ cup (6 small koftas)	240
5. *Savoury snacks*		
Bajji or pakora	8 Nos.	280
Besan ka pura	1 No.	220
Chat (Dahi-pakori)	5 pieces	220
Cheese balls	2 Nos.	250
Dahi vada	2 Nos.	180
Vada	2 Nos.	140
Masala vada	2 Nos.	150
Masala dosa	1 No.	200
Pea-kachori	2 Nos.	380
Potato bonda	2 Nos.	200
Sago vada	2 Nos.	210
Samosa	1 No.	200
Sandwiches (butter - 2tbsp)	2 Nos.	200
Vegetable puff	1 No.	200
Pizza (Cheese and tomato)	1 slice	200
6. *Chutneys*		
Coconut/groundnuts/til	2 tbsp	120
Tomato	1 tbsp	10
Tamarind (with jaggery)	1 tbsp	60
7. *Sweets and Desserts*		
Besan barfi	2 small pieces	400
Chikki	2 pieces	290
Fruit cake	1 piece	270
Rice puttu	½ cup	280
Sandesh	2 Nos.	140
Double ka meetha	½ cup	280
Halwa (kesari)	½ cup	320
Jelly/Jam	1 tbsp	20
Custard (caramel)	½ cup	160
Srikhand	½ cup	380
Milk chocolate	25 g	140
Ice-cream	½ cup	200

Preparation	*Quantity for one serving*	*Calories (Kcal)*
8. *Beverages*		
Tea (2 tsp sugar + 50 ml toned milk)	1 cup	75
Coffee (2 tsp sugar + 100 ml)	1 cup	110
Cow's milk (2 tsp sugar)	1 cup	180
Buffalo's milk (2 tsp sugar)	1 cup	320
Lassi (2 tsp sugar)	1 cup/glass (200 ml)	110
Squash	1 cup/glass	75
Syrups (Sharabats)	1 cup/glass	200
Cold drinks	1 bottle (200 ml)	150
Fresh lime juice	1 glass	60

Size of Teaspoon, Tablespoon and Cup

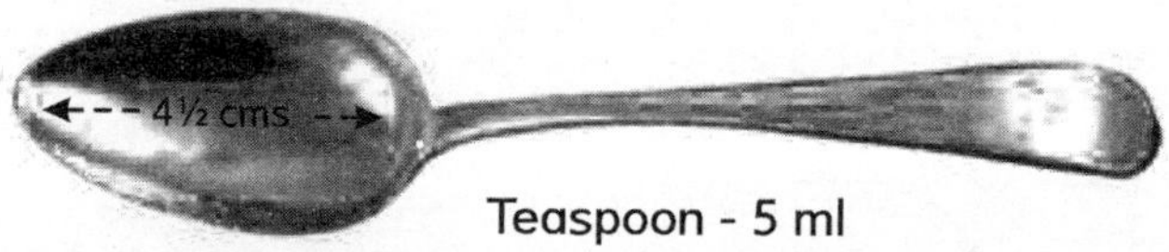

Teaspoon - 5 ml

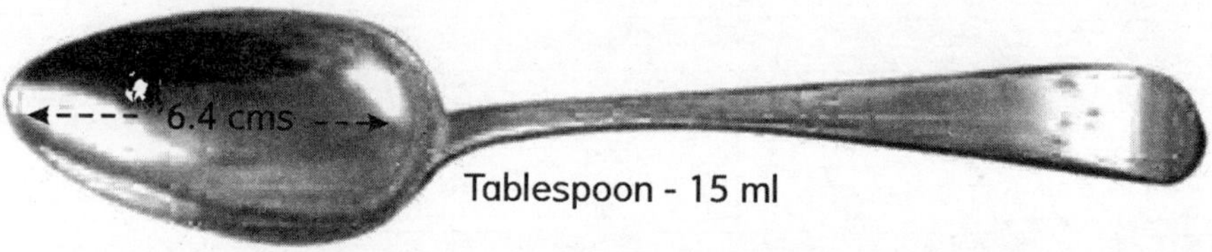

Tablespoon - 15 ml

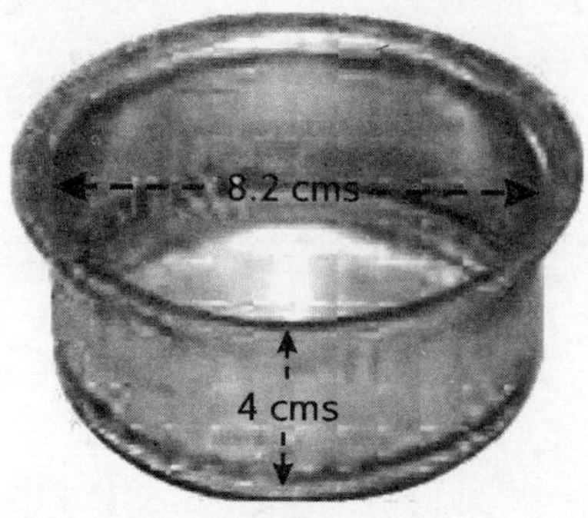

Cup 200 ml

Appendix 12

Alpha Linolenic Acid (Omega-3) Content of Foods (g/100 g)

Foods	*(g)ALA*
Cereal/Millet	
Wheat & Pearl millet (bajra)	0.14
Pulses	
Blackgram (kala chana), kidney beans (rajmah) & cowpea (lobia)	0.5
Other pulses	0.16
Vegetables	
Green leafy	0.16
Other Vegetables	0.025
Fruits	0.025
Spices	
Fenugreek seed (methi)	2.0
Mustard (sarson)	10.0
Unconventional	
Flaxseed (alsi)	20.0
Perilla seeds (Bhanjira)	33.0

Appendix 13

Glycemic Index (GI) of Common Foods

Sl. No.	*Name of the foods*	*Glycemic Index*
1	White wheat bread	75 ± 2
2	Whole wheat bread	74 ± 2
3	Wheat roti	62 ± 3
4	Chappathi	52 ± 4
5	White boiled rice	73 ± 4
6	Brown boiled rice	68 ± 4
7	Barley	28 ± 2
8	Instant oat porridge	79 ± 3
9	Rice porridge /congee	78 ± 9
10	Millet porridge	67 ± 5
11	Sweet corn	52 ± 5
12	Cornflakes	81 ± 6
13	Apple (raw)	36 ± 2
14	Orange	43 ± 3
15	Banana	51 ± 3

Sl. No.	*Name of the foods*	*Glycemic Index*
16	Pineapple	59 ± 8
17	Mango (raw)	51 ± 5
18	Watermelon (raw)	76 ± 4
19	Potato (boiled)	78 ± 4
20	French fries (potato)	63 ± 5
21	Carrots (boiled)	39 ± 4
22	Milk (full fat)	39 ± 3
23	Milk (skim)	37 ± 4
24	Ice cream	51 ± 3
25	Chick peas	28 ± 9
26	Soya beans	16 ± 1
27	Lentils	32 ± 5
28	Chocolate	40 ± 3
29	Popcorn	65 ± 5
30	Soft drinks/soda	59 ± 3
31	Honey	61 ± 3
32	Glucose	103 ± 3

Source: Diabetes care

Appendix 14

*Energy Expenditure on Various Physical Activities (Kcal/hr)

Activity	*Kcal/hr*
Cleaning/Mopping	210
Gardening	300
Watching TV	86
Cycling	
15 (km/hr)	360
Running	
12 (km/hr)	750
10 (km/hr)	655
8 (km/hr)	522
6 (km/hr)	353
Walking 4 (km/hr)	160
Shuttle	348
Table Tennis	245
Tennis	392
Volley Ball	180
Dancing	372
Fishing	222
Shopping	204
Typing	108
Sleeping	57
Standing	132
Sitting	86

* Approx. energy expenditure for 60 kg reference man. Individuals with higher body weight will be spending more calories than those with lower body weight. Reference woman (50 kg) will be spending 5% less calories.

Appendix 15

Energy Costs of Physical Activities

Activity Zones	*Examples of Activities*	*Energy (Kcal/min)*
1	Sleeping, Resting, Relaxing	1.0
2	Sitting (Light activities); eating, reading writing, listening, talking	1.5
3	Standing, standing (Light activity); washing face, shaving, combing, watering plants	2.3
4	Walking (Slow), driving, dusting, bathing, dressing, marketing, childcare	2.8
5	Light manual work, sweeping, cleaning utensils, washing clothes, other house chores	3.3
6	Warm-up & recreational activities, walking up/down stairs, cycling, fetching water	4.8
7	Manual work (moderate pace), loading/unloading, walking with load, harvesting, carpentry, plumbing	5.6
8	Practice of non-competitive sport/ games, cycling (15 kmph), gymnastics, swimming, digging	6.0
9	High intense manual work & sports activities–tournaments, wood cutting, carrying heavy loads, running, jogging	7.8

Appendix 16

Suggested food groups for a balanced diet to meet the EAR of different nutrients-ICMR 2023

Age Group	*Category of work*	*Body wt*	*Cereals/ Millets (g)***	*^Pulses & Beans (g)*	*GLV (g)*	*Vegetables (g)*	*Roots & Tubers (g)*	*Fruits (g)*	*Nuts (g)*	*Milk (ml)*	*Fats & oils (g)*	*Energy (kcal) obtained from these food groups*	*Crude protein (g) Obtained from these food groups*
Men	Sedentary	65	270	90	100	200	100	100	40	300	25	~2080	72
	Moderate		390	130	100	200	100	100	45	300	30	~2680	90
Women	Sedentary	55	200	65	100	200	100	100	30	300	20	~1660	57
	Moderate		280	95	100	200	100	100	40	300	25	~2125	72
Pregnant Women		55 +10	240	80	150	200	100	150	40	400	20	~2020	72
Lactating Women	0–6m		270	90	150	200	100	150	40	400	30	~2245	77
	7–12m		270	90	150	200	100	150	40	400	25	~2200	78
Infants	0–6m	5.8	**Exclusive breastfeeding**										
	7–12m	8.5	25	12	20	25	20	50	7	*milk	10		
Children	1–3yrs	12.9	100	50	50	100	50	50	10	350	20	~1110	38
	4–6yrs	18.3	160	60	50	100	50	75	15	350	20	~1370	46
	7–9yrs	25.3	200	65	100	150	100	100	20	400	25	~1710	59
Boys	10–12yrs	34.9	290	95	100	200	100	100	30	400	30	~2230	76
Girls	10–12yrs	36.4	250	85	100	200	100	100	30	400	30	~2060	70
Boys	13–15yrs	50.5	390	130	100	200	100	100	40	400	45	~2860	95
Girls	13–15yrs	49.8	315	105	100	200	100	100	35	400	35	~2410	81
Boys	16–18yrs	64.4	450	150	100	200	100	150	50	400	55	~3300	107
Girls	16–18yrs	55.7	330	110	100	200	100	150	40	400	30	~2490	85
Elderly	>60yrs	Man	180	80	100	200	100	150	30	400	20	~1740	62
		Woman	140	70	100	200	100	150	30	400	15	~1530	56

** 20 to 30% of Cereals (weight in raw) should be from millets for adults. 20% of cereals (raw weight) should be from millets for children upto 10 years age.

^ For non-vegetarians, 30 g of pulses may be substituted with meat. * Continue breast milk, which is roughly 580 ml per day.

- Sugar should be less than 5% of the total energy requirements.
- No added sugar children < 2 years old
- These suggested food groups are for children who are growing normally and for adults with normal BMI (18.5 to 23)

Appendix 17

Daily Nutrient Recommendations for the Elderly in India ICMR-NIN, 2020

Nutrients		*Energy (Kcal)*	*Dietary Fibre*	*Protein (g)*	*Vit-A (µg)*	*Thiamin B_1(mg)*	*Ribo flavin B_2 (mg)*	*Niacin (mg)*	*Vit-C (mg)*	*Vit-B_6 (mg)*	*Folate (µg)*	*Vit-B_{12} (µg)*	*Vit-D (IU)*	*Cal-cium (mg)*	*Magne-sium (mg)*	*Iron (mg)*	*Zinc (mg)*	*Iodine (µg)*
Men ≥60 Yrs	EAR	1700	-	43.0	460	1.2	1.6	12	65	1.6	250	2.0	400	1000	370	11	14	95
	RDA	-	30	54.0	1000	1.4	2.0	14	80	1.9	300	2.2	800	1200	440	19	17	140
Women ≥60 Yrs	EAR	1500	-	36.3	390	1.1	1.6	9	55	1.6	180	2.0	400	1000	310	11	11	95
	RDA	-	25	46.0	840	1.4	1.9	11	65	1.9	200	2.2	800	1200	370	19	13.2	140

Glossary

Absorption The uptake of the end products of digestion through the cell membranes of the digestive tract and into the blood and lymph circulation.

Abstinence avoidance

Acne Pimples

Adapt Modify or alter to suit new use

Adipose tissue Fatty tissue

Adolescence Period of years between the beginning of puberty (when the reproductive organs become functionally active) and maturity. In humans it is between eleven and fifteen years for girls fourteen and eighteen years for boys.

Agar An indigestible polysaccharide prepared by drying and purifying moss and seaweed; swells with water to form a gel and is often used to relieve constipation; also called agar-agar and is used in microbiological analysis as an inert medium to grow microorganisms.

Albumin Protein that occurs in blood plasma

Alcoholism Chronic and excessive use of alcohol and normal breathing is disturbed.

Aldehyde One of a large class of organic substances derived from a primary alcohol by oxidation; contains the characteristic group CHO.

Aleurone layer The single layer of large cells between the bran coat and endosperm of cereal grains. Rich in protein, minerals and vitamins.

Ambulatory Able to walk

Amenorrhea The stoppage of the monthly menstrual flow

Amino acids Organic compounds containing the elements carbon, hydrogen, oxygen and nitrogen. Each amino acids contain one or more amino ($-NH_2$) and one or more carboxyl ($-COOH$) group. In addition some contain sulphur. Many amino acids linked together in some definite pattern form a protein molecule.

Amniocentesis A test to determine the status of the fetus in utero

Amphoteric A compound that has at least one group that act as an acid and one group that can act as a base; describes proteins and amino acids, which carry both negative and positive charges in the molecules. At the pH at which the substance becomes electrically neutral, it precipitates from solution.

Amylase Enzymes (salivary and pancreatic) that hydrolyse starch and glycogen to maltose; ptyalin, amylopsin.

Anaemia Reduction in the number of red blood cells, packed cell volume or circulating haemoglobin, resulting in pallor in appearance.

Anaerobic Living in absence of air, a chemical reaction, which occurs in the absence of oxygen.

Angina Pectoris Pain in the heart muscle due to reduction in blood supply.

Annatto Yellow colouring matter.

Anorexia Loss of appetite.

Anorexia nervosa Loss of appetite due to psychological stress.

Antibody A protein produced in an organism as a response to the presence of an antigen (foreign body).

Antibiotic A substance produced by living organisms that inhibits the growth of other organisms, used as a food preservative in some countries.

Antifoaming Agents Substance which reduce foaming caused by the presence of dissolved proteins or other substances.

Antioxidants substance preventing damage from oxygen by retarding retard the oxidative changes (rancidity) in fats and oils.

Anthropometry The science which deals with the measurement of size, weight and proportions of the human body.

Antivitamin A substance that inactivates a vitamin or inhibits its synthesis.

Aponea suspension of breathing.

Arachodonic acid A fatty acid, containing 20–carbon atoms with four double bonds, in the body it is synthesised from the essential fatty acid, linoleic acid.

Arrowroot Starchy substance obtained from the root of arrowroot plant, almost pure starch.

Atherosclerosis narrowing of arterial walls due to deposits of fatty material (plaques), with resistance to blood flow and increased blood pressure. Increased blood pressure injures the arterial wall further, thus worsening the atherosclerosis.

Autoimmune disease occur when body's immune defenses attack the body itself, the antibodies produced attack its cells and organs.

Autolysis Process of self-digestion by the enzymes naturally present in the tissue which may lead to deterioration of quality (especially in fresh foods).

Availability of nutrients Nutrients, free to be absorbed from the intestine into the blood.

Basal Metabolism Energy used by the body, during physical, digestive and emotional rest (usually determined 12 hours after ingestion of food).

Beriberi A deficiency disease due to lack of thiamin, characterised by polyneuritis, edema (in some cases), emaciation and cardiac disturbances (enlargement of heart and a very rapid heartbeat).

Beta-carotone A fat soluble plant pigment, which is precursor of vitamin A.

Bile acids Acids (glycocholic and taurocholic) formed in the liver and secreted in the bile.

Bioavailability The degree to which a drug or other substances become available to the target tissue.

Biological value The relative nutritional value of a protein as compared to a high quality protein such as egg protein.

Blood cells (corpuscles) These include red blood cells (erythrocytes) and white blood cells (leukocytes).

Bone matrix The protein groundwork in which minerals are deposited.

Buffer Substance which resists change in pH (alkalinity and acidity).

Calcification Process by which an organic tissue becomes hardened by a deposit of calcium salts.

Capillary A minute blood vessel connecting the small arteries (arterioles) and small veins (venules). Exchange of materials between the blood and tissues takes place through the walls of the capillaries.

Calorimeter An instrument used for measuring the heat or energy produced (e.g., by oxidation of a food).

Carbondioxide Colourless, odourless gas formed by oxidation of carbon produced in tissues and eliminated by lungs.

Carcinogen A substance, which triggers abnormal cell growth.

Caries Tooth decay.

Carotenoids A group of fat-soluble, yellow-orange plant pigments.

Carrier A person in apparent good health, who harbors pathogenic microorganisms and passes these on to others.

Cassava (Tapioca) Tropical plant with edible, starchy roots.

Catalyst A substance which increases the rate of a chemical reaction without being used up in the reaction.

Cation lon with positive charge, e.g., Sodium, Calcium.

Cell The smallest structural and functional unit of plant and animal organisms.

Cellulose A polysaccharide constituent of plant which passes undigested through the human digestive tract.

Chemotherapy Treatment of a diseased tissue with chemical drugs.

Chlorophyll Green plant pigment, used to manufacture carbohydrates from simple salts and carbon dioxide using energy derived from sunlight.

Cholosterol A solid alcohol (sterol) which is synthesised in animal tissue, and is essential for normal function.

Cirrhosis Generic term for liver disease with formation of fibrous scar tissue, with loss of cells disrupting normal liver function; occurs in malnourished adults (due to excessive alcohol intake) and highly malnourished children.

Coagulate Curdle, clot form into a mass, congeal, solidity. Proteins coagulate due to heat and/or change of pH.

Coenzyme A helper needed by some enzymes to accomplish a biochemical change.

Cofactor Non-protein part required by some enzymes for their activity.

Coliform bacteria Group of aerobic lactose fermentors. Generally not harmful but their presence indicates lack of sanitation.

Complement system is a group of proteins, which interact with each other in a stepwise progression to bring about antigen-antibody reactions.

Conjunctiva Fine membrane covering eyeball and lining the eyelid.

Colloid Fine particles suspended in either solid, liquid or gaseous phases.

Colostrum Fluid secreted during the first week of lactation.

Constipation Difficulty in emptying bowels; usually due to lack of water and/or fibre in the diet.

Contamination Entry of undesirable organisms in some material or object.

Corn, opaque-2 Genetically developed corn with higher than normal amounts of lysine and tryptophan.

Cretinism Dwarfism usually caused in the infant due to severe depletion of iodine of the mother in her pregnancy resulting in her inability to supply iodine for the development of the foetus. It is characterised by low basal metabolism, muscular flabbiness and weakness, dryness of the skin, arrest of skeletal development and severe mental retardation.

Crystallisation Form into crystals, usually from a super saturated solution by the seeding of a very small quantity of the crystalline compound.

Deamination Removal of an amino group from a compound.

Deficiency disease A disease resulting from inadequate dietary intake of something required nutritionally.

Dehydration The loss of water from the body, which is not compensated by intake of water.

Dementia Mental disorder resulting in impairment of transfer of nerve impulses.

Denaturation Structural change in proteins due to effect of heat, light, change in pH, etc. Results in change of solubility. May be reversible, if conditions are mild but mostly irreversible changes occur.

Deodourisation Removal of flavour or odour of fats during refining.

DNA Deoxyribonucleic Acid Substance forming the genetic material in most organisms.

Dermatitis Inflammation of the skin.

Dextrins Mixture of water soluble compounds formed by partial breakdown of starch by heat, acid or enzymes.

Diabetes mellitus is a genetic disease of metabolism in which there is a partial or total inability to synthesise insulin; it is characterised by the partial loss of ability or complete inability of the tissue to use carbohydrates. Hyperglycemia, glycosuria and excessive urination occur.

It is a chronic degenerative disease, in which the body lacks the normal ability to metabolize glucose.

Dialysis mechanical filtration of the blood; used when kidneys are no longer able to function normally.

Diarrhoea Rapid movement of food matter through the digestive tract resulting in watery stools. Leads to dehydration and profound cellular disturbances.

Diastolic pressure Blood pressure measured when heart is at rest.

Diffusion Movements of molecules from high concentration areas to low ones.

Digestion Mechanical and chemical breakdown of food to simple substances which can be absorbed and used by the body cells.

Disaccharide Carbohydrate consisting of two monosaccharide units.

Diuretics substances used to increase the amount of urine excreted.

Duodenum First portion of the small intestine.

Edema (Odema) Excess accumulation of fluid in the intercellular spaces of the body.

Element Any one of the fundamental atoms of which all matter is composed.

Emaciation Wasted condition of body due mainly to lack of food, wherein the fat reserves and muscles to a certain extent are used up for sustenance of life.

Emphysema A lung disease in which surface area of lungs is reduced and normal breathing is disturbed.

Enamel Calcified tissue covering crown of a tooth.

Endemic disease Disease, which occurs, regularly in a given region and affects health adversely for a long time.

Endogeneous Produced within the organism.

Enteric Pertaining to the intestines.

Enzyme Protein formed in plant and animal cells, which acts as a catalyst for certain specific reactions.

Epidemic An epidemic disease spreads rapidly and affects many people of a given region.

Epithelial Cells that form the outer layer of the skin, respiratory, gastrointestinal, urinary, reproductive tract and also of eyes, nose, ears, throat, lungs, liver and kidney.

Erythropoietin A hormone produced by kidneys, which stimulates maturation of red blood cells in the bone marrow.

Esophagus Hollow muscular tube connecting the mouth and stomach.

Ester Chemical name for a compound formed by reaction of an acid and an alcohol. Fats are esters of an alcohol (Glycerol) and fatty acids such as stearic, oleic, etc.

Exchange lists Lists of foods with interchangeable nutrient and kcal contents; used in specific forms of diet therapy such as diabetic and heart ailment diets.

Excreta Products of digestion and metabolism that are discarded from the body—faeces from the intestinal tract and urine from the kidneys.

Extracellular fluid Fluid outside the cell consist of tissue fluid, blood plasma, cerbrospinal fluid, fluid in the eye and fluid of the gastro-intestinal tract.

Fatty acid Organic acids composed of carbon, hydrogen and oxygen. They combine with glycerol to form fats and oils.

Fecal matter Solid waste from large intestine.

Fermentation Breakdown of compounds without the use of oxygen, e.g., breakdown of sugar by yeast to form alcohol and carbon dioxide.

Fibrosis Development of tough, stringy tissue.

Flora (Intestinal) Bacteria and other small organisms that live in the intestine.

Fluids Liquids or gas.

Fomite An inanimate object that carries living organisms.

FAO Food and Agriculture Organisations of the United Nations, established in 1945, to improve food production, distribution and consumption in member countries, so as to improve level of nutrition of people; also publishes periodic estimates of food available and has panels, which set international recommended dietary allowances.

Food guide A guide to help to individuals to select food so as to meet their nutritional needs.

Food poisoning A general term applied to all stomach and intestinal disturbances due to food contaminated with certain microorganisms or their toxins.

Fortification Addition of one or more nutrients to a food to make it richer than the unprocessed food, e.g., Vitamin C added to fruit juice.

Free Fatty Acids (FFA) Fatty acids obtained by the breakdown of fat under adverse conditions. Thus measurement of FFA is an index of fat quality.

Galactosemia Inherited error in metabolism that prevents normal metabolism of galactose.

Gastro-instestinal Part of the digestive system made up of the stomach and intestines.

Gel Technically, a colloidal solution of a solid in a liquid.

Gelatinsation Swelling and increase in viscosity of the starch molecule due to absorption of water on heating. Each type of starch such as rice, maize, wheat has its own gelatinsation temperature. This varies between 60°C to 80°C.

Glomerulonephritis Inflammation of the capillaries in glomerulli of the kidneys.

Glomerulus Filtering unit of the kidneys.

Glossitis Inflammation of the tongue.

Glyceride Compound (ester) formed by the combination of the glycerol and a fatty acid.

Glycerol A trihydroxy alcohol formed by the hydrolysis of fats.

Glycogen Chief storage form of carbohydrates in humans and animals. Found mainly in liver and muscles.

Gram Metric unit of weight equal to a 1000 milligrammes.

Growth Generally denotes increase in the physical size of the human body as a whole, or any of its dimensions, part of tissues. This begin at conception and continues up to adulthood.

Health State of complete physical, mental and social well-being and not just absence of disease or infirmity.

Haemo Non-protein segment portion of haemoglobin which contains iron.

Hemicellulose Indigestible polysaccharide which forms the cell wall of plants.

Haemoglobin An Iron-containing protein in the blood which carries oxygen from the lungs to the tissues.

Hepatitis Inflammation of liver.

Homeostasis State of physical balance, stable condition.

Hormone Substances produced in the body (chiefly by the endocrine glands), which is carried by the blood stream, and has a specific effect on the other cells, tissues and organs.

Host Plant or animal harbouring another organism as a parasite (or an infectious agent).

Human immunodeficiency virus (HIV) a virus which destroys body's immune system leading to AIDS

Hydrochloric acid A normal constituent of human gastric juice.

Hydrolysis Splitting up of a compound into smaller units due to uptake of water.

Hypermetabolic state A state of accelerated metabolic activity.

Hypertension Higher than normal blood pressure.

Hypervitaminosis Undesirable effects produced by taking an excess of a concentrate or pure fat soluble vitamin.

Hypochromic Condition in which there is an abnormal decrease in the haemoglobin content of the erythrocytes (red blood cells) found in the blood.

Hypoglycemia Subnormal level of blood sugar, accompanied by a feeling of weakness, giddiness and fainting, if not attended to promptly by feeding sugar in some form.

Hypoproteinemea Abnormally small amounts of total proteins in the circulating blood plasma.

Hypothyroidism Condition in which thyroid gland secrets too little thyroxine resulting in slower than normal metabolic rate.

Incidence The frequency of occurrence of a situation or of a condition like disease.

Insensible perspiration Perspiration that evaporates before it can be felt as a fluid on the skin.

Insulin Hormone produced by the pancreas, essential for proper metabolism of glucose.

International Unit (I.U.) Units of measure used for vitamin A activity and Vitamin D.

I.I.U. of Vitamin A = 0.3 mcg. retinol = 0.6 mcg. beta-carotene.

I.I.U. of Vitamin D = 0.25 mcg. of Vitamin D_3

Intolerance Sensitivity or allergy to certain foods.

Intrinsic Factor (I.F.) Mucoprotein secreted by the stomach walls which is required for the absorption of Vit. B_{12}. A lack of this factor leads to pernicious anaemia.

Iodised salt Table salt to which potassium or sodium iodine and a small amount of magnesium carbonate is added.

Ischemic heart disease Lack of blood supply to the heart muscle resulting in a heart attack.

Isotonicity Solutions having the same osmotic pressure and isotonic and this condition is called isotonicity.

Jaundice Yellow colour of skin and eyes due to deposition of bile pigment, indicating liver disease.

Jejunum The middle section comprising about two-fifths of the small intestine.

Ketonuria Ketone bodies in the urine.

Ketosis Accumulation of large quantities of ketone bodies (substances synthesised by the liver in the process of combustion of fats) in the body tissues or fluids. This results from the incomplete oxidation of fatty acids by the liver.

Kilocalorie Unit of heat used in nutrition. The amount of heat required to raise the temperature of 1 kg of water from 15 to 16°C.

Kilogram Metric unit of weight equivalent to a 1000 gram or 2.2 pounds.

Lactic acid 3 carbon acid produced in milk by bacterial fermentation of the milk sugar lactose. Also formed in the body during the anaerobic metabolism of carbohydrates.

Lactose Carbohydrate found in milk, milk sugar; disaccharide composed of glucose and galactose.

Lecithin A phospholipid which occurs in nervous tissues. Also found in egg yolk. It is an effective emulsifier.

Legume Pod or fruit of peas and beans.

Lethargy State of prolonged unconsciousness from which a person can be aroused but into which he immediately relapses.

Linoleic acid An 18–carbon unsaturated fatty acid which occurs widely in plant glycerides and is an essential fatty acid needed for maintaining growth and skin health.

Lipids Term for fats including neutral fats, oil, fatty acids, phospholipids and cholesterol.

Lymph Fluid circulating within the lymphatic system. Eventually added to venous blood circulation. Arises from tissue fluid. Colourless, odourless and slightly alkaline in nature.

Macrocyte An abnormally large red blood cell.

Malnutrition An all-exclusive term for poor nourishment. May result from an inadequate or excessive intake of one or more nutrients or of some defect in metabolism, which prevents the body from using the nutrients properly.

Inadequacy in the quality of diet or insufficient intake of one or more nutrients; may also refer to excessive intake.

Maturation The process of coming to full development, maturity or adulthood.

Mcg. Microgramme.

Metastasize Spread of cancer cells from one organ to another.

Micro Prefix meaning small.

Micro-organisms Very small living beings.

Bacteria, yeast and Fungi are the common microorganisms found in foods.

Millet Small grain of Indian cereal, edible seeds of grass family which are small in size.

Monovalent Having a valence of one, e.g., the valence of the hydrogen atom is one.

Mucous membrane A membrane lining the cavities and canals of the body that have contact with the air. It is kept moist by mucous secreted by special cells and glands. The eyes, ears, nose, throat, lungs, digestive tract, genitourinary and reproductive tracts are lined with mucous membranes.

Mutations Permanent transmissible changes in genes.

Myocardial infarction Heart attack caused by the blockage of an artery leading to the heart.

NIN National Institute of Nutrition.

Neoplasm Abnormal uncontrolled cell growth of new tissue, which leads to developing mass called tumor of neoplasm.

Nephritis Inflammatory disease of the kidney.

Nephron Functional unit of the kidney containing a glomerulus.

Neuropathy Nerve damage.

Nourish To provide food or other substances necessary for life and growth.

Nucleus Part of the cell that contains the chromosomes. It is the control centre of the cell for both chemical reactions and reproduction. It contains large quantities of DNA.

Nutrient A substance essential for the growth, maintenance, function, and reproduction of a cell or organism.

Nutrient deficiency or imbalance Reduces production or maturation of T-cells or B-cells, depresses DNA synthesis, cell division or replication and thus decreases immunity.

Nutritional status Health of a person as influenced by the quality of foods eaten and the ability of body to utilise these food to meet its needs.

Organic Acid Contains one or more carboxyl groups (COOH). Simple examples are formic (HCOOH) and acetic acid (CH_3COOH).

Organic Kingdom The animal and vegetable kingdoms.

Osmosis Transfer of solvent through a semi-permeable membrane to equalise solute concentration on either side of the membrane. The walls of living cells are semi-permeable membranes, and much of the activity of the cell depends on osmosis.

Osmotic pressure The pressure that causes water or any other solvent to move from a solution with low concentration of solute to one having high concentration of solute.

Osteoporosis A disease of bone characterised by increased porosity of bones.

Oxidation The change in an atom, atoms or a molecule, which involve: (1) gain of oxygen, (2) Removal of hydrogen, or (3) loss of electrons.

Palatibility The equality characteristics (such as colour, flavour and texture) of a food product that make an impression on the organs of touch, taste, smell or sight and have significance in determining the acceptability of the food product to the user.

Parasite Animal or plant deriving nourishment from another living organism: self-interested hanger-on.

Parenteral nutrition Nutrition provided via a vein; it does not use the gastrointestinal tract.

Pathogenic Capable of producing disease.

Pectin A soluble polysaccharide (found in many fruits), which can form a gel in the presence of adequate sugar and acid. It is unaffected by animal enzymes.

Pepsin Protein splitting enzyme found in the gastric juice of the stomach.

Peristalsis Rhythmic wavelike movement caused by the muscles of the small intestine to move food forward; moves the chyme along.

pH Negative logarithm of hydrogen ion concentration, which express the acidity or alkalinity of a substance.

Phenylketonuria (PKU) An inborn error of metabolism in which the infant lacks are enzyme needed to metabolize phenylalamine, an essential amino acid.

Phospholipids Fat-like substances consisting of glycerol, 2 fatty acids, a phosphate group and a nitrogeneous base, e.g., lecithin.

Photophobia Means fear or hatred of light, a condition resulting from lack of riboflavin, characterised by rough eyelids and sensitivity of eyes to bright sunlight.

Photosynthesis The process by which the chlorophyll presents in the plant converts water and carbon dioxide into carbohydrates using sunlight as an energy source.

Phytate Salt of phytic acid (a phosporous containing compound found in the outer layers of cereals). Phytates of Ca, Mg, are insoluble and hence cannot be absorbed by the small intestine. Hence phytic acid interferes with normal calcium absorption.

Placenta Connecting tube between the wall of the uterus and the foetus—through which the foetus is nourished.

Plasma Fluid portion of blood in which formed cells (white blood cells, red blood cells, platelets) are suspended.

Polluted containing fecal matter, (the presence of coliform bacteria is an indication of possible fecal contamination).

Polyneuritis Inflammation of a number of peripheral nerves.

Polyunsaturated fatty acid (PUFA) Fatty acids containing 2 or more double bonds, e.g., linoleic, linolenic, and arachidonic acids.

Potential energy Energy in chemical form, which may be released either as heat or muscular work when the substance is oxidised.

Precursor A compound that can be used by the body to form an essential nutrient.

Proteolytic Capable of splitting or digesting protein into simpler compounds.

Radiation Is the emission of alpha, beta particles or electrons or gamma rays.

RDI Recommended dietary intake for nutrients.

Red Blood Cells (RBC) Also known as erythrocytes, contain pigment haemoglobin, which is red.

Reduction A chemical process involving removal of oxygen, the addition of hydrogen or in general gain of electrons.

Renal stone Kidney stone.

Rennin A gastric enzyme which coagulates milk.

Respiration The exchange of O_2 and CO_2 in the lungs, between the cell and its environment, which ultimately releases energy.

Retinol Equivalent (R.E.) A unit used to express vitamin a activity; 1 R.E = 3.33 I.U.

Retinopathy Damage to small blood vessels in the eye.

Rickets A deficiency disease caused by absence of vitamin D or calcium or both which affects the skeletal system.

Salmonella Genus of bacteria causing intestinal infection. Frequently contaminates foods is destroyed by heating.

Sanitary Pertaining to cleanliness.

Scurvy A deficiency disease due to the lack of vitamin C. Symptoms are bleeding gums, weakness and loss of weight.

Semi-permeable membrane A membrane which is permeable to certain solids only and is freely permeable to water.

Serum The fluid part of blood, which separates from the blood cells after clotting.

Short chain fatty acids Those with 10 or fewer carbon atoms in one molecule.

Simple sugars Are the monasaccharide—glucose, fructose and galactose.

Stearic acid A saturated fatty acid made up of 18 carbon atoms.

Sterol An alcohol of high molecular weight, e.g., cholesterol, ergosterol, etc.

Subclinical deficiency An inadequate intake of a nutrient leading to a deficiency, which cannot be detected by a clinical test.

Syndrome A medical term meaning a group of symptoms occurring together.

Synthesis A coming together of two or more substances to form a more complex one.

Systolic pressure Blood pressure taken as the heart contracts.

Thyroxine Hormone produced by the thyroid gland containing iodine (regulates energy metabolism).

Tissue A collection of cells forming a structure.

Toxin A poisonous substance elaborated by certain organisms, e.g., bacterial toxins.

Triglyceride An ester of glycerol and three fatty acids.

Trypsin An enzyme secreted by the pancreas, which splits protein.

Tyramine A vasoactive amine found in decayed animal tissue, ripe cheese and other foods.

Urea The final product of the deamination of amino acids, chief waste product of protein metabolism.

Virus A minute microscopic highly infectious organism, characterized by total dependence on living cells for its reproduction and metabolism.

Viscosity Measures of fluidity of a liquid.

Vitamin Organic compounds occurring in minute amounts in foods and essential for numerous metabolic reactions.

WHO World Health Organisation of the United Nations. The specialised agency started in 1948, located in Geneva, that is concerned with health on an international level.

Xerosis Abnormal dryness on skin and eye.

Yeast Microorganism responsible for fermentation of sugars. Convert sugar into alcohol and carbon dioxide anaerobically.

Bibliography for Further Reading

I. Nutrition and Diet Therapy

1. Antia, F.P.: **Clinical Dietetics and Nutrition,** 3rd ed., Oxford University Press, Bombay, 1986.
2. Cataldo, Corinne B., Whitney, Eleanor N. and Linda Kelly DeBruyne: **Nutrition and Diet Therapy – Principles and Practice,** West Publishing Co. St. Paul, 2003
3. Chaney, Margaret S., Margaret L. Ross and Jelia C. Witchi: **Nutrition** 9th ed. Houghton. Mifflin, Boston 1979 (Indian Reprint, Surjeet Publications, New Delhi, 1979).
4. Davidson, S.R., Passmore and J.F. Brock.: **Human Nutrition & Dietetics,** 8th ed. Churchill Livingstone, London, U.K., 1986.
5. Fleck, Henrietta: **Introduction to Nutrition:** 4th ed., Macmillan, New York, 1981.
6. Garrow J.S.S., W.P.T. James and A. Ralph: **Human Nutrition & Dietetics,** 10th ed. W.B. Saunders, Philadelphia, USA, 1999.
7. Joshi, Shubangini A.: **Nutrition and Dietetics,** Tata McGraw Hill, New Delhi, India, 1992.
8. Leverton Ruth, M. **Food Becomes You**: Better Health through Better Nutrition, Doubleday Publishing, Boston, USA, 1980.
9. Lutz, Carroll A. and Karen R. Przytuski: **Nutrition and Diet Therapy,** 4th ed. Davis F.A., Philadelphia, USA, 1995.
10. Martin, Ethel A. and Ardath A. Coolidge: **Nutrition in Action** 4th ed., Holt Rinehart and Winston, New York, 1978.
11. McDivitt, Maxine E. and Sumati R. Mudambi: **Human Nutrition – Principles and Applications in India,** Revised Edition, Prentice Hall, New Delhi, 1973.
12. Patwardhan, V.N. : **Nutrition in India** 2nd ed. Indian Journal of Medical Sciences, New Delhi, 1961.
13. Robinson, Corinne, H., Marilyn R. Lawler, Wanda L. Chanoweth & Anne E. Garwick: **Normal and Therapeutic Nutrition,** 17th ed. Macmillan Publishing Co. NY, USA, 1996.
14. Shils, Moshe S, Benjamin Caballero, A., Catherine Ross and Robert J. Cousins: **Modern Nutrition in Health and Disease,** 10th ed. Lippincott, Williams & Wilkins, Baltimore, USA, 2005.
15. Swaminathan, M.: **Essentials of Food and Nutrition,** Volume I and II, 2nd ed. Ganesh, Madras, India, 1985.
16. Townsend, Carolyn E. & Roth, Ruth A.: **Nutrition and Diet Therapy** 8th ed., Delmar Publishers, Albany, USA., 2003.
17. Williams, Sue R. **Basic Nutrition and Diet Therapy,** 3rd ed. by Stacy Nix, Mosby, 2009.

II. Food Science, Food Hygiene & Microbiology

1. Bennion, Marian and Osee Hughes: **Introductory Foods,** 8th ed. Macmillan, New York, 1985.
2. Frazier, W.C.: **Food Microbiology:** 4th ed., Tata McGraw Hill, New Delhi, 1988.
3. **Health Hazards of the Human Environment,** WHO, 1973.
4. Kawata, K.: **Environmental Sanitation in India,** Lucknow Publishing House, India, 1963.
5. Meyer, Lillian: **Food Chemistry,** Reinhold, New York, 1978.
6. Mudambi Sumati R., Shalini M. Rao and M.V. Rajagopal **Food Science,** 2nd ed. New Age International, New Delhi, 2005.
7. Peckman, Gladys C. and Jeanne H. Freeland-Graves: **Foundations of Food Preparation,** 5th ed., Macmillan, New York, 1987.

III. Publications of The Indian Council of Medical Research

1. Banerjee, S.: **Studies in Energy Metabolism,** Indian Council of Medical Research Special Report Series no. 43, 1962.
2. Gopalan, C.B.V. Ramashastri and S.C. Balasubramaniam, Revised and updated by B.S. Narasinga Rao, Y.G. Deosthale and K.C. Pant: **Nutritive Value of Indian Foods,** National Institute of Nutrition, Hyderabad, India, 2000.
3. **Manual of Standards of Drinking Water Supplies,** 2nd ed. Indian Council of Medical Research, Special Report Series No. 44, New Delhi, 1975.
4. Venkatachalam, P.S. and L.M. Rebello: **Nutrition for Mother and Child,** 3rd ed., Indian Council of Medical Research, Special Report Series, No. 41, 1978.

IV. Publications By United Nations Agencies: FAO, WHO

1. Aykroyd, W.R.: **Legumes in Human Nutrition,** Revised ed., FAO, Rome, 1982.
2. **Energy and Protein Requirements FAO Nutrition Meetings Report Series 62,** WHO Tech. Report Series No. 522, Rome, 1973.
3. **Food Composition Tables for International Use,** FAO Nutritional Studies No. 11, FAO, Rome, 1954.
4. **Nutrition and Working Efficiency** FFHC Basic Study No. 5, 1962.
5. **Calcium Requiremetns** WHO Tech. Report Series 230, Geneva, 1962.
6. **Control of Nutrition Anaemia with Special Reference to Iron Deficiency.,** Tech. Report Series 580, Geneva, 1975.
7. Jelliffe, D.B.: **Assessment of Nutritional Status for the Community,** WHO, 1966.
8. **Requirements of Ascorbic Acid, Vitamin D, Vitamin B-12, Folate and Iron,** WHO Tech. Report Series 452, Geneva, 1975.
9. **Vitamin A Deficiency and Xerophthalmia,** Tech. Report Series 590, Geneva, 1976.

Index

C

O

P

R

S

T

U

V

W

X

Y